RENEWALS 458-4574

DATE DUE

GAYLORD			PRINTED IN U.S.A.

The Myth of Pain

Philosophical Psychopathology: Disorders in Mind
Owen Flanagan and George Graham, editors

The Myth of Pain, by Valerie Gray Hardcastle, 1999.

Divided Minds and Successive Selves: Ethical Issues in Disorders of Identity and Personality, by Jennifer Radden, 1996.

Philosophical Psychopathology, edited by George Graham and G. Lynn Stephens, 1994.

The Myth of Pain

Valerie Gray Hardcastle

A Bradford Book
The MIT Press
Cambridge, Massachusetts
London, England

Library of Congress Cataloging-in-Publication Data

Hardcastle, Valerie Gray.
  The myth of pain / Valerie Gray Hardcastle.
    p. cm. — (Philosophical psychopathology. Disorders in mind)
  Includes bibliographical references and index.
  ISBN 0-262-08283-7 (hardcover : alk. paper)
    1. Pain. 2. Pain—Psychological aspects. 3. Pain—Philosophy.
I. Title. II. Series.
RB127.H38 1999
616′.0472—dc21   99-30099
                                                                      CIP

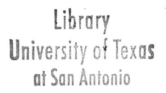

For Kiah, Cheshire, and John Quinton,
my three earth-angels

Contents

Series Foreword

The aim of the series is both interdisciplinary and uncharted: to offer philosophical examination of mental disorder, an area of intense and fascinating activity in recent years. The perspective of philosophy provides a richly synoptic vision of the forms, limits, and lessons of mental disorder, as well as its study and treatment. Potential topics include, but are not limited to, the following:

- How to explain mental disorder.
- Dissociative personality and volitional disorders and what they tell us about rational and moral agency
- Disorders of consciousness and what they tell us about selfhood and self-representation
- The lessons of cognitive neuropsychology for the nature and function of mind
- Whether disorders are "rational strategies" for coping with trauma or stress
- Relationships between dream states and psychosis
- Neural-network models of pathology and their implications for the debate over the functional integration of mind/brain
- Culture-specific and gender-linked forms of psychopathology and their lessons for both the taxonomy of mental disorder and the scientific status of the study of mental illness
- Logical and epistemological relations between theories of mental disorder and forms of therapy

- Conceptual and methodological foundations of psychopharmacology
- Ethical and political issues in definition and treatment of mental disorder

The editors welcome proposals and submissions from philosophers, cognitive scientists, psychiatric researchers, physicians, social scientists, and others committed to a philosophical approach to psychopathology.

Owen Flanagan
George Graham

Acknowledgments

Chapter 4 is a revised and expanded version of a paper with the same name published in the *Studies in the History and Philosophy of Biology and the Biomedical Sciences,* 30 (no. 1), 1999, 69–89; chapters 5 and 6 contain parts of the paper "When a Pain Is Not," *Journal of Philosophy* 94 (no. 8), 1997, 381–409; chapter 7 draws from my entry on eliminative materialism in the *Encyclopedia of Philosophy Supplement,* ed. D. M. Borchert (New York: Macmillan, 1996), 136–137, and from "Distinctions without Differences: Commentary on Horgan and Tienson's *Connectionism and the Philosophy of Psychology,*" *Philosophical Psychology* 10 (no. 3), 1997, 347–358. My thanks to the editors of these journals and book for permission to use this material.

Excerpts from chapter 7 were presented at the Mid-South Philosophy Conference in Memphis in 1998; I thank Jonathon Cohen for his thoughtful response to this paper. Part of chapter 8 was presented to the Southern Society for Philosophy and Psychology in Louisville in 1999. I am grateful to both audiences for their helpful comments and discussion.

This book began as a talk for the Society for Philosophy and Psychology in San Francisco, 1996. I owe thanks to Jim Garson for making special arrangements for me to come and to Dan Dennett for his thought- and comment-provoking commentary. George Graham was in the audience there and persuaded me that I really had a book in the presentation. I believed him. With generous support from the philosophy department at Virginia Tech and a Taft Fellowship from the University of Cincinnati, I turned that pie-in-the-sky daydream into reality.

There are many individuals to whom I am especially grateful, for, without them, this book simply would never have been finished. I owe a huge debt of gratitude to George Graham for suggesting the project in the first place, guiding me through the process, holding my hand when I needed it, and reading endless email messages, proposals, chapter drafts, and full manuscripts promptly, thoroughly, and with a balanced eye. He will give all other series editors a bad reputation by comparison. Special thanks go to Matthew Stewart and Rosalyn Walker Stewart for help in translating medical jargonese into something resembling English, Mark Gifford for talking to me about Aristotle's views on pain, Nance Cunningham for sharing her research on infant pain, Carol Bailey for her thoughts on the etiology of self-injurious behavior, Don Gustafson and Bob Richardson for their support and interest, and Gary Hardcastle for letting me blather on about psychogenic pains and self-injurious behavior at the supper table. I recognize that I rarely chose the best topic for dinner conversation, but I did have some good stories that couldn't wait about chain saws and skulls. R. Hugh Walker discussed the nature of chaos and how to understand nonlinear mathematical models with me over email; he noted that an early version of the manuscript was "readable"— high praise from my dad. Owen Flanagan engaged in and endured endless talks, lectures, dialogues, and diatribes about pain and its problems (and my problems with its problems). Patient and thoughtful, he made lots of noncommittal comments. In other words, he was a perfect help.

John Bickle and several anonymous referees made many insightful suggestions early into the project, which kept me from wandering too far astray. Nick Chater wrote detailed comments on an earlier draft of chapter 4, which made that chapter all the better. Dick Chapman and Jonathon Cole went way beyond the call of duty in going over the penultimate draft of this book with a fine-tooth comb, picking all sorts of nits and ranting about language hygiene. I probably did not change the manuscript enough to suit them in the end, but just about every page reflects their input nonetheless. I wish I could pin whatever errors remain on them, but I can't; they are due to my own pigheadedness.

Betty Stanton of Bradford Books is retired now; this book is one of the last that she personally saw through publication at MIT Press. Since one of the first books she and Harry ever published got me into philosophy and mind/brain studies in the first place, I feel thrilled and honored to have worked with her and to have been part of her and Harry's great adventure. She, her assistant Amy Yeager, and manuscript editor Kathleen Caruso are wonderful; I could not have asked for a better experience with MIT or Bradford.

Finally, I owe great thanks to my three children, Kiah, Cheshire, and Quinn. They are my fiercest passion and my finest joy. Too often in our discussions of children—the having of them, the raising of them, the disciplining of them—we fail to mention how much we do love them and with what force. My life is not only richer and deeper and more meaningful with my children in it, it could not be my life without them.

I dedicate this book to them. At first, I was worried about writing a book for my children on pain; I had thought that I might be sending the wrong message. On second thought, though, I believe that this book advocates many of the traits I hope they internalize as they grow: looking beyond what others assert as obvious, intellectual curiosity about what we are and how we work, compassion for the suffering of others, and a commitment to setting wrongs right. Even if I fail to attain these goals, and I probably have and will, I give this book to my children in the hope that they will learn from my missteps.

1

The Myths of Pain

Touch my heart so that I may repent my faults, since without this internal pain, the external ills which you inflict on my body will provide me with new chance to sin. Make me truly understand that the ills of the body are nothing more than punishment and the complete manifestation of the ills of the soul. But also make them the remedy, by making me consider, in the pain that I feel, that which I did not feel in my soul albeit it was quite ill and covered in ulcers. . . . All that I am is odious to you, and I find nothing in me that could please you. I see nothing there, Lord, apart from my pain that in some way resembles yours.
—Pascal

Philosophical interest in psychopathologies has been increasing steadily in the past few years. Unfortunately, though, attention has been focused mainly on the more bizarre and less common maladies. These make for interesting discussion, to be sure, but insofar as the disorders are rare and exceedingly complex, few conclusions can be drawn that are applicable to psychopathology as a whole, or to psychology or psychiatry in general.

I wish to rectify this problem, at least partially, by offering a philosophical and biological analysis of pain. Pain is, obviously, very common, but it is little understood. Psychogenic pains—pains for which there is no (known) organic cause—are as mysterious and frustrating as any of the more curious disorders one might observe on morning talk shows. In fact, if one looks at dollars spent or days lost from work, chronic psychogenic pain is the most disabling disease state around. Though not as glamorous as multiple personality disorder, schizophrenia, or anosagnosia, the mystery of pathological pain merits serious attention.

In particular, the problem of psychogenic pain warrants a philosophical analysis, for it raises complex questions about the relation of the mind and body (Psychogenic pains are "mental" pains—pains that have a "psychological" cause. If we be materialists, then what distinguishes pathological pain from real pain?); the relation between neuroscience, psychology, and folk explanations (Under what conditions, if any, should neurophysiological data trump psychological theories? Under what conditions, if any, should a [counterintuitive] scientific explanation supersede an intuitive account?); the relation between alleged psychological disorders and rationality (Can we explain pathological pains as a rational strategy for coping with trauma? If so, then how are we to understand the notion of rationality?); and the relation between theory and therapy (If pain is "mental" rather than "physical," does that have an impact on the treatment of pain? What are the epistemological connections between how we conceive of pain and what we know to do about it?).

But before we can begin this analysis, we need to shake loose some of our intuitions regarding pain. For example, we commonly identify pain with the sensation of pain and we believe (implicitly, anyway, since this isn't a general topic for dinner conversation) that this view of pain is (1) transparently true, and (2) the way it has always been. However, a quick glance at the history of pain tells us that we have viewed pain quite differently over the centuries and that our current understanding of pain is a recent invention. This should, if nothing else, underscore the fact that our commonsensical ideas about pain are only educated guesses about what pain is and how it functions in the body. Highlighting the contingent nature of our understanding gives us room to change our beliefs with relative ease.

A Brief and Scattered History of Pain[1]

During antiquity, pain had no real significance other than signaling specific disorders and aiding diagnosis. It was neither an alarm bell nor a watchdog, for it did not herald disease. Instead, pain was the disorder itself. Each form of pain, with its own "color," had its own treatment, and pains were individuated not only in terms of how they felt, but also by the weather, and the personality, gender, and age of the patients. Pain was seen as completely incompatible with health and physical fitness, and every effort was made to rid bodies of their pains and suffering. Of course, the remedies were rather primitive, consisting of bloodletting, vinegar and mustard plasters, oil and sulphur rubs, particular types and temperatures of foods, exercise, sexual abstinence, hot seawater baths, and various topical ointments.

Galen (second century A.D.) argued that pain is a sense, in the general category of touch. Sensory experiences occur via a psychic *pneuma* between the person's directive principle (located in the encephalon, the seat of all intellectual activity) and the sense organ itself. Continuous sensations require a continuous change in the pneuma; hence, pain could signal damage to the body, but absence of pain might indicate that the body has merely adjusted to whatever damage without a cure. There are two types of damage possible: "interruption of continuity" of the bodily tissues or the bodily humors becoming "distended, compressed, crushed, or injured," and "sudden and major" changes in individual "temperament," as the blend of hot and cold, dryness and moisture becomes imbalanced.[2] The Galenic view of pain remained in fashion up through the Middle Ages, though by then the rest of Galen's medical doctrines had been distorted, diminished, and padded.

With Christianity's new emphasis on Christ's suffering and Incarnation around the twelfth century, views of pain underwent a shift as people became more focused on bodily suffering in general. Pain became a form of divine retribution or a sign of having been chosen by God, both of which encouraged an acceptance of pain and suffering. Monastic practices of mortifying the flesh, flagellation, and performing base menial tasks increased as Christianity in turn offered salvation and healing (in the true sense of the term) through prayer and faith.

From what we do know of the Middle Ages, pain seems to have been eclipsed by larger issues at the time, though in all likelihood, treating pain qua pain with opium and various other sedatives probably continued much as it had been done since antiquity. The fact is we really don't know much about what people actually did then about their pains.

With Descartes, we return to a Galenic view. Galen's pneuma become Descartes's animal spirits, both moving through the nerve tubes in the body. Pain for Descartes is a perception of the soul. As with Galen, it is part of our sense of touch, though it is an aspect of a sensation (as was pleasure) instead of a perceptual quality like hardness or warmth. Still, our understanding of pain becomes more complex in the seventeenth century, as the "English Hippocrates" Sydenham hypothesized that there was an "internal man" who could sense pain consciously though reason. Pain then had a dual role: it subconsciously produced reflex reactions and flight through neuromuscular interactions, and, if it crossed a certain threshold, it became a conscious sensation perceived by our inner life. As we shall see below, this view isn't far from the truth.

At the same time, the Christian mystical attitude toward pain remained. Since we are supposed to be on this Earth solely to serve God, then health is no more important a good than any other Earthly good. Indeed, pain could be seen as beneficial, as Pascal's prayer quoted at the beginning of the chapter indicates. Nevertheless, from a practical perspective, doctors and patients alike struggled to relieve pain in all its manifestations, whether a gift from God or not, for even divine pain hurts.

By the eighteenth century, particularly the latter half, pain had become secularized. With the advent of the experimental method, the study of pain could be divorced from the problems of sin, evil, and punishment. Medicine in general became focused on symptomology and not purported etiology. Physicians prized careful observation, precise descriptions, and practical medicine over any unsubstantiated theoretical pronouncements.

Pain was now seen as a warning, alerting us to danger toward our bodies. It warns us of immanent harm and suggests that we change our ways before it is too late: "This bitter fruit of nature hides the seed of a great blessing; it is a beneficial effort, a cry of sensitivity through which our intelligence is warned of the danger menacing us; it is the thunder which rumbles before crashing. . . . It wounds us in order to serve us."[3] The pain of gout protects against other infirmities; the pain of gangrene prompts amputations and so saves the rest of the body. Though patients consistently tried to rid themselves of pain, both the medical community and lay society understood it to be largely a beneficial bodily voice.

There was some discussion at the time over whether it might not be better to feel the pain so that one could understand and treat whatever was happening in the body. Silencing the pain would also silence the messenger. Medicine itself also inflicted pain, through cauterization, moxibustion (the practice of burning a stick made from fabric and vegetable fibers on the skin), surgery, and the like. Doctors began calculating the value of life against the extent of suffering. Some pain and suffering were worth continued existence; some weren't. The question and debate were over where to draw the line. The ambivalence over the value of felt pains contributed in part to the slowed acceptance of the idea of anesthesia among doctors, discussed in chapter seven. If doctors numbed their patients, then how would the patients be able to communicate what was wrong?

There was also disagreement over what pain was exactly. The mechanists, who believed that the body was a simple machine, explained pain in terms of the stretching or separation of neural fibers. The vitalists believed sensibility, which was both physiological and psychological, somehow played a role in the pain. The animists were conflicted; they believed that pain was both a purely mechanical matter and a message of internal strife for the soul.

By the end of the eighteenth century, the vitalists were in the majority, and science then strove to understand the detailed mechanisms involved in producing the sensation of pain. Two theories about how pains are produced were in the offing: specificity and summation. Those who championed specificity held that each sensation corresponded to a particular sort of nerve or neural configuration. The job of physiologists was to map organic structures to particular perceptual experiences. This approach did not produce many positive results by the end of the nineteenth century. The summationists believed that pain required more than particular structures; it resulted from the summation of effects at a central level. Both views are reflected in twentieth-century research, which sees us trying to figure out exactly how pain as both a biological phenomenon and a psychological one must work, both as a specific response generated by particular nociceptive neurons and as a central reaction to the nociception. Though in many ways pain research is still in its infancy, its general theoretical foundation has remained unchanged for about a century.

However, there is a disconnection between our theories of pain and the treatment of pain, especially chronic or psychogenic pain. Our theoretical foundations may be progressing, albeit slowly. But (excepting the advent of morphine) our methods of curing chronic pain, or of otherwise helping those in intractable pain, have not advanced as much over the past several centuries. As pain historian Roselyne Rey concludes, "There was no decisive progress between the methods available in Graeco-Roman times and those in use at the beginning of the 19th century; . . . [in fact,] there may actually have been some regression." In addition, "If the opening of the 19th century enjoyed a major leap forward with the discovery of morphine and its close with the advent of aspirin, our own century has yet to have produced anything of such revolutionary moment."[4]

A Vague Road Map and Preview

As I shall discuss in the following chapters, this failure in treatment is at least partially connected to our beliefs about pain. Our notions of pain are wrong; consequently, our methods of handling pain patients suffer from an inadequate theoretical foundation. Correcting our beliefs should lead to better treatment. I make some suggestions about how to do this toward the end of this monograph.

More generally, in this book I argue that how the professional community and laypeople alike understand and define pain is wrongheaded. Both identify pain with a sensation. I view this move as most unfortunate, for it mischaracterizes pain completely. Defining pain in terms of how it feels is both philosophically and empirically mistaken. Moreover, it has dangerous implications for philosophy of mind in general and for the study of mental disorders in particular—it has interesting philosophical implications for materialism, reductionism, eliminativism, and our regimentation of scientific explanations, as well as profound consequences for how psychological malfunctions are explicated, for how pain and pain patients are treated, and for how we care for infants and children.

In place of medicine's current articulation of what pain is, I offer a biologically based complex theory of pain processing, pain inhibition, and pain sensations. I then use this theory to help us understand some of the larger issues surrounding pain processing, including levels of explanation in the brain sciences, the ontology of psychological entities, when a mental disorder is really a disorder, and how our language should map onto our world.

There are two myths about pain I hope to debunk in my discussion. The first is that pain is a subjective state of mind. That psychopathological pains actually exist is the second myth. In doing these things, I argue that there is no such thing as psychogenic pain, defend an eliminativism about pain talk, and articulate a complex but purely materialistic theory of pain and pain inhibition. To motivate these claims, I defend a notion of mental causality, illustrate how we should individuate systems within the brain, and discuss the relation between lower-level disorders and higher-level cures. Most of these arguments are tied to exposing a pernicious dualistic mind/body distinction lurking in psychopathology. In short, I argue that all pains are physical and localizable and that all are created equal.

I conclude by sketching some of the implications my view has for how we understand mental disorders and the people who have them. I believe that the sort of analysis of pain I present—even if it is wrong in its details—could and should serve as a model for how other psychological disorders are analyzed in philosophy and psychiatry. You would not be misunderstanding my project if you took this book as an extended argument by example for how philosophers (or scientists, for that matter) should analyze the disorders found in psychology, psychiatry, or neuroscience.

For the purposes of truth in advertising, let me close this chapter with a brief disclaimer. This book provides an analysis of some of the issues that I, as a philosopher, find important and interesting. Its goal is not to provide a balanced technical writer's summary of pain research. Pain researchers, especially those who concentrate on understanding nociception, might find my picture of the field distorted. I don't believe it is, but it is a view from above (or the side) and not from the trenches, and that fact can make a great deal of difference in what is emphasized and what is glossed over.

2

Pathological Pains

My pain is a screech against an open, ripped, upside down sky. And the sky is my head, jagged and tearing, tearing, tearing. Sometimes I think it's on backwards because my teeth are in the wrong place. How can your own teeth gnash your own temple otherwise? The same way your temple is a fist all doubled up to really smash you with those steel knuckles, first icy cold, then fire hot; then flashes out in tough, ragged mandarin nails to scrape that same spot over and over. And there's a bruise—blue and purple and blood red—in the back of your eye. Your ear is being ripped off and the blood isn't blood but fire, stabbing in centimeter by centimeter down the back of your neck. And your neck fights back. It wants to be the sky so it sends the lightning back boxerlike in stiff jabs and explosion punches. Your teeth erupt and pelt you in the face; your ear bursts open and pastes itself against your eye; your eye recoils and shoots out through your temple and the blades and the whistles and the symbols and the blackboard chalk and the bombs and the jets all go off at the same time in a piercing scream. Then the rocket attached to the electric drill attached to the razors zooms down exactly on target to the temple. And a minute has passed.

—A forty-two-year-old woman's description of the headaches from which she has suffered for a decade (as quoted in Bresler and Trubo, *Free Yourself from Pain*)

Chronic pain is an enormous and costly industry. Somewhere between 11 percent and 34 percent of all adults in the Western world suffer from some form of debilitating and ongoing pain at any given time.[1] Persistent pain costs the United States somewhere between $40 and $100 billion a year in medical services, loss of productivity, and compensation payments.[2] It is the primary reason for missing work and the primary cause of disability.[3] It is the second most frequent illness—the common cold is the first—and affects about four-fifths of all people.[4] It is the most prevalent symptom in patients seeking medical assistance and the primary motivation in seeking a physician in 80 percent of all doctor visits.[5] In short: pain is the most disabling disease around.

These statistics should be shocking. In comparison, the Center for Disease Control has verified only 641,086 cases of AIDS in the nation from when the disease was first reported in 1981 to 31 December 1997. Total deaths number 390,968. Even New York City, which has the highest concentration of AIDS patients in the United States by an order of magnitude, numbers only 101,670 total reported cases. Citizens are rightly demanding proper treatment and care for this disease; why don't we find similar efforts for pain? Where is the social outrage? Why aren't there thousands of citizens demanding better from modern medicine? Where is the national campaign to fight against pain?

The very commonness of pain, and the enormous numbers and costs associated with it, allows us to minimize the actual suffering of the individuals in pain. Lots of people have it and there is no easy cure, so it is all too easy to sweep the personal aspects of pain aside. Nonetheless, the damage done to pain patients and their families is very real and, for all practical purposes, incalculable. Persistent pain is demoralizing, frustrating, depressing, and wearisome. It destroys one's emotional and psychological resilience to the vagaries of life. It depletes the reserve strength of the sufferer's family, friends, colleagues, employers, health-care providers, and society at large, for (though they may try) they cannot provide adequate relief or support. Pain hurts, along many dimensions. Its impact on our quality of life cannot be underestimated and should not be ignored.

Unfortunately, for all the prevalence of pain, we know remarkably little about its nature, causes, and treatment. The past few decades have seen tremendous advances in our knowledge of anatomy, physiology, biochemistry, and pharmacology. New medical and surgical techniques and innovative treatment strategies abound. Yet still, basic pain relief eludes us. A majority of chronic pain sufferers have an affliction for which there is no known cause, little or no medical help, and no good explanation for why they have the condition they do.

Quite often these pains are diagnosed as being a type of psychopathology—they are either psychogenic, some sort of conversion or somatoform disorder, malingering, or hypochondriasis. In other words (at least in the eyes of some of the medical establishment), a significant proportion of pains suffered are not genuine pain states at all. They might be pathological, imaginary, feigned, or delusional, but they are not real pains. These sorts of chronic pains (or pseudopains) are, by and large, a mystery. Otherwise perfectly normal people—with no serious (or even superficial) injury—live their lives feeling constant pain.

Few parallels for this situation exist with our other perceptual systems. Rarely do otherwise normal individuals have ongoing visual, auditory, or olfactory experiences without some determinate cause or explanation. Chronic hallucinations by themselves are quite rare. So why are "unreal" pains so common? And how should we understand them?

The philosophical difficulty here is how to explain (or to approach explaining) such phenomena within the materialist framework of the mind/brain sciences. If the mind is just the brain or is at least related to the brain in a metaphysically deep way, then there is an important sense in which all pains are "in the head," as it were. Real pains and psychogenic ones are both the product of the firings of certain neural pathways. If this be the case, then how can we differentiate pathological pains from real ones? What sort of marker would we be looking for? More generally, what is the relation between our minds and our bodily pain or suffering?

Articulating the relation between mental states and physical pains is a large project, and, to a certain extent, it shall occupy us for the rest of the book. In order to answer that larger query, though, there are a range of issues that need to be considered and responded to. Three case studies briefly sketched below introduce some of these puzzles and questions as well as a bit of the variety of pain phenomena that needs to be explained and understood before we can get clear on what a pathological pain might be and what its place is in our mind/brain ontology.

Setting the Stage

Case 1[6] Mathieu Froment-Savoie was born in Canada in 1978. He began playing the violin at age four and then switched to the cello at six. Also at six, he auditioned and was accepted into a music conservatory.

By age ten, he was receiving the highest marks given in the Québec Conservatory exams and was destined to be the protégé of Yo Yo Ma, with whom he carried on an active correspondence. Sadly, Mathieu was diagnosed with cancer of the central nervous system a short time later. Despite aggressive treatment, the disease progressed and Mathieu was unable to continue playing music. These were devastating blows, but Mathieu persevered and flourished in defiance of his illness. He shifted his attention to writing, completing his autobiography before he died.

Though we may stand in awe of this little boy's creative accomplishments, what is important here is that he also used his talents to control his pain. Though he felt his pains intensely, both emotionally and physically, and often demanded assistance in coping with them, Mathieu generally refused any sort of medication when it was actually offered. Instead, he wrote about his life, what music meant to him, what it feels like to have cancer as a child, and his eventual death. He preferred to be "awake"—as lucid and as in touch with his unpleasant world as possible—rather than relieved of pain by artificial means. He chose to live out his life creatively and to use his psychological resources to diminish pain.

And, to a large extent, he was successful. According to a Parent Inventory given after the onset of illness, Mathieu lived in a safe, supportive, and stimulating environment. He was exposed to a wide array of literary and musical efforts and had been introduced to a number of creative people. His special talents were nurtured and protected by his parents. Scores from the Piers-Harris Children's Scale and the What I Think and Feel personal inventory indicated that Mathieu had a strong concept of self. He liked himself, liked other people, was confident, and learned new things well. He believed that he had lots of friends, was loved, and felt just as good as other children. These sorts of self-reports are fairly atypical in children coping with a terminal disease. Health records show that Mathieu dealt with his illness in original and unconventional ways, often analyzing his bouts with pain after the fact and suggesting ways that they could be avoided in the future.

Mathieu died at the age of thirteen, barely a month after his life's work, *Le Cancer à 11 Ans,* was published.

Questions: What can we learn from this little boy's life? What exactly about his intellectual life or the process of writing kept his pain at bay? Could it be that all pains are, in some sense, figments of our imagination that a proper attitude can overcome? Is there a genuine and generalizable therapy here for chronic pain patients, or is Mathieu a special and unique hero, a child to be appreciated but not emulated?

Case 2[7] A middle-aged construction worker woke up one morning with a headache and blindness in his left eye. Upon seeking care at the hospital, he discovered that no treatment was effective. After three weeks of headache and blindness, a nurse encouraged the man to try to count her fingers as she stood about six feet from him. Eventually, he could. The next day, his visual acuity measured 20/20 and his pain was gone. For five years after that, his vision remained normal, but his headaches returned with regularity. Then, his blindness abruptly returned and started to recur with his headaches. Extensive testing could never pinpoint any abnormalities whatsoever. The patient endured pupillary, funduscopic, and ophthalmodynamometric examinations; several blood counts; urinalysis; skull X rays; an electroencephalogram; magnetic resonance imagining of the head and an arterial biopsy; plus tests of his sedimentation rate, his spinal fluid, antinuclear antibodies, and his rheumatoid factor. All were normal. The only item doctors noticed as being even remotely out of the ordinary was that he was easily angered and frustrated during his stay at the hospital. Since his latest bout, he has remained blind and consumes large amounts of over-the-counter analgesics for his headaches. He admits that emotional distress intensifies his pain, but he adamantly refuses to entertain the possibility that his problems are in any way psychological.

Interestingly enough, his son suffered a similar affliction. He developed a severe one-sided headache and two days later his visual acuity measured 20/400. Again, all tests came back normal and no treatment produced any lasting results, though his ophthalmologist could talk him into seeing for a brief period. Over the next few months, his blindness would fluctuate but would always recur with intense headaches. After seven months, the symptoms suddenly ceased and he has had no further relapses. The son also rejected psychological difficulties as the cause of his illness.

His daughter too experienced frequent headaches and blindness attacks, with blindness lasting up to three and a half months. Since childhood, she has suffered from severe headaches accompanied by a great sensitivity to light. Preliminary tests were all normal, but she refused any follow-up examinations, claiming that they had not helped her father. She believes her illness is due to an allergy to monosodium glutamate and some sort of hormonal imbalance.[8]

Questions: How are we to understand this family's headaches? Are they psychogenic, unusual but purely organic migraines, or merely large-scale confusions about what pain behavior amounts to? Is this mass hysteria or an inherited and subtle brain disorder? Should these patients receive psychiatric counseling, undergo more costly medical tests, or be dismissed altogether?

Case 3[9] An eighteen-year-old boy had a horrible accident while waterskiing, damaging several nerves in his cervix and spine. As a result, he lost all sensation and function in his right hand, arm, and shoulder. However, he continued to feel severe and unremitting pain in his damaged limb, which is not unusual with this sort of injury. While in the hospital, morphine, sleeping pills, and various analgesics were administered. He also tried transcutaneous nerve stimulation, physiotherapy, and acupuncture. None of these measures provided any degree of relief. He described his pain as tingling most of the time, with intense burning and stabbing peaks every few minutes. Any movement or other activity increased the severity of the pain. He spent most of his time at home, trying not to move. Though he knew that his pain was "phantom" because his arm was completely paralyzed, the pain certainly felt very real to him.

Hypnotic relaxation techniques and the use of mental imagery helped decrease his sensations of pain. Positive suggestions and discussions designed to build his confidence—made both during hypnosis and as part of psychotherapy—helped him realize that other chronic pain patients can lead fairly normal lives and that he too could do the same. Over the course of several weeks, his perceptions of his pain continued to diminish: he no longer needed a sling to brace his arm, and he was able to return to normal life activities. After only two months of therapy, he was working part-time for his father and training others to water-ski. He felt happier and very busy—too busy to feel pain.

Questions: Is a perception of pain the same thing as being in pain? How could one lose all sensation but, at the same time, still feel intense pain? What is the relation between positive thinking and feeling a pain? What are the psychosocial dimensions to pain? Is hypnosis a serious treatment for pain, or is this youth just being duped into believing that he is better?

We can group the questions I ask into three categories. First, there are questions concerning whether there are such things as pathological pains. Are there normal and abnormal causes of pain? What criteria should we use to distinguish the two? Does the cause of a pain affect how it should be treated?

Second, there are questions concerning the relationship between our sensations of pain and other psychological states. We want to know whether and how other mental states can affect our perception of pain. And, for those who suffer from chronic pain, there is the need to know whether one can learn to manipulate one's own mind so as not to suffer from intractable pain. If we could do this, would this constitute curing a disease or merely learning to ignore what is still present?

Third, there are questions concerning the ontological status of pain itself. Is pain an incorrigible mental state? Could we be in pain but not know it? Conversely, could we believe we are in pain but be mistaken? How exactly should we understand pains: are they attitudes? bodily states? mental events? a relation? some sort of combination or hybrid of these ideas?

This chapter concerns itself primarily with the first category of questions. Here I shall outline my reasons for why I believe diagnosing pain as a mental disorder is mistaken. I am going to present an empirical argument that the pains suffered by Mathieu, the construction worker, and the waterskiing accident victim are all essentially the same. The next chapter will outline some philosophical considerations for the same answer. My main claim there will be that evidence for psychogenic pains being some sort of mental aberration is weak to nonexistent. Chapter four will then argue that there is no metaphysical distinction between mental and physical pains, but I am getting ahead of myself. Let us begin at the beginning.

Are Pains a Mental Disorder?

A Brief Tour of the Official Line

Psychiatrists and other mental health professions have long believed that pains could be caused by various and sundry emotional difficulties. As early as 1871, physicians were asked to render their opinions regarding whether injuries were real or imagined, prompted by third-party insurance companies over disputes in railway accidents. In 1889, Oppenheim introduced the term "traumatischen Neurose" (traumatic neurosis) for delusional pain.[10] Whether that title named anything real was debated in the academic and medical establishments until 1930, when Liniger and Molineus concluded definitively that "eine traumatische Neurose gibt es nicht"[11] (there is no such thing as a traumatic neurosis). That conclusion remained in force, and the medical community rejected any notion of psychogenic pains until 1959, when George Engel produced a then seminal report on otherwise unexplained pains that resist treatment.[12] He labeled these pains "psychogenic." Patients suffering from such disorders were "pain-prone," and he outlined a specific psychodynamic personality profile that allegedly fit them. Thus began the rather large cottage industry in psychiatry of searching for the basic psychiatric or psychological features underlying chronic pain.

As a direct consequence of this movement, the second edition of the *Diagnostic and Statistical Manual of Mental Disorders* (DSM-II) included psychogenic pains under the heading of "psychophysiological disorders."[13] Interest in this phenomenon grew, as did empirical support for it, and the next *DSM* distinguished psychologically induced pain as a separate disorder officially called "Psychogenic Pain."[14] These are pains for which there is evidence that psychological factors played some sort of etiological role and for which no other pathology could account for the degree of pain suffered.

It soon became clear that these criteria are problematic. Too often the history of chronic pains is difficult, if not impossible, to establish. Furthermore, some pains have a completely understandable physical cause but then persist for unknown reasons after the physical abnormality is fixed. Pains with this sort of psychopathological dimension should also be considered. Concerns that there is a genuine mental disorder associated with chronic pain but that the *DSM*-III criteria prevented successful diagnosis led to a serious revamping of how pain disorders were approached in the revised version of *DSM*-III (*DSM*-III-R).

DSM-III-R broadened the mentalistic approach in three ways: psychological factors no longer had to be part of the etiology; other mental disorders could play an influential role in producing the sensations of pain; and patients had to be "preoccupied with pain for at least six months." It renamed the disorder "Somatoform Pain Disorder."[15] These changes increased the scope of the diagnosis of pathological pain disorders and so served to expand the number of cases that could be counted as a mental disturbance.

However, problems with the criteria remained.[16] In a recent literature review of the use of the Somatoform Pain Disorder diagnosis,[17] only five of over two thousand articles surveyed on pain, its psychogenic components, and issues involving classification applied *DSM*-III-R criteria to patients. And none of those articles diagnosed any patients with a somatoform pain disorder. They were concerned primarily with anxiety, phobias, or major depression and its relation to pain. (Since the time of the survey, there has been one article that used the criteria to estimate how many people actually suffer from Somatoform Pain Disorder. The authors of the study concluded that only 0.6 percent of the general population are so afflicted.[18])

The authors of this literature review speculate that one reason for the paucity of use is the vagueness of the criteria. For example, how one is to determine whether someone is "preoccupied" with pain or whether pain is in "excess" of what would be expected is left up to the individual practitioner. Furthermore, clinicians could not use the diagnosis to describe those with both psychological factors and medical conditions contributing to pain or involved in maintaining it. They also could not describe those who exhibit abnormal pain behavior even though their pains have a well-understood physical etiology. Most people with chronic pain and many with acute pain (for which there is no diagnostic category at all) fall into one of these three categories.

Others surmise that, in addition to these considerations, it is possible that a medical cause just has not been detected yet and that even though the pain itself might be explained entirely in terms of physical circumstances, it still might diminish using psychiatric techniques.[19] Though perhaps not enough time has passed to determine fully the value of the *DSM*-III-R criteria, it does appear that several of the problems that plagued *DSM*-III carried over into *DSM*-III-R.

Once again, the description of pain disorders was completely redone for *DSM*-IV, the latest diagnostic manual for mental disorders.[20] The name was changed once again too, this time to "Pain Disorder." The definition was broadened even further so that it now covers medical conditions contributing to the etiology of pain. Moreover, it no longer requires that pain be in excess of what is expected, so long as psychological factors play an important role in its etiology or maintenance. Two types of Pain Disorder are currently recognized: Pain Disorder Associated With Psychological Factors and Pain Disorder Associated With Both Psychological Factors and a General Medical Condition. (A third officially sanctified possibility—Pain Disorder Associated With a General Medical Condition—is not considered a mental disorder.) Not elegant names, I will agree, but they do cover the possibilities.

The box below reproduces *DSM*-IV's diagnostic criteria for Pain Disorders. Pain becomes a mental disorder when it is the primary focus of clinical attention or treatment and if psychological factors comprise an important aspect of the experience. Pains that are part of the normal course of other afflictions—including other mental disorders—are not diagnosed separately as an illness in itself unless the pain is unusually severe or long-lasting. As the *DSM*-IV Guidebook stresses, it is very important to "always rule out substance use or general medical conditions in the differential diagnosis of all presenting symptoms," for these items are "missed surprisingly often in clinical practice."[21]

Though the *DSM*-IV changes have been hailed as a step forward,[22] their real utility is still unclear. It is true that the new criteria are clearer and simpler and that they are more consistent with how clinicians actu-

---

DSM-IV's Diagnostic Criteria for Pain Disorder

A. Pain in one or more anatomical sites is the predominant focus of the clinical presentation and is of sufficient severity to warrant clinical attention.

B. The pain causes clinically significant distress or impairment in social, occupational, or other important areas of functioning.

C. Psychological factors are judged to have an important role in the onset, severity, exacerbation or maintenance of the pain.

D. The symptom or deficit is not intentionally produced or defined....

E. The pain is not better accounted for by a Mood, Anxiety, or Psychotic Disorder and does not meet criteria for Dyspareunia.

Code as follows:
307.80 Pain Disorder Associated With Psychological Factors: psychological factors are judged to have the major role in the onset, severity, exacerbation, or maintenance of the pain. (If a general medical condition is present, it does not have a major role in the onset, severity, exacerbation, or maintenance of the pain.)....

Specify if:
   Acute: duration of less than 6 months
   Chronic: duration of 6 months or more

307.89 Pain Disorder Associated With Both Psychological Factors and a General Medical Condition: both psychological factors and a general medical condition are judged to have important roles in the onset, severity, exacerbation, or maintenance of the pain. The associated general medication condition or anatomical site of the pain ... is coded on Axis III.

Specify if:
   Acute: duration of less than 6 months
   Chronic: duration of 6 months or more

Figure 2.1
The American Psychiatric Association's Definition of Pain Disorder. (From American Psychiatric Association 1994, 461–462.)

ally conceptualize the pathological aspects of pains. However, some worry that it will lead to overdiagnosis of pain as a mental disorder;[23] others believe that the criteria are not open enough.[24]

This may all be moot, though, since, as of July 1997, *no one has published a single article that makes use of the* DSM-IV *criteria for Pain Disorder* (except for commentaries on the criteria themselves).[25] Though perhaps it is too early to determine exactly how fruitful the official American Psychiatric Association's definition for psychopathological pains will be, it is striking how remarkably underused the criteria are, especially in light of the prevalence of inexplicable persistent pains. I conclude that whatever one might think about the veracity of psychogenic pains, the *DSM* definitions are not terribly helpful to clinicians or scientists. Though they may clarify some of our intuitions about when pains are abnormal, they do not meet the need for differentiating normal from abnormal cases of pain phenomena.

The Psychology of Chronic Pain

However, examining the official definitions for pathological pains may not be the best approach to take, if our goal is to elucidate a framework for understanding them, because official definitions and diagnostic tools already assume a certain perspective on the phenomena. Far better is to examine what we all can agree are paradigm cases of psychogenic pains directly without worrying too much over exactly how to define their characteristics. From these, we should be able to cull some basic psychological characteristics of the pains belonging to the putative "pain-prone" patients. We should not expect to end up with a list of necessary and sufficient conditions for being an abnormal pain, but we should at least get some sense of the family resemblances among the cases or—as a best-case scenario—a list of the exemplar traits for our phenomena. Consequently, the next few sections look at recent research aimed at uncovering the psychological profiles of chronic pain patients and the psychodynamic dimensions of psychogenic pain.

I am not promising an exhaustive review in this chapter. That is beyond the scope of this chapter and would be far too unwieldy to be of any use. Instead, although I have tried to be as thorough as possible in locating the relevant literatures, here I only cite cases or studies I believe exemplify current trends and positions.

What follows is my view of the state of the art with respect to clinical psychiatric research on psychogenic pains. To summarize what is to come: It is not a pretty picture. In fact, things are in quite a state of disarray. Experimental protocols are poorly conceived and poorly analyzed. Clinical diagnostics do not measure what the researchers claim they do. And all correlations between hypothesized mental doodads and abnormal pain are weak at best. We have no other choice but to conclude that there is no solid evidence for alleged psychopathological pains being any different than real pains. It looks as though all pains are created equal after all.

Methodological Ills   Our task of summarizing the unproblematic mental dimensions of psychogenic pains is made more difficult by the severe methodological problems of many studies in this area. In particular, inadequate control groups, selection biases, and overinterpretation of positive correlations hamper analyzing pain data. For instance, one study notes that of 654 men who had some form of an anxiety disorder, 5.5 percent had transferred negative emotions into physical symptoms (otherwise known as a somatoform disorder) and that those with a general form of anxiety were more likely than the others to have it.[26] The authors conclude that these facts support the contention that somatoform disorders frequently co-occur with anxiety disorders. But, despite the authors' assertion to the contrary, it is in fact impossible to make this inference without additional information: we have to know what the incidence of somatoform disorders is in a population without anxiety disorders (though otherwise similar to the one studied).

Moreover, we have to know that there is not anything special about the 654 men such that we would antecedently expect them also to have somatoform disorders. One would expect that psychiatric patients enrolled in clinical studies form a particular breed. At the least, they are driven to seek treatment for some reason, something that not all who are ill do. This latter point is frequently overlooked in psychiatric pain research. Scientists perform much of their pain research using patients enrolled in pain clinics receiving treatment for chronic psychogenic pain as subjects. They then generalize results to the population at large.[27] However, to be most effective, a control group of chronic pain sufferers who do not seek treatment in a clinic should be included, for pain clinic patients in fact differ on a number of psychological variables—as well as in socioeconomic status—from nonclinic sufferers.[28]

To be fair, because Pain Disorder is a clinical diagnosis, using traditional scientific experimental protocols is probably not feasible. The best we should expect is a series of correlational studies. Of course, a positive correlation alone does not indicate a causal relation, a fact that many researchers in this domain overlook. One experimental report notes that immigrant workers who are diagnosed with conversion and pain disorders following a work-related injury are more anxious, depressed, and socially dysfunctional than uninjured or psychologically normal immigrant workers.[29] What are we supposed to conclude from these data? That is difficult to discern, for there are too many confounds. Are the depressed workers depressed because they were injured, because they are socially dysfunctional, because their pain does not respond to treatment, because they are unable to work, or because they have always been depressed? We have no way of telling. Some studies even argue that *poor* correlations among different measures of pain for a subject demonstrate the presence of psychogenic pain.

Most troubling, though, are studies that confuse or confound cause and effect. For example, a group at the University of Iowa College of Medicine examined women with pelvic pain. They discovered that, of the women studied, those with a history of sexual abuse and a high rate of somatization were more likely to have pelvic pain for which doctors could not find an organic cause. From this, they concluded that previous sexual abuse predisposes women to somatize and to experience psychogenic pelvic pain.[30] However, they did not show that sexual abuse precedes tendencies to somatize. Nor did they show that sexual abuse, as opposed to physical abuse, was a crucial determining factor. (Indeed, preliminary data suggest that physical abuse is a better predictor than sexual abuse.[31]) They also fail to consider that abuse and neglect could cause physical injuries that result in chronic pain, as well as in psychological abnormalities. Most important—and more alarming—they did not compare the women with chronic pain to those without, so we have no way of knowing what the incidence of sexual abuse, somatic tendencies, but no pelvic pain is in the general population. Without this information, we are prevented from drawing any definitive conclusions regarding the relationship between childhood abuse and pain.

For another example, consider the various hypothesized relationships between depression and chronic pain. We know that selective serotonin re-uptake inhibitors work to decrease pain sensations in some cases of intractable pain and that pain patients have lower concentrations of serotonin markers in their spinal fluid. We also know that a decrease in serotonin is linked to depression. Moreover, persons diagnosed with psychogenic pains are more depressed than those with coronary heart disease or normal controls. They also have greater difficulty adjusting to loss and change.[32]

So far, so good. But then some scientists have erroneously concluded that depression is an important etiological event in pathological pains.[33] Others infer that chronic pain is a variant of depressive illness.[34] However, it is clear to me at least that having intractable pain could cause the depression. The scientists overlook the fact that having what feels like a legitimate illness attributed to a mental disorder is extremely stressful, especially when you are not convinced of this fact yourself. Or, as an alternative possibility, both chronic pain and depression could affect serotonin levels independently.[35] We know very little about what regulates serotonin and how it is connected to depression; it stands to reason that more than one CNS process could influence its concentration.

In considering these possibilities, it is interesting to note that depressed chronic pain patients show considerable differences in their reported thoughts and emotions from depressed individuals without chronic pain.[36] Whatever emotionality chronic pain patients have, at least some of their depression is not a typical clinical depression as indicated by changes in sleeping habits, weight loss, eating abnormalities, or sexual desires.[37]

Some researchers interpret the emotional state of a patient after years of pain to reflect the emotional state of the patient before the onset of pain.[38] But severe distress is a reasonable reaction to unremitting pain, especially to pain for which doctors can find no cause. Still others cite some psychological factor—for example, hostility—as being correlated with psychogenic pains. However, since a significant proportion of patients is not evidently hostile, researchers conclude that those pain patients are repressing their true feelings such that they cannot be detected.[39] Here again, though, hostility and the other psychological variables purported to be causal factor in psychogenic pain are also natural reactions to the very existence of chronic pain.

Several studies indicate that most chronic pain patients have completely normal life histories until the onset of the pain.[40] Neither hostility, depression, nor sexual abuse appears disproportionately. Whatever the psychological results after the onset of chronic pain, we can draw no general inferences from those facts to what the patients' lives were like before the onset. And we certainly can draw no useful inferences without the proper experimental controls and a careful analysis of experimental results. Clinical difficulty or not, researchers studying psychogenic pain must be careful about the morals they draw and how they arrive at them.

Diagnostic Tools   That psychogenic pain is a clinical beast also creates trouble for the clinicians and their traditional diagnostic tools. Getting clear on what is "merely" pain and what are (other) mental disorders is no easy task with what turn out to be the sledgehammer-like tools clinicians must rely on. The *DSM*-III criteria, which are used far more often than the new *DSM*-IV definitions, do not differentiate among all various mental disorders completely. The diagnostics for pain contain substantial overlap with depression.[41] And measures of somatization can be influenced by depression or anxiety.[42]

A second tool in psychiatry often used in diagnosing psychopathological pains is the Minnesota Multiphasic Personality Inventory (MMPI). The traditional MMPI marker for psychopathological pain is the "conversion V"—lower scores on the depression scale and higher scores on hysteria and hypochondria.[43] However, chronic pain sufferers can receive scores indicative of neuroses even if their only aberrant responses are regarding their pains.[44] Not surprisingly, neurotic scores increase as age, the number of surgeries, and the number of doctors consulted also increase, though it isn't prima facie clear that more activity to relieve pain—over perhaps a greater period of time—is in itself substantially neurotic behavior.[45] Moreover, when we look at the results from the NEO personality inventory instead of the MMPI, we find that most psychogenic pain patients score as having normal personalities.[46] (On the other hand, these same patients might test positively for schizophrenia, since schizophrenia diagnostics include somatic complaints and complaints regarding difficulties in living, though I have been assured by one psychiatrist that this does not in fact happen.)

Most important, even though the MMPI shows differences between persons diagnosed with psychogenic pains and controls without pain, it shows no differences between "real" pain patients and those diagnosed with psychogenic pains.[47] The traditional psychiatric diagnostics are too crude to distinguish the different pain states, even differences that the psychiatric community itself defines and endorses! (None of this should be too surprising, though, since the MMPI is designed to measure personality traits, not occurrent psychological states.)

One would expect that with inadequate psychiatric protocols, medical testing would be correspondingly more precise. Such is often not the case, though. For example, many gynecologists generally use only laparoscopy to diagnose women who complain of chronic pelvic pain. If the examination is normal, then the pain is diagnosed as being psychosomatic. By one estimate, this means that an astounding 91.8 percent of all cases of pelvic pain should be considered mental disorders![48] However, a laparascopic exam only shows the exterior of organs; it is used primarily to look for endometriosis. If the pain is generated from something happening within the uterus or fallopian tubes, its causes will not be visible.[49] Whatever the difference between psychogenic pains and physical ones, it is going to be quite subtle and difficult to detect.

Two factors make medical diagnoses difficult.[50] First, multiple causes are generally at work, which makes the precise etiology much harder to pin down. Usually, the best that can be done is to rule out the frank and more obvious pathologies. Second, it is often impossible to examine directly the parts of the body in which the pain is located. In these cases, doctors have to resort to imaging techniques and other indirect measures of anatomy. Unfortunately—though the resolution in imagining technology has greatly improved in the past few years—it isn't perfect, especially when one must examine soft tissue. Even the Cadillac of imaging technology, MRI (magnetic resonance imaging), cannot capture, for example, the lining around the vertebral joins (known as the synovial fold) that contains lots of tiny blood vessels and nerve endings, any of which, when irritated, can contribute to pain.

To see the limitations of imaging in living creatures, as well as to illustrate the complex but minute deformities that can lead to chronic pain, consider figure 2.2, which shows tissue samples taken from an adult female cadaver. What is important to note in these illustrations is that while (a) shows bony projections and a small slipped disk, either of which can cause back pain by pressing on the spinal cord, other nerve roots, or blood vessels, (b) shows these items plus an irritated joint lining, probably from being compressed between the cervical joints. This too can also cause pain. Any of these abnormalities can cause pain; it is likely that a combination of all of them did. And none of these features are easily detectable on routine tests—or even more sophisticated ones.

There are numerous different ways pain can be caused internally: little lesions in joint capsules, slight compressions of autonomic nerves, deformed blood vessels, general degeneration of an area of the body, or some combination of all four. We have no good way to identify any of these problems conclusively prior to autopsy. Standard tests do not discriminate what needs to be studied in order to rule out biological causes of pain. Consequently, we should not automatically label patients as psychologically abnormal when the usual diagnostic tests fail to produce definitive evidence of pain.

Moreover, as physicians dig deeper into the exact causes of different chronic pain syndromes, it is gradually becoming clearer that many disorders originally believed to be purely psychological actually have organic etiologies—in spite of the limitations in our diagnostic technologies. For one example, consider the case of a 54-year-old man who complained of a low back pain that radiated to his left thigh following a serious automobile accident.[51] CT, MRI, myelography, X rays, bone scan, EMG, nerve conduction velocity, and thermography failed to show any abnormalities in his back. Psychological testing, including the Luria-Nebraska test, the Symptom Check List 90, and the MMPI showed postconcussion syndrome, dysthymia, hysteria, hypochondriasis, and depression. Several surgeons evaluated his case and concluded that his pain

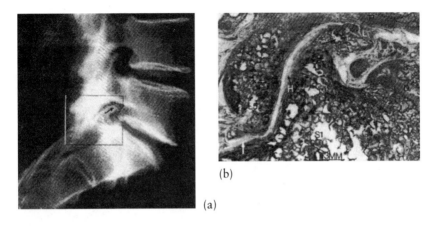

(b)

(a)

Figure 2.2
(a) Side view X ray of lower part of the spine in an adult female cadaver. Two malformations affect the spinal cord: there are several bony projections pressing on the spinal cord (one occurs at the arrow), and one vertebra has slipped relative to another, putting additional stress on the cord. The rectangle shows the region where a 100 mm histological sample was taken. (b) This section shows a very small slipped disk (D) with a bone spur (S). There is also another bony spur at the top of one joint (black arrow), which presses on the spinal cord as well as the motor and sensory nerve roots and their blood vessels. The cartilage on the joint surface of the sacrum is worn or damaged (H). Finally, the lining of the joint (the synovial fold) is irritated and wrinkled (white arrow). L5 is the lumbar joint; L is the ligamentum flarum, one of the ligaments running along the back of the spine. P is the pedical (wing) of the L5 vertebra. (Reproduced from Giles and Kaveri 1990. Reprinted with the kind permission of the publisher.)

was psychogenic. And there his case normally would have ended. However, in this case, a research team from the Mensana Clinic in Maryland created a special three-dimensional reconstructed CT scan of his lumbar spine. It indicated two small bone fractures. (See figure 2.3.) The patient then had a spinal fusion, which reduced his back pain by 75 percent.

The moral of this story is that creative (and often expensive) testing can produce results. Consider recurrent abdominal pain. Its pathogenesis is unknown, and it is usually diagnosed as psychogenic, especially in children with no other obvious health considerations. However, one hospital was able to diagnose sixty-six out of seventy-one children complaining of recurrent abdominal pain with some sort of inflammatory lesion in their gastrointestinal system using tests not normally done on children.[52] Another example: people with burning mouth syndrome also

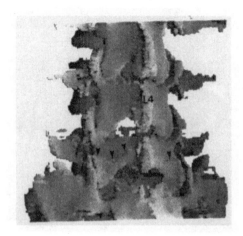

Figure 2.3
L5 laminar fracture (three arrows on left) and L5 right inferior facet fracture (single arrow on right) as seen in a three-dimensional reconstructed CT scan. (Reproduced from Hedler, Zinreich, and Kozilowski 1993, 92. Reprinted with kind permission of the publisher.)

have an increased sensitivity to heat pain on their tongue and lips, which suggests that specific changes in the peripheral pain pathway might be responsible for disorder.[53]

However, even taking these sorts of success stories into account, if physicians can't find a physical cause for a pain and it continues despite repeated medical interventions, they generally persist in attributing it to something "psychological."[54] In my opinion, how we diagnose pain—or fail to—is a serious and embarrassing social and scientific issue. In an analysis of one pain clinic, researchers discovered that 70 percent of laboratory studies indicated significant abnormalities, even though these patients were ultimately diagnosed with pain of a psychological origin. They estimate that fully two-thirds of the diagnoses at referral were either wrong or incomplete.[55] A follow-up study conducted three years later found that 40 percent of patients were incompletely or inaccurately diagnosed, 76 percent of diagnostic tests showed significant abnormalities, and an organic cause for pain was found in 98 percent of the cases.[56]

We have little direct medical evidence for the existence of any psychogenic pains. Much of this deficit can be blamed on our woefully inade-

quate capacity to perform the definitive tests on living, breathing creatures, to be sure. But until technological innovations catch up with our
theoretical knowledge, diagnoses of psychogenic pain in the face of
purely negative tests can be at best an unsupported hypothesis. At worst,
it is a euphemism for our own ignorance.

A different tack is required. Perhaps we should approach this problem
from a different direction. We cannot distinguish "real" from psychogenic pains medically, but if pains are driven by psychological factors,
then we should be able to isolate what those factors are. Can we do this?

The Pain Personality   Isolating the relevant psychological factors in producing psychogenic pain challenges the best of empirical research. Headaches and backaches are the most common complaints at pain clinics,[57]
with almost half the cases of acute back pain becoming chronic (that is,
still in evidence after six months).[58] These ailments would seem to present
a fertile ground for investigation. And they do. But, according to a recent
review of the literature on back pain, exactly no psychosocial differences
between organic and psychogenic backaches have been documented.[59] In
addition, there is no difference in psychological tests between organic and
psychogenic lower back pain patients, including differences in tests for
hysteria, pain duration, physical functioning, or depression.[60]

Indeed, the psychological tendencies that one can find with back pain
are not all what one might expect. If one imagines or feigns or exagger-
ates pain, or if one works oneself up into a painful state in response to
some emotional difficulty, then we might expect an increased sensitivity
to real pains. This pain is exaggerated, so that one will be too. However,
contrary to these sorts of reasonable expectations, instead of being overly
sensitive to pain, or misreading pressure as pain, back pain patients
regularly underpredict laboratory-induced pressure pain relative to normal controls.[61] Victims of back pains expect life to be less painful than
it actually is, despite their experiences otherwise. In sum, we have thus
far been remarkably unsuccessful in discovering any psychological trait
or ailment that is correlated with sensations of back pain.

When we expand our data pool to also include studies from myofacial
disorders, migraine, abdominal pain, and temporomandibular pain, we
still fail to pinpoint any psychological traits that correlate with tendencies

to any sort of pain disorder. Pain sufferers score the same on tests of anxiety, phobia, obsessionality, and somatic preoccupation, regardless of the diagnosed etiology.[62] Some pains can feed depression, fearfulness, and nervous tension. Upon reflection, this should not be surprising at all.

Moreover, psychogenic pain is not a difficulty with pain behavior or with expressing painful feelings. There is no difference in patients diagnosed as having a *DSM*-III-R Pain Disorder on self-reports of pain sensitivity or number of pain locations between those with alexithymia—the inability to verbalize emotional feelings—and those without (though there are differences between those with pain and normal controls).[63] The emotional reactions of persons with psychogenic pains fall in line with those suffering from a diagnosed physical problem: some have problems emoting, and others do not.

Finally, there are no obvious connections between large-scale psychiatric disorders and psychogenic pains. Some studies show *no* differences in the lifetime history of any psychiatric disorders among the different types of pain sufferers, including the incidence of major depression, somatization disorders, or anxiety.[64] It turns out that increased sensitivity to anxiety does increase anxiety itself, as well as negative emotions, cognitive disruption, fears associated with chronic pain, and use of analgesics and other treatments; however, it is not clear that it increases the intensity of the pain sensations themselves.[65] Anxiety can feed negative judgments about being in pain, but it might not affect the pain itself.

In particular, a special connection between pain and depression is not supported. Pain is a common complaint in all psychiatric illnesses—about three-quarters of all nonpsychotic psychiatric patients complain of pain upon admittance.[66] Major depression is found in equal proportion in pain and nonpain psychiatric patients.[67] It is true that serotonergic activity is significantly different in patients with pain than in normal controls. However, no correlation exists between levels of serotonin markers and chronic and acute pain, or among those diagnosed with psychogenic pain, sympathetic pain, somatic pain, or pains of central origin. Finally, no differences in depression (as evaluated by the Zung scale) have been found among types of chronic pain patients.[68] Though robust studies on the relationship between depression and pain are quite limited—only thirteen published during past twenty years[69]—we cannot at this time use degrees of depression to differentiate among pain mechanisms. (Things are even less clear with other personality disorders. I have found studies that suggest that they are more common in medical illnesses than in diagnosed somatoform pain disorders,[70] and those that claim that they are less common with medical illnesses than with diagnosed somatoform pain disorders.[71]).

In general, we have not been able to isolate any psychological factors relevant to psychogenic pain. Studies have tried to relate psychogenic pain to family size, birth order, socioeconomic status, abuse in childhood, and a variety of personality disorders, all without success.[72] In each case, we find no difference between persons diagnosed with chronic psychogenic pain and normal controls. Once we control for confounds, poor instruments, and faulty reasoning, we see that there is no good reason to hypothesize that any psychological factor or trait causes pain.

In short, we have found precious little evidence that pains differ from one another in a fundamental or significant way. In all likelihood, all pains are physical in origin. At least that is where the data currently point. This is not to say that psychological factors do not influence our perceptions of pain. I am quite certain they do, and this topic is explored in later chapters. But we should not oversimplify this role for psychological effects either. Great individual variability exists in the relationship between personality traits and pain. Some people amplify their symptoms, others minimize.[73] A set of complex interactions between physical and psychosocial factors probably best explains each token sensation involved in chronic pain.[74] Whether one can create useful and explanatory generalizations out of the complexity remains to be seen. However, there is no solid evidence that pains amplified by some cognitive or emotional reaction are any different than pains not so amplified; that psychological factors have some impact on pain processing does not differentiate abnormal pains from normal ones.

Others concur with this view. In her review of pain literature, Ann Gamsa concludes that "the body of psychological research into pain has failed to yield compelling evidence for a direct causal relationship between psychological factors and pain in the general population of pain patients."[75] Hendler and Kozikowski note that "if a patient has a disorder that escapes detection by standard objective measures of organic pathology (e.g., EMG, MRI, nerve conduction studies, X ray, myelogram, CT), then the diagnosis of psychogenic pain becomes a self-fulfilling prophecy" as "hypocondriasis, depression, and hysterical features emerge as the result of pain."[76]

But despite an astonishing lack of evidence for any psychological factors correlated with chronic pain, the diagnosis persists. Though the *DSM* criteria are not used very often, some doctors regularly label pains psychogenic or the result of malingering, much to the dismay, frustration, and consternation of their patients. It should be a question of importance why this is the case.

I believe that a large part of the blame can be laid at the feet of these medical doctors and other health-care providers. Part of the problem is health care's general assumption that its medical obligation is to treat pathologies and not to relieve pain. Pain becomes only a somewhat useful marker for the true underlying problem, and once pain's medical usefulness is exhausted, then it is no longer of concern to the medical profession. Many doctors and surgeons consider chronic pain patients "difficult and demanding,"[77] and the medical workups "costly and frustrating."[78] (One wonders how the patients must find them.) Consequently, they recommend the diagnosis of Pain Disorder or Malingering when patients have atypical symptoms or when they do not respond to treatment.[79] They recommend this even when some of the symptoms correspond to specific syndromes, for example, reflex sympathetic dystrophy.[80]

The doctors in turn blame our pop culture for encouraging people to take vague symptoms as evidence for real illness and for popularizing certain trendy, relatively new diseases.[81] As a consequence of making chronic pain a social problem, they do not entertain their patients' complaints of pain seriously, especially when the symptoms do not fit any clear and well-articulated etiological profile. Studies have shown that both doctors and nurses are biased against what they perceive to be psychogenic pains, ranking the discomfort of those pain patients to be substantially less than what the patients in fact report.[82]

Children and women are marginalized the most, with the diagnostic presumption being that their pains are purely psychological.[83] Doctors note, for example, that chest pain in teenagers usually gives rise to no abnormalities in routine tests and that their pains usually disappear on their own. Consequently, their recommendation is not to bother with testing since the pains are not significant. Instead, physicians should provide "support."[84] Often, too, the caregivers (usually women) are blamed for exacerbating the situation, for they generally believe that there remain undiscovered physical causes for their children's pain.[85]

In addition, there are no statistically significant differences between children with recurrent abdominal pain and children without on variety of psychological variables.[86] Somatization scores were higher in recurrent abdominal pain patients as compared to those with a diagnosed organic etiology or well subjects. However, chronicity of abdominal pains was not associated with level of somatization symptoms.[87] And, no relation has yet been found between psychological profiles and the resolution of abdominal pain.[88]

Chronic pelvic pain in women is generally written off as reflecting some previous (maybe forgotten or repressed) sexual trauma.[89] Indeed, attempts to find an organic cause for the pains are seen as counterproductive because they might "reinforce the belief" that the pain is physical.[90] Far better, it is thought, is to provide psychological assessments for women with pelvic pain, reserving medical tests only for the cases in which psychiatric treatment isn't helpful.[91]

But there is little evidence that this approach is warranted. For example, there is no difference in mood disorders between women diagnosed with endometriosis and those with unexplained pelvic pain. (Indeed, social dysfunction is greater with endometriosis.[92]) A recent review of the relation between psychological factors—especially childhood sexual abuse—and chronic pelvic pain was inconclusive. The conclusion was that there is no medical advantage in differentiating psychogenic pelvic pains from organic ones.[93]

Those who claim that some pains are purely subjective or psychological are being too facile.[94] They are not appropriately valuing their patients' ability to report their own bodily states, and they are relying too heavily on the routine diagnostic tests to ferret out any real problems. A more sophisticated and sensitive approach is called for, one that does not demean or dismiss patients' legitimate complaints. A fair start would be to rid the health community of the notion that some pains in themselves are mental disorders. This diagnosis misses the mark and marginalizes chronic pain patients in the medical community. It allows many people to suffer for years, perhaps needlessly, in pain and in relative silence.

In conclusion, empirical attempts to distinguish psychological pain from physical pain have not been successful. Certainly, as I have mentioned, psychological states can aggravate feedback cycles and increase frustration and depression if not diagnosed or treated effectively.[95] But whatever distinctions we make with respect to pain, the psychogenic/organic one should not be it. To put it starkly, no pain is a mental disorder simpliciter.

3

Mind over Matter?

. . . we are not ourselves
When nature, being oppress'd, commands the mind
To suffer with the body.
—William Shakespeare

Common sense would tell us that it is exceedingly difficult for a materialist—that is, someone who believes that our universe is composed only of matter (and its transformations)—to maintain a real distinction between the mental and the physical. Materialism, by its very definition, collapses one into the other. Any mental cause will ultimately be some physical cause or other. Let us assume so much as given.

The assumptions underlying a diagnosis of psychogenic pain are that (1) there are two sorts of causes for pain: organic (or physical) and psychological (or mental), and (2) if pain has no physical explanation, then it has a psychological cause. The last chapter argued that taking (2) as a default assumption is mistaken. I concluded that whatever distinguishes normal pains from abnormal ones isn't going to be physical versus mental etiologies. In this chapter, I tackle (1). The medical establishment's traditional approach to pathological pain appears confused metaphysically as well as being dismissive. What exactly are we doing when we distinguish between the physical and the mental?

Psychiatry is beginning to move away from a rigid physical/nonphysical distinction. (Other disciplines have already moved, more or less.) The last DSM[1] retired the term "organic." Previous DSMs had distinguished between brain malfunctions and various types of mental disorders. But, as the new DSM-IV Guidebook points out:

The accumulating knowledge about the biological factors that contribute to the traditionally nonorganic mental disorders has made this "organic" versus "nonorganic" dichotomy foolish and obsolete. . . . In fact, a literal interpretation of the *DSM*-III-R definition of organic mental disorders and syndromes might dictate that the majority of the disorders in the manual be considered organic. Furthermore, the variety of factors (biological, psychological, and social) that contribute to the origins, onset, and presentation of virtually all of the mental disorders has made it essentially impossible to make very clear distinctions between organic and nonorganic. In a sense, all of the *DSM*-IV disorders are organic; all are also related to psychological factors and to the environmental context.[2]

DSM-IV now only distinguishes between disorders due to a general medical condition and those due to substance use or abuse. Nevertheless, *DSM*-IV still clearly retains a distinction between the organic and the psychological. The psychiatric community does recognize and appreciate the complex and multifarious factors that can produce psychiatric symptoms, but they also divide those causes into biological, psychological, and environmental conditions. Can they do this and still be good materialists? If so, how?

The Terms of the Debate

There are two ways in which we can understand the claim that the mental is different from the physical. It could be the claim that there is a fundamental ontological difference between mental and physical entities, or it could be the claim that there is a fundamental explanatory difference between theories that explain mental phenomena and those that explain physical phenomena. This chapter will be mainly devoted to discussing differences between mental and physical things, for those who hold to a difference in theories generally do so because they believe that some sort of important difference between mental and physical entities forces a difference in the way the sciences of them are practiced.

It will be helpful if we have a simple example of pain before us to guide our thinking about how and whether mental states are physical ones. Here is my example: I drop a hammer on my foot. Among other things (and assuming everything else is equal), this event will cause great writhing, cursing, and gnashing of teeth. It will also cause in me a sensation of pain, and it will lead me to believe that I am now currently in pain. I will come to believe, in some sense, and maybe only in a very crude and nonreflective way, that there is damage to my foot.[3]

The question before us is whether something important distinguishes my sensation of pain and concomitant beliefs from the hammer, my foot, and my pain behavior. Most want to say that yes, it does; sensations and beliefs are mental, while hammers, feet, and bodily movements are physical. *DSM*-IV claims that pains with a purely mental cause are defective, while those with a purely physical cause are normal. It is important to know what this important thing is so that we can evaluate this claim properly. What makes mental objects or properties "mental"? And does this thing distinguish them from the physical?

A materialist must answer that the hallmarks of the mental do not serve to separate it from the rest of the physical world, for the world only contains physical things. Though it is easy to endorse this quick claim, it becomes more difficult to maintain an even somewhat detailed version of materialism. In defending a materialist view of the mental, one is in serious danger of denying that anything at all is mental or that the mental is material after all. To keep both the mental and the physical in place in a material world requires skating a very thin line between the two. Doing that and then also holding that the mental, as opposed to the physical, can uniquely cause other events requires even more navigational skill. In the final analysis, I remain unconvinced that one can or one should distinguish mental from physical causes, though that point need not detain us here.

Mental Causation

There are two sorts of sticking places in defending any sort of materialism of the mind: the problem of mental causation and the problem of naturalizing content. The difficulty with mental causation is roughly as follows. If I drop a hammer on my foot and subsequently experience pain, *that experience* is the proximal cause of my writhing, cursing, and gnashing of teeth. Dropping a hammer on my foot only leads to pain behavior if it causes in me the sensation of pain and the belief that I am in pain. If I were unconscious or otherwise oblivious to my surroundings, then I could not sense any pain, nor could I believe that I were in pain. I could manifest no pain behaviors either.

On the other hand, if we take a neurophysiological view of the entire hammer-dropping incident, then it seems as though we should be able to explain exactly the same events without appealing to mentality or any sort of psychological entities at all. We might talk about the intense pressure of the hammerhead on my foot stimulating various nerve endings, which causes action potentials to travel up my leg to my spinal column, where other nerves are then stimulated to fire. These nerves transmit the firing pattern to other nerves, and so it goes until nerves that cause muscles to contract are likewise stimulated and you get the writhing, wincing, and teeth-gnashing behavior. Why wouldn't the possibility of this sort of more precise, purely physical explanation not rule out the higher level, more general mental account? Or, why wouldn't it make the mental account nothing more than a place-holder until we get the details of our central nervous system figured out? Willard van Orman Quine certainly believes that it does:

If there is a case for mental events and mental states, it must be just that the positing of them, like the positing of molecules, has some indirect systematic efficacy in the development of theory. But if a certain organization of theory could be achieved by thus positing distinctive mental state and events behind physical behavior, surely as much organization could be achieved by positing merely certain correlative physiological states and events instead. . . . The bodily states exist anyway; why add the others?[4]

The last chapter told us that some believe that depression is somehow related to pain processing. For the sake of argument, let us assume that one of the views I mentioned earlier is correct and that untreatable chronic pain leads to depression, which can in turn increase the sensation of pain. This is a brief, probably grossly oversimplified, mentalistic explanation of how a mood causally interacts with other events. At the same time, we also know that depression is correlated with—if not identical to—a decrease in the neurotransmitter serotonin. Persons suffering from chronic pain also show a decrease in serotonin. But, if depression is just an imbalance in serotonin, and sensations of pains are some neural state or other, then why shouldn't we (someday) explain (what we now call) the relation between depression and pain in terms of neurotransmitters affecting neural firing patterns? Why isn't the cartoon story I told above just a stand-in until we have all the more basic neurophysiological details under control?

Mental events causing other events seems to be a natural part of the fabric of our universe. At the same time, accounts of mental causation seem to be nothing over and above a sloppy characterization of more fine-grained and little understood physical details. The difficulty for materialists who would like to keep their minds intact is explicating how it is that mental causation has a legitimate place in our understanding of the universe, above and beyond being a surrogate for the real causal story. Why doesn't materialism lead to pure and simple *eliminativism*? If we take materialism seriously, then why wouldn't we claim that our ultimate goal in explaining psychogenic pain is to reduce our pain states and other related mental events to their instantiating cellular interactions, thus eliminating the former for a discussion of the latter?

Naturalizing Content

Naturalizing content, showing how it is that mental states can refer, point to, or be about other things in our world without begging the question is the second large unfinished project in the materialist's version of the world. Jerry Fodor notes: "Sooner or later the physicists will complete the catalogue they've been compiling of the ultimate and irreducible properties of things. When they do, the likes of *spin, charm,* and *charge* will perhaps appear on their list. But *aboutness* surely won't; intentionality simply doesn't go that deep."[5] "Content" is not a primitive item of our universe; it is composed of some other primitive elements or relations. Explicating what these things are—explaining how mental content is neither mysterious nor mystical—is the problem.

This problem becomes particularly acute when we recognize that quite often our mental states refer to events or things that do not exist and that we can have mistaken, though contentful, beliefs about the world. For example, suppose I believe that a grag flung the hammer at my feet, when, in actuality, grags don't exist. My belief would still be about the behavior of a grag. I could even have particular beliefs about grags' appearances and dispositions. The difficulty is explaining what these mental states refer to, what they are about, without taking representation or reference as primitive.

Most theories of reference or content rely on some sort of causal connection or nomic covariation between an object in the environment and the corresponding mental state about it. My belief that it was a hammer that dropped on my foot is a belief about that hammer, and we know this because we can trace a direct causal pathway from the hammer through my foot to my brain. My belief that I am now in pain covaries with the hammer dropping. I believed that I am in pain now when the hammer dropped, and I didn't believe it before that incident, and presumably I won't believe it after I recover (at least I won't believe it until I have another painful experience). These sorts of connections between the world and my head form the basis for easy stories about reference. This mental state refers to that event or object because of a lawful connection between the two.

But there does not seem to be anything similar that we can say about beliefs about grags, or Santa Claus, or unicorns, or any number of other false propositions we might entertain. What is it that my belief that a grag is responsible for my pain supposed to coincide with to make it that belief and not some other false belief—the belief that a ghost dropped the hammer, say? Being unable to answer this question prevents us from having a satisfactory theory of reference. And without a theory of reference, we cannot explain how it is that mental states can refer to other things. And if we cannot explain content in purely natural or physical terms, then we cannot legitimately claim that the mind really is just another physical object after all. Or so the usual claim goes.

Though most philosophers of mind treat mental causation separately from issues concerning reference, I think explaining the causal powers of the mind piggybacks on the problem of naturalizing content. At bottom, we understand important aspects of the mind as a set of contentful states plus various and sundry operations and transformations involving those states. Being contentful might separate being minded from not. (At least it is a necessary condition.) Any science of the mind is going to have to address the mind qua operations over contentful states.[6]

If we ignore the fact that mental states are contentful, then the question of mental causality becomes no more than the problem of explaining causal interactions among midsized objects. If mental states are really just patterns of neuronal firing patterns (say), then we should be able to account for any mental interaction just in terms of the firing patterns.

But neuronal firing patterns are nothing more than the influx and efflux of ions across cell membranes. So we should be able to account for the interactions of the firing patterns in terms of ionic flow. But the movement of ions across membranes turns on the physico-chemical structure of the ions and the channels. And that depends on the arrangement of electrons, neutrons, and protons . . . And so on down. From this perspective, any sort of causal interaction above those at the very lowest levels of organization should be in principle eliminable, for it seems not to be doing the actual causal labor. Instead, discussions of the higher-level arrangements of matter merely stand in for the complexity of the underlying causal work. Mental states, from a materialist's point of view, would fare no better and no worse than any other potential causal item. This may be a problem, but it wouldn't be a problem peculiar to the mind.

Actually, I don't believe that causality presents much of a problem. Though popular, the sort of reductive metaphysics I outlined above stands on the unwarranted prejudice that the smaller the object, the more "real," or the more ontologically basic, it is. Molecules somehow seem more tangible than our ephemeral sensations of pain; therefore, they get assigned to do the actual stuff of interacting. The rest is mere reflection or appearance. This means that most of what we think of as a simple causal interaction in our everyday life—pressure on a foot causing pain—isn't causal at all. Maybe it isn't even a true interaction. All that stuff takes place between things too small to be seen.

However, I see no reason to give priority to the small in exchange for such uncomfortable consequences, especially when there are other, more plausible strategies immediately available. Our intuitive view of the world is to find causal chains everywhere: the hammer dropping caused my pains; the firing neurons caused more neurons to fire; the concentration gradients caused ions to move in and out; and so forth.[7] Why not just stick with that?

The real question, then, for causality is not locating it properly because it resides all around us, at every level of organization. The real question is deciding *which* causal chain to choose in our explanations and theories of the world. This is not a metaphysical question, but an epistemological or pragmatic one. Of the indefinitely many causes embedded in the universe that underlie each particular change, only a few will best serve our explanatory needs in accounting for this event or events like these at this time. How do we choose?

What makes the question of mental causality peculiar, and more than an epistemological or pragmatic choice, is that the content of the mental states is relevant to their efficacy. I wince and nurse my foot because my corresponding mental states are about my foot. If they were about something else, then I would most likely be doing something else. To explain exactly how it is that mental events cause other things, we are first going to have to explain how it is they refer. That is, to justify privileging a mentalistic explanation of sensations and beliefs over a lower-level physicalistic one of neuronal firing patterns or ionic flow in our scientific explanations, first we have to have a clear grasp of what we mean by mental events being contentful since their content is what is causally relevant to our subsequent behavior.

The question about the power of the content of beliefs and other mental states is quite important to understanding pain processing. We can see this most clearly if we return to the original three case studies of pain from chapter 2. Mathieu, the boy with cancer, used his natural creative and analytic talents to diminish his suffering at the end stage of his illness. Exploring the content of his own beliefs about and reactions to death, disease, and pain reduced Mathieu's sensations of pain. Coming to understand and appreciate the details of his interactions with the hospital staff also helped Mathieu control his pain. In both instances, what his beliefs refer to—death, disease, recent conversations, and so forth—are causally relevant to pain processing. Not just any belief would do. Mathieu needed to have belief states that were explicitly about the nuances of his life story.

In contrast, the construction worker and his children refused to entertain the belief that their pains were at least in part caused by other psychological or psychiatric factors. As a result, treatments were slow in coming, if at all. Health professionals had to work around, or in spite of, the family's conviction that its pains had purely physiological causes. (I leave to the side the question whether the ineffectiveness of medical remedies was due to the doctors' insistence that there was nothing physically wrong with the family or due to the family's denial of their doctors' diagnosis.) Again, the content of the mental states is what is causally most important to explaining the family's and the doctors' behavior. Had either the doctors or these patients believed something else regarding their chronic pains, then the story would have gone very differently, I am sure.

Finally, the teenager with the phantom limb pain learned how to live with his injury in part by learning to believe that he could lead a normal life even though he had lost the use of his arm and shoulder. By shifting his general beliefs about the sort of person he could be, the youth either eliminated his pain or learned to pay less attention to it. Whether these amount to the same thing is a topic for a later chapter. But again, the content of his beliefs, what he believed about himself and what he was capable of doing, was directly relevant to his ability to manage his own pain.

If we are going to understand how it is that merely believing something else—how it is that changing the content of our beliefs—alters pain processing, then it looks as though we need to understand how these states are about things in the first place, since what the mental states are about is the only thing that changes (or is held constant, as in the instance of the construction worker) in these cases. The changes in mental content are causally responsible for enormous changes in pain processing. If we want to understand the etiology of chronic pain, it seems we need to understand how beliefs have content.

Explaining how to naturalize reference, explaining content as a natural and nonmysterious part of our physical world, is an important plank in the materialist's program. Jerry Fodor and others take the project of naturalizing the intentional categories, of showing that things like pain sensations and beliefs about pains are legitimate parts of the physical world as understood by science, as one of fundamental importance.[8] They believe that if representational content cannot be explicated as part of the physical world, then the idea of semantic content and the rest of commonsense psychology are surely false. Furthermore, they hold that if it is true that nothing represents, then some horrible consequence will obtain. To wit: Fodor writes that "if it isn't literally true that my wanting is causally responsible for my reaching. . . , and my believing is causally responsible for my saying, . . . then . . . it's the end of the world," and that the collapse of intentional psychology "would be, beyond comparison, the greatest intellectual catastrophe in the history of our species."[10] In moments less prone to hyperbole, Fodor suggests that "if it turns out that the physicalization—naturalization—of intentional science . . . is impossible, . . . then it seems to me that what you ought to do is do your science in some other way."[11] Fred Dretske concurs: "If reasons aren't causes, one of the chief—indeed (for certain people) the *only*—motive for including them in one's inventory of the mind vanishes."[12]

It appears that if we want to be materialists and we want to maintain the causal efficacy of mentality qua mental, then we need to maintain a defensible view about how content is really part of the physical world we know and understand. If we want to claim that some pains have a mental cause, then we first need a detailed story about how it is that mental states (at times) reflect the external world.

The Real Question

The above, at any rate, is the standard line in philosophy of mind. I don't buy it. Quite often, philosophers muddle metaphysical issues together with logical and empirical ones, much to the detriment of their arguments. I believe that these confusions are occurring here. Actually, in order to understand the mind's place in the world, we can be quite lazy in what we have to explicate. What is not so simple is using this information in our scientific explanations, but that is a topic for another time.

As I mentioned above, the true sticking place in defending any sort of materialism is the question of how to explain the aboutness, the content, of mental states in purely physical terms. How can we demonstrate that the referring state is part of the ordinary natural world, without taking reference itself as metaphysically primitive (and hence suspect)? The *real* difficulty is that so far, nothing has worked. The *real* question is what conclusion we should draw from this fact.

The failure to naturalize content after so much effort has been expended has led some at least to give up on the project itself.[13] Stephen Stich, for example, maintains that the naturalizing project in philosophy of mind itself is ill-conceived. This is bad news for those who want to defend the causal efficacy of the mental in a materialistic framework, for reasons that should now be clear.

I disagree with this assessment. In what follows, I defend one perhaps idiosyncratic view of what naturalism amounts to and, in doing so, I shall set out exactly what is involved in being a materialist about the mind and how this should affect distinctions between biological and psychological causes of pain.

The usual tack to take in defending a materialist vision in philosophy of mind is to outline some sort of metaphysical connection between the mental and the physical. There are several alternatives from which to pick: type-type identity, token-token identity, type-token identity, multiple realizability, determinates and determinables. . . . The list goes on. But, it is my contention that this general strategy is misguided if our goal is to outline the requirements for understanding the mind as being part of the furniture of the physical world. The usual approach is much too ambitious, or so I think. Instead, a very minimal sort of materialism is all that is needed when worrying about whether and how the mind is physical.[14]

In Defense of Lazy Materialism

Stich argues that the naturalizing project itself is misguided, but no horrible consequences follow from that fact (except perhaps that "practically everything that [Fodor] believe[s] about anything is false."[15]). He makes his point by showing that none of the canonized methods for naturalizing representations or content can satisfy a pair of reasonable constraints. In particular, (1) any account will have to "sustain an argument from the premise that intentional notions can't be naturalized to the conclusion that intentional irrealism is true," and (2) there will have to be "some reason to think that, when 'naturalizing' is unpacked along the lines proposed, it is in fact the case that the intentional can't be naturalized"; that is, the claim that content can't be naturalized must be "intuitively plausible" or "supported by a convincing argument."[16] In other words, materialism can't be trivial; it has to have some metaphysical bite. Stich urges that no coherent conception of materialism can simultaneously meet those demands.

Nevertheless, Stich is quick to admit that he is only presenting a survey of three of the possible ways to understand what it is to naturalize content. He allows that "of course, it is always possible that there is some other account that will satisfy the constraints."[17] However, he points out that the onus is on "the other guy" to provide such an account, and until such an account is given, his conclusion—that it is not helpful to worry whether representations are part of the physical world—is the more rational.

Let us take Stich up on his challenge. Our aim is to sketch a version of intentional naturalism that is intuitively plausible, meets his two constraints, and would have rather dire consequences if false (though I strongly doubt it would be the end of the world). I shall proceed first by setting out some simple distinctions I believe have been overlooked in this dialectic—distinctions that help clarify what our goals are in naturalizing some concept—and then by outlining my own account of what naturalizing content amounts to.

Distinctions and Definitions

We can distinguish two questions that fall under the heading of naturalizing content. Many discussions regarding content in philosophy of mind run them together. On the one hand, we can ask whether representations are part of the physical world (and what the question itself means). (More generally, we can ask whether x's are part of the physical world [and what the question itself means].) On the other hand, we can ask: if representations are part of the physical world, then what exactly would the relationship between the semantic and things that (intrinsically) represent be? (More generally, we can ask: if x's are part of the physical world, then what exactly would the relationship between the x and the properties of the things that instantiate x be?) Obviously, these questions differ. I shall be concerned only with the former, since answering it should come before attending to the latter. But first let me illustrate how the two questions can be confused, since keeping them separate will be important for my purposes.

Stephen Schiffer gives us a clear case of confounding the issues. He suggests that how the semantic and the psychological are related to the physical should be "an urgent question" *because* "we should not be prepared to maintain that there *are* semantical or psychological facts unless we are prepared to maintain that such facts are completely determined by, are nothing over and above, physical facts."[18] Notice, though, that we can maintain that representational content is completely determined by the physical facts—we can even maintain that unless content is nothing more than something physical, then semantic facts do not exist—without answering Schiffer's "urgent question" of *how* they are related. To believe otherwise is to confuse a metaphysical question with an empirical one.

Consider an analogous example: the phenomena of gravity. We can (and do) maintain that gravitational attraction is completely determined by physical facts; however, we have little knowledge of the ties between mass and attraction. Notice also that if gravity were not part of the physical world, then we would have to reshape our current fundamental views of the structure of the universe; it would be a fairly serious discovery that gravity is immaterial. However, if we discovered that some particular Grand Unified Theory (or any other theory that specifies how gravity is related to the rest of the world) is false, then the results would not be so dire. We simply would have to try again to state the relationship; our basic ontology need not change. To presume otherwise would be to confuse answering whether x's are part of the natural world with specifying the relationship between x and properties of things that instantiate x. Scientists believe gravitational forces are physical; however, it is perfectly coherent that they also have no beliefs regarding, for example, *how* a change in mass induces a change in gravitational field.

Similarly, we know that anxiety exacerbates chronic pain.[19] We can be quite convinced of this fact and can hold this fact as true without knowing exactly how anxiety does it. All evidence points to some sort of important causal interaction between anxiety and the severity of pain, but the data are not fine-grained enough to cull out the precise causal mechanisms. I can believe that anxiety and other such mental states are part of the physical world and that they have important and real physical consequences without knowing exactly what anxiety is in the brain, how to understand mental states in terms of neuronal interactions, or how to articulate their causal interactions either psychologically or neurophysiologically. To presume that I am required to answer fully the latter before I can believe the former is to confuse answering whether x's are part of the natural world with specifying the relationship between x and properties of things that instantiate x. It is to hold that one needs a completed science before metaphysics can even begin, instead of considering a metaphysical framework prior to empirical investigation.

Setting this issue aside for the moment, let us turn our attention to exploring the affirmative answer to the first question, which materialists must give unequivocally. What do materialists take "nothing over and above [the] physical" to be? Quite simply, I think the following: For each instance of x, x is part of the physical world if and only if x is nothing more than a set of electrons, quarks, kaons, lambdas, etc. (or whatever most basic units are currently in vogue). So, then, chairs are part of the natural world just in case we could specify each instance of a chair in terms of electrons and quarks and so on. This is not to say we would explain *chairness* in terms of the basic quantum elements, but only that we can pick out the space-time region that is this chair using only the basic elements. Similarly, representations and sensations are part of the natural world just in case we can specify each instance of a representation or sensation in terms of electrons and quarks and so on. We don't have to explain what representations or sensations *are* in terms of field inter-ference, or whatever; we just need to be able to pick out the space-time region that comprises this mental state via the basic elements.[20] I take this answer to be little more than an unproblematic materialist position.[21]

In contrast, Stich tries to draw a parallel between the current natural-izing project and logical positivism.[22] He suggests that both take physi-calism and mechanism as *starting* assumptions and then go on to try to specify a legitimating relation R between the thing in question and a set of more basic physical properties. The logical positivists took being a sensory experience to be their more basic physical property. What mod-ern naturalists take as their foundation is unclear, or as Stich asserts; hence the difficulty he sees with the project. Indeed, he holds that because our scientific ontologies are enormously diverse, it would be surprising if there were only one R-relation and set of basic properties. So, for example, we might connect the mind to the brain via the relation of supervenience, but then connect neuroscience to biochemistry via a more straightforward reduction relation. ("Supervenience" names a logical relation between objects. Perhaps the simplest criterion for supervenience is to say that A supervenes on B if a change in A entails a change in B).

Contrary to Stich, though, let me suggest that we qua materialists are restricted to only *one* thing as the R-relation—token identity—and to a *single* set of basic units—the set of electrons, quarks, kaons, lambdas, etc. In other words, there is only one answer to the first question of whether representations are part of the physical world. The more complex ontology and the myriad of relations among all scientifically interesting events and properties that Stich highlights pertain to how to answer the *second* question: if representations are part of the physical world, then what exactly is the relationship between content and the things that are doing the representing? And here I agree with Stich that it is entirely likely that there will be many different but correct answers to that question depending on how it is posed.

This space-time worm of gravitation attraction is composed of basic physical elements and nothing else. This hammer-dropping instance of pain is likewise composed of nothing more than electrons, lambdas, quarks, and so forth. It could be that in our completed sciences, we would understand and explain all cases of gravity as abstractions of particular configurations of our basic elements (whatever they turned out to be), but we would not be able to abstract over pain in the same way. Pain might turn out to be some sort of higher-level object or property that only decomposes into a messy and uninteresting disjunction of basic element descriptions: hammer-pounding-on-toes pain would be described in one way; heartburn in another; tension headaches in yet another. In this case, we would say that gravity is reducible but pain isn't. So be it. This would not cut against our belief that pain still is purely physical in just the same way that gravity is. Each token instance of gravity or pain is identical to some set of basic elements or other. It is a further question whether we can create interesting and explanatory generalizations across our token identities.[23]

I should emphasize that I am not claiming that what makes chairs, or representations, sensations of pain, or whatever, *what they are* is specifiability in terms of more basic units. What makes a chair a chair in part turns on how we use it; a chair is a functional unit. Though I can only guess what makes representations and sensations what they are, I am quite sure that, whatever it is, it will be some relational property as well.

Furthermore, these sorts of relational properties will *not* be capturable in terms of the fundamental elements, for they hold only at the macrolevel. To take a simple example, consider the relation "taller than."

I am taller than my children. At bottom, I am this lattice of molecules, and molecules are composed of quarks, lambdas, etc. Consequently, you should be able to specify me in terms of the fundamental units of physics; that is, you should be able to specify the space-time region that makes up my time worm. From this perspective, there is not a lot of difference between me and my children. You can specify their time worms in the same way. However, from the perspective of massless fields in a Hilbert space, "taller than" loses its meaning. To be "taller than" something, you have to be at least oriented in a particular direction relative to some frame of reference. This is a descriptor that applies only to midsized observables.[24]

For a slightly more complicated example, consider the (probably false) claim that a history of sexual abuse in childhood is correlated with psychogenic pelvic pain in women.[25] Childhood sexual abuse is causally related to later pelvic pain. Each instance of abuse and each time-slice of pain are composed of nothing more than the basic elements of the universe. But so far as physics is concerned, the specification of one set of fundamental particles is pretty much like any other set. From the vantage point of quantum mechanics, there really is nothing to distinguish an instance of sexual abuse from appropriate sexual behavior from physical abuse, nor is there anything to distinguish pelvic pain from shoulder aches from indigestion. Sexual abuse requires at least two people, at least one of whom is cognizant of what he or she is doing to the other person. To be in pain requires being a living organism. But being cognizant, affecting another person, and being alive are properties that inhere only in organized macrolevel objects. They require suitably animal-like bodies.

Some have suggested that we still should be able to reduce relations and properties to lower-level physics (for otherwise these properties would be completely mysterious, harking back to the emergentists of the twenties). I do not believe that they are correct, at least not in any straightforward way (nor, however, do I think higher-level properties are inherently spooky; they are just relations among macrolevel objects, specified in terms of those macrolevel objects). In order to discuss my height relative to that of my children, you not only have to specify my space-time region and the space-time regions of my children, but you also have to specify some common observational frame. In order to discuss abuse, you are going to have to account for both the interaction of alive animal bodies and some awareness of social mores. I don't see how you are going to do any of this without smuggling in a higher-level perspective. Observational frames are defined in terms of observers, who exist at a macrolevel. Comprehension is also defined in terms of an "observer," namely, the thing doing the comprehending. The requirement for observers means that macrolevel properties are confined to macrolevel objects. Hence, they aren't reducible to sets of quarks or whatever. Nevertheless, individual instances of the macro-objects—including any observer—are "nothing over and above" sets of micro-units.

I should point out though that in suggesting this as an admittedly simple-minded version of what a materialist's position amounts to, I diverge from Stich's construe of the project. He understands naturalism as relating *properties;* I see it as relating *objects.* This is no trivial distinction. Properties are not reducible in the sense in which objects are. And if naturalism is about properties, then I don't understand what it is either, except perhaps as the position that the individual objects in which properties inhere are nothing more than sets of micro-units.[26]

I recognize that this simple-minded position does little to answer the second question above, namely, how to understand the relationship between the higher-level objects to be naturalized and various lower-level units. This is a complex and difficult issue. Fortunately though, *this* issue does not have to be settled either to be a materialist or to answer the first question.

Defining Mental States

Nevertheless, our work is not yet finished. It is not enough to posit that sensations of pain or beliefs about pain sensations are part of the physical world in the weak manner above without attempting to elaborate upon this position. Materialism as I construe it literally falls out of the assumption of physicalism. What is more interesting and more difficult is to articulate how we should understand representations and sensations once we have adopted a materialist framework. This question too may differ from the second one above in that how we should *understand* content may be orthogonal to how lower levels of organization actually *instantiate* content. Understanding something is an epistemological concern; how that thing actually *is* is a metaphysical question.

This second inquiry, also fundamental to the materialist's project, can also be divided into two parts. First, we can ask: What are representations? How should we conceive of representational content in a materialist, mechanistic world? Second, we can ask: How are we to understand this particular representation? What conditions in the world make it true that *r* represents *s*? Again, I maintain that I shall only be responsible for answering the first (or trying to, at any rate) in order to justify a materialist's perspective. Nevertheless, philosophers confuse responding to the first, which revolves around whether semantic content is a scientifically respectable notion, with responding to the second, which turns on whether individual instances fall under the extension of "content."

We can see an instance of this confusion in Stich's own discussion of conceptual analysis as a contender for the naturalizing project. He intimates that because there are plausible accounts of representation that do not involve necessary and sufficient conditions, for example, Eleanor Rosch's prototype theory,[27] then any approach that presumes to define concepts in terms of necessary and sufficient conditions is outdated. But this suggestion confuses the two questions.

Rosch's research in prototype theory and other related projects are directed in part toward explaining what mental representations are (they are prototypes) and how to understand them in a naturalist framework (they are directed vectors in a multidimensional state space[28]). Her research is in service of the first question. However, Stich takes her to be answering the second question and explaining how the scientific term "concept" is supposed to work, what conditions in the world are required for it to refer to a concept. This is a separate issue, unless you can show that terms in scientific theories represent in the same way as our brains represent.[29]

Despite the fact that our brains might represent the world using prototypical vectors, as scientists, we can still give a list of necessary and sufficient conditions for being a prototype, a directed vector, a state space, etc. Stich is just wrong when he claims that "if Classical theory [of content] is wrong, then terms like 'force', 'mass', and 'gravity' won't be definable."[30] Of course, they will be definable. Science is in the business of defining them for us. To wit: Force is the condition necessary to bring about a change in the state of motion of any material object. Mass is the measure of resistance by a material object to any change in its state of motion. Gravity is the observed phenomena of identical change in the state of motion of different material objects at given fixed locations independent of the particular object's mass, when no other change in environmental conditions is observed.[31] If something like prototype theory is right, then we may not *recognize* a force, the mass of some object, or gravity in terms of necessary and sufficient conditions. In all likelihood, we will use some sort of similarity matrix to distinguish force from mass on the fly. However, *how we represent these ideas in our head in our daily lives is a separate question from how we represent them scientifically or on paper.* To presume all instances of representation are exactly alike is to presume that any answer to the first question is also an answer to the second.

Cognitive science is charged with telling us what representations are in our species. It will tell us what is going on in my brain when I believe that I dropped a hammer on my foot and am now in pain. Neurology is charged with telling us with what happens in my foot when I drop a hammer on it. It may represent the hammer-dropping events in some sort of diagram, as a flow chart of neural firings, perhaps. Linguistics might then tell us how it is that neurology's illustration appropriately abstracts and reflects the actual events. But it is highly unlikely that the sheet of paper that contains the rendering of low-level nociceptive processes in any way resembles what is required in our brains for beliefs, what cognitive science will ultimately tell us is going on. The sorts of representing occurring here are simply different. And it is up to science to sort out how we should conceive of both cases of representation, for these are empirical questions that turn on the domains of the individual disciplines.

"Content" and "representation" are terms that scientists will presumably use in their hypotheses and laws about us existing in our world. This would make them natural kind terms. A "natural kind" refers to all the objects that fall under some law. All natural kind terms (in all disciplines) aim to refer to the "essence" of a set of objects; science does want to carve nature at her proverbial joints. Each discipline that uses the notion of representation as a natural kind should define the idea using the terms and methods appropriate to that domain. Whether these notions will ultimately have something interesting in common is something yet to be determined and relatively unimportant from the perspective of the individual sciences.

What also varies across the disciplines is the relative scope of their scientific laws. The domain of physics and chemistry, for example, is quite large; in general, their laws range over the entire universe. The old chestnut, "water is H_2O," is a law of chemistry that picks out the underlying nature of water, regardless of where or when in the universe you happen to be. (That is, the necessary and sufficient conditions for being water is to be H_2O, at any place and at any time.) In other cases, the natural kind terms are not so broadly defined, even though the "essences" are still thought to be captured. *Homo sapiens* as a creature with a particular evolutionary history is one such example. Though a necessary and sufficient condition for being *Homo sapiens* is to have a certain evolutionary history, hypotheses concerning the evolution of man refer only to one planet at a particular time. Still other cases have even smaller scopes. These natural kinds might be operationally defined. The "special" sciences are replete with instances of this sort. "I.Q. is the score on an I.Q. test" is but one such instance.

Despite some philosophers wanting all scientific laws to range over the entire universe, psychological laws generally range over a particular species (or set of species). I suspect that the notion of mental content will fall in the latter category: psychological laws involving mental representations will have a fairly narrow scope and will be defined in virtue of some operation we could perform to test whether something is a representation. Nevertheless, they will still (intend to) articulate the essence of what it is to be representational in the mind.

The answer to the (second) first question is that semantic content is whatever science understands it to be, and this answer may differ across domains. It is then a further question whether any particular instance of putative representation should fall under some particular definition of the term. I would expect that my sensation of pain and my belief that I am now in pain should fall under the laws that cognitive science develops concerning mental activity. I would not expect that neurology's drawing of nociception in the foot should be an expression of the same laws. But these questions are best left to the details of the individual empirical enterprises.

Of course, it is entirely possible that science ultimately will not use the notion of semantic content in any of its laws. If this were to occur, we would have to conclude that representations are not scientific entities and any explanations of behavior that rely on the intentional in the *explanans* will have to be dismissed as incorrect just as we now dismiss explanations that use witches or phlogiston. However, serious repercussions would occur if we could not use content in our scientific explanations, for much of current psychology explicitly assumes the mind's representational capacity. The prototype hypothesis discussed above is just one case in point. Indeed, much of modern biology, neuroscience, computer science, and cognitive science explicitly relies upon content as a natural kind. For a short list of examples, consider discussions revolving around infant cognitive development, our folk sciences, the binding problem, mnemonic associations, clinical disorders, neural ethology, strong artificial intelligence, our sensory processes, language, socialization, learning, differentiating our memory systems, and cognitive neuroscience. Theories from these areas would not just have to be revised if content turns out not to be a natural kind; the areas themselves would have to be replaced, for we would have to find another way to conceptualize an organism's behavior and interactions—a way that does not rely on contentful states of any sort. I suggest that this type of fundamental change in the ontology of the special sciences would be comparable to discovering that gravity is not physical and to the alterations in the basic ontology of the physical sciences that would ensue as a result.

If the intentional is not part of the natural world (which in a materialist's framework would be tantamount to saying that content does not exist), then scientists would have to reconceptualize how to explain purposeful bodily movements, higher-level brain states, patterns of activation in connectionist nets, social interactions, and so on. And because content and related ideas are so embedded in theories in the special sciences, I maintain that the magnitude of the shift in our Weltanshauung would not be on a par with the mere denial of witches or phlogiston; instead, it would be as drastic as the Copernican revolution.

Nonetheless, Stich is quite right when he asserts that if science does not use the notion of representation in its theories, then perhaps it would still be a perfectly legitimate interest-relative term, similar to our notions of dirt or germ. So far as I can tell, content not being a scientific term will have little impact on our common sense explanations of one another. "Folk" psychology, like other folk "sciences," need not be concerned with facts of the matter. It could function as well (or as poorly) as it ever did, regardless of whether intentional states really exist.

However, recognizing that point says little about how science proper should react. And since there are many significant and influential theories that assume the existence of content, demonstrating that content does not exist should force a fundamental shift in our scientific ontology. Though I do not believe the consequences are as dire as Fodor and others paint them to be, the ramifications would still be far-reaching.

Meeting Stich's Challenge: Philosophy's Place in Science

I read Stich as holding that if our scientific conception of the intentional does not line up with our first-pass or commonsense intuitions, then any new more radical view of natural representations cannot meet his second criterion for naturalizing the intentional, that materialism has to be nontrivial.[32] Since most of the arguments about whether representational content is part of the physical world turn on our folk views, ridding ourselves of those views and the concomitant arguments leaves us little reason to believe that whatever concept science ends up using can't be naturalized. (Indeed, since we do not yet have something that approaches a completed science, speculating on what is and is not a true scientific term is premature, to say the least.) Philosophy then should remain silent until science has made up its mind about how to conceptualize representations.

It is my position that science should help us understand representational content. Like Stich, I believe that "if there is good science to be made out of the intentional categories, that's all the legitimization they need."[33] Moreover, I do expect that this scientific conception will differ from our ordinary folk accounts. So, "pure" conceptual analysis of our notions would be rather useless. But this does not mean that philosophy is out of the game; I disagree with Stich that working science alone will settle the issue. An important part of philosophy revolves around analyzing good science, and one component of that task is deciding whether (and in virtue of what) the terms scientists use in their theories and explanations are kosher. Philosophically analyzing a scientifically informed view of concepts could still be enormously useful in that it could tell us whether the concept that science either implicitly or explicitly defines is free from troubling counterexamples. Philosophy can aid in setting the parameters of defining a scientific term. One should not be duped into believing that just because science makes use of a concept, the concept is therefore coherent or legitimate.

For example, Hilary Putnam's and Tyler Burge's well-known Twin Earth puzzles demonstrate that our first-pass intuitions about how to understand content in a rigorous manner have to be incorrect.[34] We learned that if reference to the larger environmental or social surrounds are required for assigning representational content, then molecule-for-molecule identical brain states (or whatever) could differ in what they represent if they are located in significantly different contexts. Hence, any scientific conception of content will not be able to individuate mental states "widely" (in terms of environmental or social context), else we lose supervenience (and with that our materialist mechanistic view of the universe). And if a wide causal theory of reference were the only way to explain content, then the Twin Earth thought experiments would show that content as we think of it cannot exist, for we would lose token-token identity between the "mental" and its instantiators. However, similar to the failure of Grand Unified Theory with respect to gravity, these thought experiments really only show we should try again to articulate how to understand the intentional. We now know that a scientific conception of content will have to be more "narrow" than our folk conceptions.

Nevertheless, even at this stage of infant scientific and philosophical speculations, there is at least one reason to suspect that content may not be part of the natural world. That is simply that even though many people have tried to define representations naturalistically, no account has succeeded. Moreover, the failures are not explained by the fact that philosophers may not have a clear idea of what naturalizing amounts to. A quick survey of the field tells us that the lack of success turns on problems intrinsic to the proposals themselves. To wit, wide-content accounts belie supervenience, teleological and information-theoretical accounts fall prey to the problem of error, causal historical "narrow" accounts turn out to be interest relative,[35] and so on. The death of a thousand failures may be upon us. If so, then content should not be considered a proper notion at all, much less something suitable for scientific inquiry. Currently being unable to articulate exactly what content is keeps materialism from being a trivial claim.

In fact, both of Stich's constraints are met. We do have a serious reason to believe that the naturalizing project may not work: so far, we cannot get it to work. Our failures prevent materialism from being an easy and obvious position. This meets the second challenge, that materialism be a real and interesting position. Moreover, despite philosophy's abject failure thus far, science continues to use the notion of representation unabashedly and in all sorts of ways. If our failure is complete, then we would have no choice but to become irrealists about content, for eliminativism—our only other option—is already out of the question. This meets the first challenge, that a failure to naturalize sustains an argument to the conclusion that we cannot be realists about mental representations.

Mental versus Physical Causes

It makes perfect sense to adopt a serious materialism yet also to profess ignorance regarding the details of any particular physical interaction. Claiming that everything is physical is a stance we take about our universe prior to empirical investigation.[36] It is the framework into which we then fit our more detailed analyses of the world around us. We do not need to answer all of science's ontological questions before being able to discuss issues philosophically. Philosophy sets the stage for science—it can provide useful frameworks for inquiry—but it cannot and should not settle the important empirical issues regarding the particular connections among levels of objects and their properties. We can understand mental states are being purely physical without having to explain exactly how their representational capacity occurs.

The psychiatric community is justified in claiming that all pain is organic, with both psychological and biological events contributing to the pain process, since that is what our best science tells us at the moment. That is all the justification that they need. This is not to say that science's pronouncements are the end of the story: each claim should be subject to philosophical and empirical scrutiny. However, that we cannot at this moment spell out exactly what we mean by a psychological event and exactly what distinguishes it from biological ones does not mean that the distinction is a useless one or that we should not draw it.

Indeed, even though a sharp list of necessary and sufficient conditions for being mental eludes us, the distinction between mental and biological causes is prima facie clear in the study of pain processing. To illustrate what I mean, consider physician Paul Brand's memory of confronting his first patient suffering from the inability to feel pain. His description underscores both the central role of pain in our everyday lives and the so-very-important connection between incoming pain information, what we believe about the world and ourselves, and how we act.

Tanya was a four-year-old patient with dark, flashing eyes, curly hair and an impish smile. . . . Testing her swollen left ankle, I found that the foot rotated freely, the sign of a fully dislocated ankle. I winced at the unnatural movement, but Tanya did not. . . . When I unwrapped the last bandage, I found grossly infected ulcers on the soles of both feet. Ever so gently I probed the wounds, glancing at Tanya's face for some reaction. She showed none. The probe pushed easily through soft, necrotic tissue, and I could even see the white gleam of bare bone. Still no reaction from Tanya. . . .

[I]t seemed apparent that Tanya suffered form a rare genetic defect known informally as "congenital indifference to pain." She was healthy in every respect but one: she did not feel pain. Nerves in her hands and feet transmitted messages about changes in pressure and temperature—she felt a kind of tingling when she burned herself or bit her finger—but these carried no hint of unpleasantness. Tanya lacked any mental construct of pain. . . .

Seven years later I received a telephone call from Tanya's mother. . . . Tanya, now eleven, was living a pathetic existence in an institution. She had lost both legs to amputation: she had refused to wear proper shoes and that, coupled with her failure to limp or to shift weight when standing (because she felt no discomfort), had eventually put intolerable pressure on her joints. Tanya had also lost most of her fingers. Her elbows were constantly dislocated. She suffered the effects of chronic sepsis from ulcers on her hands and amputation stumps. Her tongue was lacerated and badly scarred from her nervous habit of chewing it.[37]

That Tanya could not sense pain as we do is truly unfortunate. However, that fact could have been mitigated a bit by an awareness of how pain information functions in the production of movement and beliefs. It is a belief that pain sensations should be avoided or that pain sensations should provoke certain protective movements that could connect the tingling sensations that Tanya receives to appropriate behaviors. Her lack of these mental states contributed to destroying her body. One of the tragedies of Tanya is that she could not or did not form appropriate beliefs about pain and bodily preservation.

The story of Tanya and what she was missing relies on a rough-and-ready distinction between mental states—the things with content—and physical states—the things without content—that we can use in further investigations. And that is probably as good as it is going to get for now. Psychology, psychiatry, cognitive science, and biology all recognize a distinction between the mental and the physical, and they have constructed elaborate theories based on this distinction. Whether the distinction will ultimately be maintained is another question, but it need not be answered to do the science today, just as the ultimate truth of any posit need not be concluded before any theory is adopted.

Even though I do not believe that pains for which we can find no physical cause should be presumed to have a mental one, I do believe that distinguishing the mental from the physical makes sense from the perspective of contemporary science, even though the mental and the physical are comprised of the same basic stuff. And how the mental and the physical interact in our pain processing is the subject for most of the remainder of the book.

4

What We Don't Know About Brains:
Two Competing Perspectives

To the theoretical question, can you design a machine to do whatever a brain can do? the answer is this: If you will specify in a finite and unambiguous way what you think a brain does . . . then we can design a machine to do it. . . . But can you say what you think brains do?
—W. S. McCulloch

Pains can have a multitude of causes. Some of these are "physical"; some might be "mental." But regardless of type of cause, they will all be organic, biological, neural. Hence, understanding the details of pain processing is ultimately going to turn on how well we understand the brain. What do we know about brains in general? And what do we know in particular about pain processing in the brain? We just finished living through President Bush's Decade of the Brain. What did it teach us?

Though our knowledge of the brain did increase by leaps and bounds, we still do not know as much as we would like. Most everyone knows that we don't know everything there is to know about the brain. Most everyone also probably knows that we really know very little about it. However, what is less known is that we don't even know how to conceptualize the brain in the most general way. We don't know what the relevant processing units are, much less how they operate.

This chapter serves as a warning to those continuing on to the rest of the book: We know not whereof we speak from here on out. I give you educated guesswork and piecemeal investigation held together by dogma and faith. But I cannot give you any definitive answers, for we cannot even be sure that we are on the right track in our empirical testing of the brain.

Negative arguments are difficult to make. My approach in illustrating the depth of our ignorance in neuroscience is to outline the guiding doctrines in brain research and highlight their weaknesses and fundamental points of conflict. These doctrines shape how we interpret the data—indeed, they determine what we call data in the first place. Their respective merits and liabilities are currently being debated in journals, laboratories, conferences, barrooms, and hallways around the world. And these perspectives are in deep conflict, over what counts as evidence for a claim, over what counts as a good scientific explanation, and over what the fundamental unit of cognition is. That there is more than one fundamental doctrine in neuroscience and that they cannot agree on the most basic points in science tell us something about what we do not know about the brain. In particular, they tell us that we do not agree on the units of organization in the brain, the methods by which we should investigate these units, and when we have a successful explanation in neuroscience.

However, as we shall see, which perspective is correct—or, at least, which one is better than the others—is not going to depend much on conceptual issues, as one might have expected. Rather, the resolution of this conflict will probably have to wait for future technological developments. It is a trivial observation that technology changes how we see things, that different devices give us different perspectives on the world. Though undoubtedly true, there is more to the story of explaining psychoneural phenomena than this. This is a story of a missing technological infrastructure in neuroscience that prevents us from being able to determine what the basic cognitive currency is in the brain, including how to understand pain.

The Feature-Detection Perspective

There are three competing perspectives in neuroscience: feature detection, dynamical systems, and dendritic microprocessing. The first, most popular, and most intuitive approach maintains that the firing neuron is the basic brain unit. The second, less popular, but rapidly expanding approach holds that large-scale patterns found within neuronal activity is most basic. The third and decidedly minority view is that dendritic networks form the most basic unit.

In this chapter, I focus on only the first two approaches, for the power of dendritic microprocessing has not yet made it to the pain literature. Both of these perspectives operate on the cutting edge of technology, and scientists from both camps have pioneered their own techniques to advance their investigations and further justify their approach. Moreover, both theoretical orientations offer solutions to the same general problem in neuroscience, that of how we should explain mental processing in the brain. But there is currently no good way to adjudicate between the views. As a result, our understanding of pain, such as it is, will be a hodgepodge of data, bolstered by different experimental techniques and theoretical orientations, held together only by the belief that all will be made into a coherent account someday.

The Organization of the Brain[1]

The neurons that make up the brain are essentially identical across all animals in the kingdom. As is now almost common knowledge, the human brain contains about 10^{11} neurons and 10^{14} synapses (give or take an order of magnitude). Simple subtraction tells us that the average number of synapses per cell is about a thousand, eight orders of magnitude less than the total number of neurons. If each synapse were connected to a different neuron (which is unlikely), then each cell would communicate directly with only about one out of every hundred million cells, which is but a tiny fraction of the total brain. This means that the brain is not fully distributed, as cognitive scientists often pretend. In fact, though distal connections are important, information processing in the brain is largely local, for most neuronal connections are made within a millimeter of the cell body.

In any event, our neurons are arranged in a dense mass (called a neuropil) in the cranium, with only about two tenths of a μm separating each cell. On average, each cell has a cell body (or soma) somewhere between 5 and 100 μm across. At one end of the soma, a single axon radiates outward, then bursts into a veritable forest of branches. At the other, we find a multitude of dendrites extending from the cell. Incoming

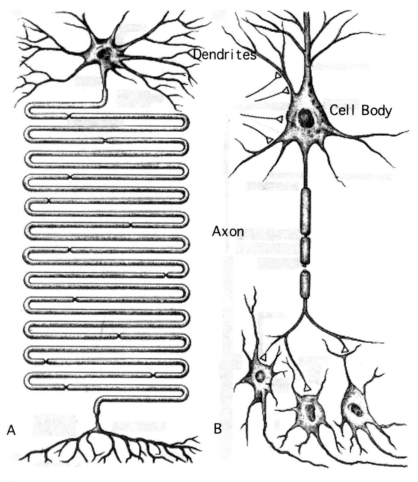

Figure 4.1
Main Features of a Neuron. (A) A neuron scaled relatively proportionally, though axons can vary greatly in length—some measure longer than a meter—and are thinner relative to the soma than pictured here. (B) Neuron drawn to illustrate points of contact with other neurons (drawn as triangles). Most synapses join the axon terminals of one neurons with the dendrites or cell body of another neuron. Thus dendrites from a single neuron might receive signals from hundreds or thousands of other cells. (After Kandel and Schwartz 1985.)

action potentials from other neurons pass through the dendrites to the soma, or impinge directly upon the cell body itself. (See figure 4.1.) The cell body computes a weighted "average" of the incoming pulses (quotes are used because the computation is actually more complicated than mere averaging) and then the axon transmits the result to new cells. For all this to occur takes about one-thousandth of a second, which is pretty slow in computational time.

In 1908, Brodmann discovered that there were six major horizontal layers across cortex.[2] Our description of this laminar pattern became more complex in 1943, when Lorente de Nó found vertical columns transecting the horizontal layers.[3] We now believe that these columns form processing modules in the brain within which complex computations occur. The results are then broadcast to neighboring modules and across cortex via pyramidal cells. The connections within layers III, IV, and V of each module are similar, as are the connections in layers I and II.

The view of brain processing that results is one of a linear, hierarchical, and locally distributed information flow. Data comes in through the sensory transducers and then flows more or less in a direct path to cortex. As it flows, it is being computed over and transformed along the way. Each sucessive transformation or computation is more abstract, more removed from the actual stimulus itself, and more closely tied to some sort of conceptual representation of what that stimulus might mean. This process occurs across many neurons; we can't identify the one neuron that represents this experience of pain. At the same time, however, not all the neurons in your head are involved in each thought; only a few are, and those few live close together.

In the same year that neuronal columns were discovered, McCulloch and Pitt published their seminal work on cognition in the brain.[4] On the basis of their research, they hypothesized that axonal discharge is the currency of cognition. The advent of microelectrode studies in 1957, which allowed scientists to study single neurons in their natural environments, provided data that corroborated the conjecture. Vernon Mountcastle showed that each column in the brain has a similar response pattern to very specific inputs and differs from other columns.[5] His data fed the view that neuronal columns are the basic processing unit in the brain.

The final linchpin in developing what is now the dominant approach in understanding the brain's computations was Hubel and Weisel's isolation of the receptive fields for individual neurons.[6] They showed that different neurons respond differently to different stimuli, and more important, that individual neurons prefer to respond to specific features in the world. Cells located close to one another in a column exhibit similar response patterns. The basic presumption of "feature detector" cells, organized into computational clumps, was born.

In brief, the feature detector approach assumes that (1) each sensory stimulus causes a few neurons to react radically, while having little influence on the rest of the neurons in that sensory modality; that (2) neurons respond to basic features in the world (movement, tilt, pressure, sweetness, etc.); and that (3) we go from simple to complex responses up a neuronal processing stream. The general schematic is of a "pontifical" hierarchy in which information travels from the periphery up to cortex (and then back out again), with the highest levels of cortex responding to the most abstract and complex inputs.

This perspective is what inspires the computer/information processing metaphor and reductionist methodologies so prevalent today. Neuroscientists who buy into this view believe that understanding the mind/brain means decomposing cognitive processing tasks into a series of simpler and more basic manipulations.[7] Patricia Churchland and Terence Sejnowski provide a nice statement of this perspective in the opening sentence of their book *The Computational Brain:* "Major advances in science often consist in discovering how macroscale phenomena reduce to their microscale constituents."[8]

What I am calling the "feature detection" perspective includes a wide range of hypotheses and experimental approaches, including most computational neuroscience. By the name, I do not mean to suggest that this approach requires seeking only feature detectors in our nervous system or that we can isolate the units of cognition independent of how the rest of the system is functioning. Instead, I use this name to call attention to the fact that what all the hypotheses and experiments have in common is a commitment to the belief that cognition and our mental life is composed of computations of a variety of sorts over simple representational units.

According to this view, what is important for understanding pain processing is understanding how information is sent or damped along simple neuronal tracts running from the tissues to cortex. Sensory information is initially registered at the periphery in terms of mechanical or chemical features and then transformed into information about sensory-discriminations or affective-motivations higher up (details of this view are given in chapters five and six). This transformed information then feeds into our motor response areas, which cause us to act a particular way.

The Feature-Detection Perspective on the Dorsal Horn

This guiding theoretical orientation has supported much extremely profitable research into the details of pain processing. For one example, let us consider the challenge of understanding the connection between the reflex most animals share to withdraw a limb quickly when stimuli become painful and the dorsal horn. The dorsal horn is located in the spine and is universally regarded as the first important relay-processing station in pain information traveling from the nerves endings in our skin to the brain (cf. figure 4.2). Since withdrawal occurs even when animals are decorticated, we know that there is a more or less direct connection between the dorsal horn and the limbs of rats.

If we record from the dorsal horn neurons in the lumbar and sacral segments of anesthetized rats (who still react behaviorally to noxious heating in the hind paw or tail), we can see that neurons linearly increase their rate of firing as the temperature of the stimuli goes from 40 to 52 decrees centigrade. The effect maxes out at about 52 degrees, and the firing rate simply plateaus for temperatures above that.[9] These data tell us that the dorsal horn neurons are keyed to nociceptive information, and that, within limits, the more intense the stimuli, the more the neurons fire.

If the dorsal horn is in fact an interneuronal relay station, then the neural activity there should (slightly) precede the withdrawal reflex, as information travels from the limb, through the dorsal horn, and then (eventually) to neurons that control our motor response. Experimental

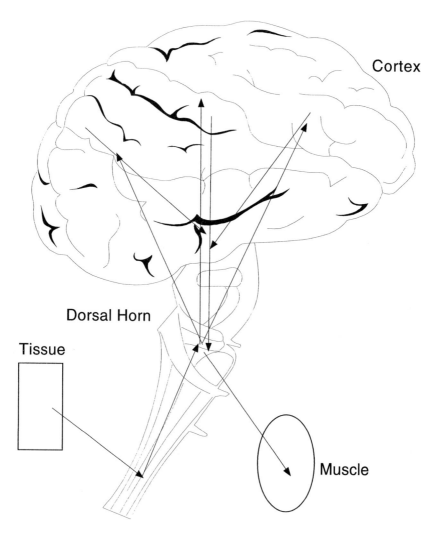

Figure 4.2
Subset of pain processing tract commonly assumed in most mammals. Information travels from the tissue through the dorsal horn and on into cortex. Information flows back out from cortex to the muscles, though there are probably direct
connections from dorsal horn to the efferent pathways as well.

studies bear out this conjecture. If we record simultaneously from a dorsal horn cell, a bicep motor unit and the actual hind paw withdrawal reflex, we can see that dorsal cells respond first and then overlap with the motor neurons' firing and the reflex activity.[10]

This sort of experimental protocol in which scientists record from the single cells of rats or other animals in the known nociceptive tract is quite common in studying the neurophysiology of acute pain. It also exemplifies the feature detection perspective. Each cell in the tract, from the nociceptors (the cells in our tissues that would be the first to note any painful events) to the dorsal horn and on up, is assumed to take information about the state of our bodies, transform it in some way, and then pass it along to the next step in the processing hierarchy. Our dorsal horn neurons respond differentially to the different sorts of nociceptive stimuli one might receive and then transmit that information to the brain—or perhaps directly to our motor response system—which then presumably initiates our avoidance behavior. We have a nice, neat, easy-to-understand story about how information regarding pain travels along our spine and then determines our output.

However, developing animal models for chronic pain, which is what we care about here, is a bit more complicated. Part of the difficulty is that the term "chronic pain" stands in for several different pathological responses to stimuli; see figure 4.3. These include the responses one would naturally expect, such as pain in the absence of any stimulus at all. They also include things like pains that last for a longer time than what is predicted should occur under normal conditions (hyperpathia), pain in response to what otherwise should be nonpainful stimuli (allodynia), pains of greater intensity than would be expected for stimuli exceeding the pain threshold (hyperalgesia), and pain and hyperalgesia spreading to uninjured tissue (referred pain and secondary hyperalgesia). Some or all of these effects occur in the case of chronic pain.

It is important to stress that chronic pain is not the same thing as a long-lasting acute pain. This point will become clearer in later chapters as we look at imaging studies of both sorts of pain. However, one should keep in mind that, relative to the processing that goes on in our sensory systems and other neural pathways, chronic pain is deeply weird, and we really don't understand much about it at all.

Allodynia	Pain from a stimulus that does not normally cause pain
Anesthesia dolorosa	Pain in an anesthetized region
Causalgia	Syndrome of continued burning pain, allodynia, and hyperpathia resulting from a nerve lesion
Central pain	Pain associated with a central nervous system lesion
Deafferentation pain	Pain caused by the loss of sensory input into the central nervous system.
Dysesthesia	An unpleasant abnormal sensation, either spontaneous or evoked
Hyperesthesia	Increased sensitivity to stimulation
Hyperalgesia	An heightened response to a normally painful stimulus
Hyperpathia	A painful syndrome characterized by an increased reaction to a repetitive stimulus
Neuralgia	Pain in the distribution of nerves
Neurogenic inflammation	The release of peptides that increase inflammation via efferent activity in afferent nerves
Neuropathy	A pathological change in a nerve or nerves
Referred pain	Pain localized to an area adjacent to or distant from the site of its cause

Figure 4.3
Terminology associated with chronic pain. (After Chapman and Stillman 1996.)

It is fairly clear that at least some aspects of chronic pain are modulated centrally; that is, changes in the nerve cells above the peripheral nociceptors are responsible for the abnormal responses. Hyperalgesia, for example, can continue even when the skin is anesthetized. The initial nociceptive inputs need to reach the central nervous system, but once increased sensitivity to pain begins, it does not require inputs from the injured area to continue.[11] The dorsal horn is probably responsible for some of the central sensitization effects, for dorsal horn neurons fire increasingly faster if repeatedly stimulated from nociceptor inputs.[12] Moreover, repeated stimulation of dorsal horn neurons causes them to continue firing for up to a few minutes after the inputs cease, a phenomenon called "wind up" in the pain literature.[13] Finally, repeated stimulation causes the neurons' receptive fields to expand, though whether the expansion is in any way connected to hyperalgesia is still unclear.[14] Even disregarding the changes in the dorsal horn neurons' receptive field, it is very clear that the dorsal horn is at least partially responsible for some of the symptoms associated with chronic pain. Others are willing to go further in this conclusion: Terence Coderre and Joel Katz assert definitively that "hyperalgesia ultimately depends on the net activity of dorsal horn neurons."[15]

Earl Carstens has addressed whether the animal model for acute pain discussed above could be modified so that it could also be used in studying chronic pain. He notes that in most models, hyperalgesia is defined as a decrease in the time it takes an animal to respond behaviorally to a noxious stimulus. However, latency measures alone could only index a decreased threshold for pain; it would not show in increased sensitivity to stimuli above the pain level under normal circumstances.[16] It would be better to measure intensity of response as well as rapidity.

He induced chronic pain in rats by severing up to one-half of the rat's sciatic nerve. This results in faster limb withdrawals to heat and an increased sensitivity threshold to pressure pain.[17] A couple of weeks after the operation, he tested the rats with damaged sciatic nerves and those that had had a sham operation. Surprisingly, there were no significant differences in the intensity or threshold of pain response for either the severed versus the unsevered side in the neuropathic rats or the neuropathic rats versus the sham-operated ones.[18] At the same time, the mechanoreceptive fields of the dorsal horn neurons on the ligated side were larger, which is what one expects with chronic pain.[19] Consequently, it is unclear that the rats actually suffer from chronic pain, even though their dorsal horns are acting as though they are.

A good animal model for chronic pain still eludes us. I mention Carstens's ongoing research program because, while not yet successful, it appears to be the best game in town at the moment. Notice too that it follows the feature-detection paradigm precisely. Carstens has shown that particular neurons in the dorsal horn react quite strongly to noxious heat stimuli, while other cells in surrounding areas react weakly, if at all. The firing of these neurons correlate directly with the withdrawal reflex, even though the intensity levels between assumed sensation of pain and the threshold of response do not match as hypothesized. The nociceptors transduce noxious stimuli and tell the dorsal horn neurons about it. The dorsal horn takes that information and then feeds it to the motor output system. This forms a small processing hierarchy, but it is a hierarchy nonetheless.

Carstens's current project is to account for the mismatch between prediction and observation within the feature-detection paradigm. He has already determined that there was no damage to the motor neurons, that the hind paw does not have an elevated temperature, and that the electrophysiological properties of the dorsal horn neurons remained unaltered for the neuropathic rats.[20] Each of these items could have changed how the information was passed from the dorsal horn to the motor neurons or how the motor neurons might interpret the information they received; that is, each could have reshaped our view of what should be included as relevant in our description of the pain processing hierarchy.

Problems with the Perspective

As we can see from these few examples, the feature detector perspective presents us with a powerful research program. It aims to provide robust explanations for pain phenomena in the form of an hierarchical processing stream, with the relevant computational attributes of cells at each level detailed. As long as we can translate across homologies, this sort of theory should generalize across humans and across species, which would make for a potent theory. Finally, this approach allows for computer simulations in testing hypotheses. As long as we can quantify what we think are the important response properties of the neurons in each processing tract, then we can write programs that will mimic what we think our nervous system is doing. Computer modeling allows for quick and dirty testing of rough hypotheses, something necessary if science is to proceed apace, but also something very difficult to do if restricted to experimentation on live animals.

However, this approach is not without substantial criticism. In general, the critics focus on the fact that we have scant evidence that whatever feature-detecting or transformational properties we uncover are actually connected to the computation of cognition. First and foremost, the problem is that it is based largely on single-cell studies. These provide sparse coverage of the nervous system at best. A column in the brain is on average about a tenth of a millimeter square (though the size varies considerably from being only about 25 µm wide to being as large as 0.3

millimeters wide[21]). Each cubic millimeter of cortex contains approximately 100,000 neurons. Obviously, single-cell protocols can record from only a tiny fraction of the cells involved in any computation, even within a single column. The study that demonstrated that dorsal horn neurons fire slightly before motor neurons was based on the activity recorded in a few dozen dorsal horn-motor cell pairs. We have little guarantee that the neurons being recorded from are not anomalous.

Second, neurons are noisy. They jitter around even when not being stimulated. Sometimes it is difficult to tell whether they are responding to some incoming stimulus or are firing spontaneously, especially when their responses are not strong. Unambiguous action potentials correlated with some specific stimulus are not the norm. Moreover, the difficulty in sorting automatic activity from externally caused IPSPs (inhibitory postsynaptic potentials) and EPSPs (excitatory postsynaptic potentials) is compounded by the fact that our so-called individual feature detectors really respond to several different features, though all not equally strongly. It is difficult to tell whether a cell is responding weakly to some input, or whether it is not responding to the input at all but firing spontaneously.

Finally, single-unit studies generally get their results by "massaging" the raw data. In the main, the published results show the responses of several cells with similar receptive fields averaged together. Though this move will diminish the magnitude of any positive response, it also washes out perhaps important individual differences as unimportant noise. Averaging similar response patterns together assumes that the general trend across the responses is the most important effect. However, given the paucity of coverage in single-cell recordings and individual neurons' propensity to fire weakly to lots of different stimuli, searching for the single common response patterns might obscure more complex and unexpected reactions.

The bottom line is that a feature-detection approach is based on perhaps weak correlations among only a few neurons at best. This is not enough to establish their actual contributions to cognition. Contrary evidence, cells that don't respond as predicted, are discounted or ignored. Assuming a feature-detection orientation means significant responses to individual stimulus features are what is most important, and the techniques we use to gather data feed into that assumption.

I want to stress that these are not merely technical difficulties. Adopting a feature-detection perspective means that we are assuming that the response patterns of individual or small groups of neurons are where cognition occurs. The problem is that once we assume that and then embark on our studies, the methods we use do not allow for contrary evidence. We will always get what we are looking for using single-cell recordings to support feature detection theories.

Perhaps the powerful technology of single-cell recordings has enamored us. We can record from single cells, so we conclude that single cells must be the important level of organization in the brain. However, it could be that this way to explain perception and cognition is simply the wrong one.

The best, and maybe only, way to overcome this criticism is by somehow measuring neuronal activity at the network level. We need to know that the few neurons that were hit in the single-cell measures reflect the general pattern of activity of most of the neurons in the isolated processing stream. We also need to know that the averaged or dominant pattern is what the next level in the hierarchy responds to. That is, we need to know that the single-cell experimental techniques and assumptions do indeed winnow the noise and leave the signal. Faster firing rates, wind up, and increased receptive field size in the dorsal horn all correlate with hyperalgesia. But we have little information regarding whether any of these effects are *causally* responsible for the increased sensitivity to noxious stimuli, even as operationalized in terms of withdrawal response. We need to know which areas of the brain are responsive to any of these effects, in virtue of what they are responsive, and how those areas lead to the phenomena of chronic pain.

The difficulty is that no one knows how to do that exactly. There are no experimental techniques currently available that permit recording at that level of organization in the brain. Magnetic resonance imaging (MRI), the best noninvasive recording device we have, only has a spatial resolution of about 0.1 millimeter—the size of one column. Moreover, each scan samples about five seconds of activity. (Positron emission tomography [PET], in contrast, can resolve brain activity only down to about 10 millimeters and takes a bit longer.)[22] In addition, most of the fluctuations recorded with MRI come from machine noise, subject movements, and heart and breathing rhythyms instead of the task at hand.[23] While using MRI to record during ongoing cognitive processing (fMRIs) can be very informative, it is not up to the challenge we have before us. We cannot tell what specific properties of cells different areas of the brain are responding to, nor can we tell how these responses translate into higher-order phenomena.

Worse, there are few new methods on the horizon to do so. One possibility is to wed fMRI or magnetoencephalography (MEG) recordings to simultaneous electroencephalogram (EEG) scalp recordings. EEG recordings can track neuronal events down to the millisecond range, but this method provides abysmal location information. Scientists are currently working out mathematical techniques for using both recordings to pinpoint where in the brain EEG waveforms were created. Results are promising, but not yet definitive. A second possibility is using the light-scattering properties of neurons to record event-related optical signals. However, experimental machines can detect light reflectance only a few centimeters inside the skull, so they are not sensitive to the neurons buried deep in the cortical folds or to the lower brain structures. Consequently, the technique is currently little better than the EEG. Still, some are confident that this difficulty can be overcome within the next decade. Bruce Rosen claims that his "eye is on optical techniques in terms of the next wave."[24]

For the foreseeable short-term future, though, our problem remains. We need to be able to chart the activity of specific populations of cells in milliseconds if we are to show that a feature-detection approach is the appropriate one to take in explaining perception and cognition. We just don't know how to do this yet.

The Dynamical Systems Approach

There is an alternative perspective, however. Instead of emphasizing the role of the individual component, the dynamical systems approach assumes that our rich web of interconnections and consequent wide (though not massively parallel) sharing of information leads to collective activity in the brain. Consequently, we can think of the currency of cognition as the messages emerging from brain areas and not as those contained in the interactions among single neurons.[25]

Though this perspective on the brain has only come into its own as of late, its conceptual history dates back at least to the cybernetics movement in the 1950s. In particular, Ashby's *Design for a Brain* outlines most of the dynamical systems program for understanding the brain being adumbrated today.[26] (At least, the "sound-bite" descriptions remain unchanged.) Then, as now, proponents of a dynamical systems perspective claim that we should understand brain activity as the product of an adaptive, embedded system operating in real time. The focus is on the larger self-organizing structures that are produced by the seemingly almost random interactions of the underlying individual components. As Aharon Katchalsky, the inspirational force behind much of this movement, remarked: "The possibility of waves, oscillations, macrostates emerging out of cooperative processes, sudden transitions, prepatterning, etc. seem made to order to assist in the understanding of integrative processes of the nervous system."[27]

This approach, too, is technology-driven in many ways. The dynamical system conceptual framework may be older, but it is only recently that scientists have been able to integrate these ideas into their research, for they had to wait until they had recording techniques that would allow them to uncover and measure embedded neuronal patterns. In general (though not always), extracellular recordings over masses of cells support this theoretical perspective. These sorts of recordings cover a far greater area than do the single-cell recordings, and many more electrodes, or other sorts of recording points, can be maintained simultaneously. What scientists are looking for with the more diffuse recordings over larger brain areas are larger patterns piggybacking on top of the activity of individual neurons. They believe that these higher-order patterns emerging from the underlying microactivity, and not the interactions of the single cells per se, are responsible for the mental life of organisms.

A Primer on Dynamical Systems

(This section provides an overview of dynamical systems theory. For those already familiar with the notions involved, it can be skipped without loss of continuity.[28]) Fundamental to analyzing the dynamics of a dynamical system, which is just any system that changes over time, is quantifying its *phase space*. The phase space is an abstract representation of all possible changes the dynamical system could undergo over time. Each dimension of the space is associated with one variable of the dynamical system; any point in the space corresponds to a possible state of the system as a whole. We can plot changes in the system by following the path the point representing the actual state of the system takes over time through the phase space. This movement is known as the *phase trajectory*. Sometimes we can find simple mathematical equations that describe a point's trajectory. These equations would then also describe the behavior of the system over time.

Some trajectories follow readily discernible patterns in space. They might settle into some sort of repetitive cycle, regardless of where they began in the space. These cycles are called *attractors,* for, if you are graphing the phase space, it looks as though the region of the space that contains the cycle is attracting the moving point to its area. A *point attractor* refers to a system that always settles into the same state, and activity in the system then ceases. The trajectory converges on a single point in space and stays there. *Limit cycles* are looping attractors. These systems forever repeat themselves, switching regularly among a set of fixed states once they are up and running. *Strange attractors* refer to chaotic behavior. When systems are chaotic, they never repeat themselves exactly. They are also very sensitive to initial conditions; the transitions they go through can vary widely almost immediately even if the initial inputs differ only slightly. Nevertheless, we can still talk about attractors in chaotic systems because the trajectories generally remain in one corner or another of the phase space.

What is unsettling about chaotic systems is that they are effectively unpredictable. Jacking up precision in measuring the initial conditions of the system will only allow for a marginal increase in accuracy in predicting the precise trajectory of the point in phase space and that accuracy will remain only for a short while. Though we may be able to describe the strange attractor or point to the hot spot in phase space, we cannot say which path the point will take within the anointed region.

Another way of putting this point is to say that there is no simple way to describe the system's behavior; these systems are unavoidably complex. As a result, we should not look for rules governing the specific transformations the system undergoes. If we are extremely lucky, we might be able to uncover some equations that describe the strange attractors, but given sensitivity to initial conditions, these equations will not let us predict how any particular trajectory corresponding to the behavior of some physical system will unfold.

However, because these systems are still well-behaved, even if unpredictable, they produce coherent and stable macrostructures. What seems to be radically jumbled behavior on a microlevel appears well organized when seen from a distance. These large-scale structures simply emerge from the underlying activity. Order, not confusion, is the natural consequence of chaos.

A Reason to Switch

The impetus for adopting a dynamical systems perspective in the brain sciences comes from several quarters. First, it is clear that information in the brain is transmitted by far more than action potentials and neurotransmitters. Hormones and neuropeptides impart data through the extracellular fluid more or less continuously in a process known as "volume transmission."[29] We are now familiar with about fifty of these chemicals, most of which are connected to our sensory systems (perhaps to act as global filters?), and more are being discovered all the time. They allow for communication over both short and long distances. Some transmission is quite slow, as in the diffusion of peptides in cerebrospinal fluid; some is rapid, up to 120 meters per second in axonal fluid. What is important is that these additional ways of communicating among cells in the central nervous system mean that simple (or even complicated) linear or feedforward models are likely to be inaccurate. The model of the brain as a serial processing computer ignores much important computation and communication in the head.

Decomposing such a system into simpler component pieces—as the feature-detection perspective would have us do—would not be easy, since there are large-scale global effects from the various messenger "baths" of hormones and peptides that have to be taken into account. Take one slightly unusual example: immune disorders are strongly correlated with the ability to do higher mathematics and left-handedness in men.[30] It could be that all these attributes are in some way related to a single (or a few) global aspects of brain processing. (It could also be that these traits are independently expressed from linked genes.) Any theory of cognition that relied on a simplified feedforward processing stream would not only be unable to account for this sort of regularity; it would miss it entirely, for each attribute would be explained in a separate mode with different processing units. Discovering the importance of global communication in the brain has led some to conclude that it is better to see our brain as a system that works together as a complex interactive whole for which any sort of reduction to lower levels of description means a loss of telling data.

A second factor in prompting the switch in perspectives is coming to appreciate the importance of timing in the brain.[31] Neurons pay attention to when events occur and respond differently to different time sequences. Incoming signals can only depolarize a cell and cause it to fire if they arrive at the soma at more or less the same time; the tendency to depolarize builds up until the neuron fires in a burst of release. After an action potential, though, the cell's membranes cannot respond at all to incoming signals. There is a period of enforced silence, and then another gradual buildup occurs. Inputs arriving immediately after a neuron has fired will have a drastically different effect on that neuron than if it arrives as it is getting ready to fire.

Moreover, neurons respond differently when signals arrive simultaneously than when they arrive merely close together. Nabil Farhat compares the response to simultaneous signals to the light and dark interference pattern one gets when two beams of light shine together. Signals arriving precisely at the same time through different dendrites cause a similar periodic modulation in the neuron's membrane. This electrical oscillation affects how the neuron can respond to other inputs.[32] And small changes in the frequency of the oscillation (caused by changing the input signals ever so slightly) can produce large changes in a neuron's output pattern.

A third factor, and the final one I shall discuss here, concerns the brain's ability to organize itself. Quite often, events in nature are very well organized. Our usual impulse in explaining that order is to presume some sort of external coordinator who makes it all happen. Our models, of course, are our own artifacts. Harking back to William Paley and his argument for God by design, we seem to believe intuitively that a creative force is required to make something out of nothing. Watches, wagons, and washing machines could not spontaneously appear in our world. We are needed to design and build them out of the disordered raw materials found lying in disarray around us.

However, Nature need not bow to our intuitions. In many instances, it has the power to organize itself, using nothing more than the properties of the materials themselves. For example, when we heat a liquid to boiling, very nice rolling convection patterns appear from what was previously randomly moving molecules. This sort of cooperative activity arises without any external organizer there to issue coordinating commands.

Similarly, at sports events in large stadiums, fans can create a large-scale waving pattern rippling through the stands without a leader on the field pointing out who should be standing and moving next. All that is required is for a few fans to stand and wave together and for those to induce the fans next to them to stand and wave. Adopting the rule "stand and wave if someone next to you is standing and waving" is the only thing that is needed to get a stadium-sized wave to generate itself.

Our brains might operate in a similar fashion: a few simple rules governing individual interactions might produce all or some of the wonderful higher-order complexity we find in our heads. With these rules, our brains could cooperatively organize themselves, without any detailed master plan. In fact, self-organization is probably necessary for our central nervous system, for we simply do not have enough genetic material to code for all the connections in cortex. At best, we have only a rough blueprint for how a finished brain should look. The rest of the coordination and organization we know is there has to fall out of the (nonmagical) properties of the brain itself.

For example, given the limits of what wiring information could be coded in our DNA, the neuronal columns that I mentioned above have to form as a consequence of neural activity and change (either internally generated or exogenously produced) and not of hardwiring. How could the brain do this? Since the columns form very early in life and can form without external stimuli, spontaneous action potentials must be the cause, though presumably environmental stimuli in the form of sensory input somehow finishes or speeds the task. But how the simple order of neuronal columns could arise from essentially random emissions seems deeply mysterious.

It is mysterious, that is, until we realize what so-called Hebbian learning among neurons produces.[33] The basic idea, going back to Donald Hebb's work in the 1940s, is that the connection between two neurons is strengthened if the neurons fire simultaneously. If we assume that Hebb was right and our brains learn by making neurons that have previously fired more likely to fire in the future (and neurons that have not fired less likely to fire), then a columnar arrangement is almost guaranteed.

Consider, for example, ocular dominance columns. Suppose an initial state in which neurons are randomly connected to one another. On average, they would receive roughly the same amount of stimulation from the right and the left eye. But because cells are more likely to be connected to their near neighbors, each time a cell fires from a retinal ganglion input, then its neighbors are likely to fire as well. All that now has to happen is for one eye to be ever so slightly more successful in getting a cell and its neighbors to fire and, voilà, an ocular dominance column emerges.[34] (I have to confess that this is a just-so story; neurons are not connected completely randomly in the beginning. Actually, contralateral connections are predominant.[35] We should keep in mind that, my caricatures aside, whatever final story we accept about brain processing is going to be very complicated.)

With the brain, as with baseball fans and boiling water, a slight perturbation of an otherwise balanced system causes it to settle quickly into a simple, stable, and coherent pattern. Our central nervous system organizes itself via its own firing patterns. No external wirer is required.

A Dynamical Systems Perspective on the Dorsal Horn

The dynamical systems approach for understanding the brain holds that emergent patterns driven by weak local correlations are the proper currency of cognition and perception. Common "carrier" waves emerge from the background noise of a sea of immense activity. If we can uncover these waves, then we can plot them on maps, which develop and change with experience and learning over time. This approach is beginning to make itself felt in pain research.[36]

J. Sandkühler and his research group study dorsal horn neurons that respond to two different types of pain input.[37] The cells they examined responded both to electrical shocks and to heat administered to the hind paw of a rat. About two-thirds of these cells fired more or less continuously, even without any stimulation whatsoever being given to the rat's paw. This background activity is pretty typical of most neurons in the central nervous system. To determine whether there were any dynamical firing patterns embedded in the background noise, Sandkühler recorded several thousand action potentials from each jittering neuron. He then constructed a phase-space portrait by calculating the differences among neighboring interspike intervals (D_n) and plotting D_n on the x-axis versus D_{n+1} on the y-axis.[38]

To illustrate: suppose a neuron fires at 0, 10, 35, 45, 72, and 82 msec, where recording begins at 0 msec. The interspike intervals—that is, the time between individual firings—are $10 - 0 = 10$, $35 - 10 = 25$, $45 - 35 = 10$, $72 - 45 = 27$, and $82 - 72 = 10$. The differences between the neighboring interspike intervals are $25 - 10 = 15$, $10 - 25 = -15$, $27 - 10 = 17$, and $10 - 27 = -17$. We could then plot on a two-dimensional graph the ordered pairs $(15, -15)$, $(-15, 17)$, $(17, -17)$. This graph would then illustrate the phase-space portrait of that particular neuron's background activity. If we connected the dots in the order that we charted them, then we could be tracing the trajectory of the neuronal firing pattern in phase space.

Small changes in the firing pattern can lead to large changes in the trajectory, so this sort of phase-space portrait of the dynamics of neuronal discharges can be used to uncover structures within the timing of action potentials that might otherwise be overlooked. A random series of firings would appear as a cloud of points with no noticeable structure. However, even a fairly subtle and complex deterministic pattern in the cell's discharges would appear as a definable structure in the phase-space portrait. Of the 90 dorsal horn cells whose background activity Sandkühler and his colleagues recorded and analyzed, sixty-six of them showed

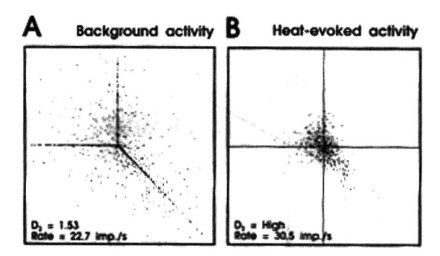

Figure 4.4
Acute noxious skin heating affects the nonlinear dynamics of the discharges of multireceptive spinal dorsal horn neurons. A phase-space portrait of the background activity recorded in the absence of any skin stimulation is shown in (A). Noxious skin heating (46° C for 100 s) destroyed the deterministic pattern in the phase-space portrait and strongly enhanced the complexity of the discharge pattern as revealed by the increase in the D_2 correlation dimension from 1.53 to a value larger than ten (High). (After Sandkühler and Eblen-Zajjur 1994.)

obvious patterns in the phase-space portraits of their neighboring interspike intervals. Figure 4.4a illustrates the pattern seen in one of their cells.

One can also quantify the complexity of the patterns seen in the phase-space portraits by calculating what is called the D_2 correlation dimension.[39] The details of the mathematics need not detain us here; we just need to know that the D_2 correlation dimension gives us the minimal number of independent variables required to get the pattern observed.[40] This number is taken to be a measure of the complexity of the dynamics of the system studied. Changes in its value would indicate changes in the underlying structure of the firing patterns. For the sixty-six dorsal horn neurons that Sandkühler identified with a relatively simple phase-space pattern, the D_2 correlation dimension was generally not more than five. This means that the background activity of those dorsal neurons is not random at all; instead, it is a deterministic process with low degrees of freedom.

When an acute noxious stimulus is applied to the appropriate spot on the rat's hind paw, the deterministic patterns in the vast majority of the neurons are eliminated. Figure 4.4b shows how the phase-space portrait changes with noxious inputs. Heating the rat's skin, for example, causes the D_2 correlation dimension to jump to values greater than ten. (After ten, the Grassberger-Procaccia algorithm used to compute the value becomes inaccurate and so the D_2 correlation dimension is classified merely as "HIGH.") This tells us that the number of degrees of freedom in the discharges increases with acute pain.

Interestingly enough, when something resembling chronic pain (prolonged skin inflammation) stimulates the dorsal neurons, we find a completely different pattern of response. As you can see in figure 4.5, the complexity decreases sharply. This change was quite robust and continued until the end of the recording session (up to six hours), often outlasting changes in the rate of firing from the neurons themselves.

An increase in the number of degrees of freedom in the neuronal firing pattern with acute pain stimuli and a decrease in the number of degrees of freedom with chronic pain stimuli adds weight to the claim that acute pain and chronic pain are two very different things, even though they are contained in the same neuronal system. Though we may not be able to differentiate organic pains from psychogenic ones, it looks as though we can distinguish acute from chronic pains as two fundamentally different neuronal transactions.

It also tells us that chronic pain, as perceived by the dorsal horn at any rate, is highly regimented and ordered, features that are generally associated with pathology and breakdown in the human body. You don't want your bodily responses to be locked into a periodic limit cycle, for then they are not free to respond appropriately to environmental vicissitudes. Reactions become stereotyped and hence dysfunctional. All things considered, the flexibility of chaos is preferred.

This is an entirely different tack in understanding the distinction between acute and chronic pain than what the feature-detection rubric provides, and whether it will ultimately be more successful is not yet clear. Though this approach cannot distinguish between physical pains and psychogenic pains, it does suggest that pain is not just a simple feedforward processing chain that the simple feature detector view posits. In-

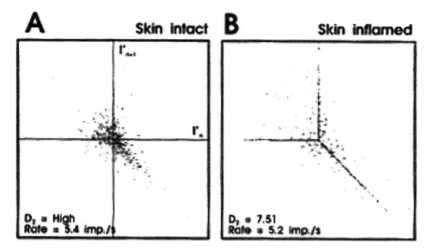

Figure 4.5
Inflammation of the skin has qualitatively different effects on the nonlinear dynamics of the discharges of multireceptive spinal dorsal horn neurons than acute stimuli. One representative example is shown here. Phase-space portraits of background activity before and one hour after noxious radiant heat-induced inflammation of the skin within the neurons' receptive field are shown. (After Sandkühler and Eblen-Zajjur 1994.)

stead, it pinpoints the difference between acute and chronic pain as a difference in the timing of action potentials for the same inputs, whose causes are many, complicated, and largely unpredictable. In contrast, the feature-detection perspective looks at mean discharge rates and holds that the difference turns on spelling out the very causes the dynamical systems approach abstracts over. What the dynamical systems approach takes as data, the feature-detection approach assumes to be noise, and vice versa.[41]

Problems with the Approach
Just like the feature-detection perspective, a dynamical systems approach to cognitive phenomena offers us robust explanations, an honest theory, powerful generalizations, and the prospect of computer simulations. In short, both perspectives offer the same theoretical promise. However, the methodological criticisms of the dynamical systems approach are very similar to those of the feature detector as well: we find the limit cycles

and other higher-level patterns by "massaging" the data; consequently, we cannot tell whether the patterns we find are causally relevant to cognition or are merely accidental features of processing brains.

To get a nice phase portrait from raw single-cell data, the waveforms have to be digitized and filtered first in order to determine when the actual action potential begins and ends. Given the natural jitter of cells, this is not always an obvious task. Analysis of EEG waves is more complicated; they are filtered for high and low frequency, then the trials are time ensemble averaged. Next a fourier decomposition and principal component analysis is performed on the resultant ERP waveforms, and finally spatial pattern classification techniques are used to determine the time periods of the oscillations.

The bottom line is exactly the same: the abstraction that a dynamical systems approach focuses upon might be the wrong one because it is based on weak correlations among small groups of neurons. This immediately and automatically discounts any cells that don't fit the projected pattern, so contrary evidence is difficult to find. In the example discussed above, Sandkühler did not analyze any spike trains that had fewer than 5,000 interspike intervals or that did not have stationary discharge rates. The approach might be receiving support simply because we know how to make these analyses. We assume that because we can map neuronal activity to chaotic bifurcations (or whatever), this activity must be an important level of organization in cognition.

Dynamicists assume that the larger patterns riding the firing patterns of individual neurons comprise the basic unit of cognition. In order to support that assumption, they need to show robust correlations between the patterns and its alleged products. So far, they have not done this.

As before, to overcome these criticisms, the best and probably only thing to do is to devise some measure of the network level that would show that the patterns discovered really are important products of neural interactions (even if single cells are discounted) and are not merely artifacts of the statistical method chosen to analyze the data. We need a better handle on how these patterns are internally generated and then how they are used within the system, but we have no clear and systematic method for measuring network behavior in the brain. The technology simply isn't available.

The Moral of the Story: Incompatible Approaches

It is worth noting that neither side denies the results of the other. The data that the two perspectives generate are real; the effects they find are robust and reproducible; and the interpretations they give appear to be correct, given the data. The point of controversy is over whether the other side has picked the appropriate changes in neuronal activity to study. Each questions the explanatory emphasis on the events themselves and claims that the object that the other chooses to study is not where the real action is. Because each side asserts that it has isolated the important interactions for cognition, both cannot be right. In addition, each approach fosters a different sort of explanation, incompatible with the other, so that even if we could somehow meld the data together, what sort of story gets to count as a good explanation is still undecided.

A Difference in Explanatory Strategies

Part of the differences between the two camps turn on how they understand the nature of explanation in science. More particularly, it turns on what they consider to be a good or complete explanation. The feature-detectors believe that whatever the events one relies on in the brain for explanation, they will have to support the extremely predictable behaviors of organisms. Dynamical systemists err in thinking that outputs are too complex or unpredictable to make statistical explanations useful. With enough time and effort, the details connecting neuronal activity with action will become clear and the rules governing the details will be uncovered. Appreciating the details and understanding the rules are both required in a reductive, feature-detection explanation.

In contrast, the dynamicists believe that no amount of effort will clarify the exact route stimuli inputs take to behavioral outputs, for the information is encoded in such a way that it cannot be usefully approximated. A narrative account that highlights the sort of phase-space attractors and then tells a story that connects that type of attractor to the general behavior of the system will be enough to count as an explanation. These explanations will not allow for predictions, but they can retrospectively account for behavior as well as categorize the system into one of several possible types.

To see the conflict in these approaches, consider two ways of explaining the dripping pattern found in a leaky faucet.[42] Physicists can devise a classical or Landau model for any dripping faucet that fits the data better than any chaotic model. The Landau models are very complicated and do not generalize from one faucet to another. In contrast, a chaotic model is relatively simple and can handle many different leaky faucets equally well. Jim Garson, a proponent of the dynamical systems view, concludes that "classical faucet modeling appears to achieve its accuracy by compounding epicycles, rather than by cutting nature at its joints. The moral is that the cost of better prediction may be immense complexity and a failure to generalize."[43] If feature-detectors want a theory that will successfully predict an organism's pain behavior, then they will probably end up with a theory that describes only one organism. From the feature-detection perspective, this might not be so bad—indeed, if they could predict the behavior of only one organism, that would be hailed as an enormous scientific triumph. But from a dynamical systems point of view, a failure to generalize spells failure of the entire project.

If we return to the two examples regarding the dorsal horn, we can see exactly this conflict. Carstens is thus far unable to get his animal model of chronic pain to work as it should. His solution is to add an additional layer of complexity onto the model: a previously overlooked neuronal connection, another relevant parameter, feedback from something else in the system, and so forth. If he can succeed in his quest, then he will have a complicated but causally detailed account of hyperalgesia in rats. In contrast, Sandkühler relies on no causal mechanisms in his story. Instead, he points to differences in measures of complexity for different types of pain. This will not allow us to chart specific reactions in the manner that Carstens does; but it does provide us with a way to classify pain in a gross way—and in a way that Carstens cannot yet do.

The impulse from a feature-detection perspective is to say that Sandkühler is only beginning; that the explanation will not be complete until we have a predictive account of what leads to the differences in the order of the interspike intervals in the dorsal horn. Noting that they are there is a first step. Explaining the causal path the brain takes to get there would be the last.

Dynamicists are not moved by that impulse, though. The causal details would simply bury the discovered correlations in a deluge of unhelpful data. Moreover, the details would vary from organism to organism, for they depend upon the precise structure of each individual neuron and its local environment. Outlining that would be no more helpful, and no more explanatory, than accounting for rising inflation in terms of points in Hilbert space. It might be accurate, but it won't help economists.

This is not to say that a dynamical systems perspective is never causal. However, the causes will be located elsewhere, in the etiology of the system. Changes in weather are famously chaotic. We cannot predict with any degree of accuracy what the weather will be like beyond a couple of days, because there are simply too many relevant factors for us to measure and we cannot measure them with enough precision anyway. Nevertheless, no one believes that our weather is uncaused, and after each atmospheric event, we can give a rough accounting for why things ended up the way they did. It rained today because the cold front from the north ran into a warm front from the south. That "because" is causal. However, giving the causal story for why the cold front ended up where it did, why the warm front ended up where it did, and why the precise amount of moisture in the air was located where it was so that we got rain (and not hail) will not be forthcoming, for those stories depend upon things we cannot track. We just know that our chaotic weather system sometimes exhibits this sort of trajectory.

A dynamical account of pain would function similarly. No one would claim for a minute that our mental events or subsequent behavior is not caused. And we would strive to give retrospective simple accounts of why something exhibited the behavior it did. However, detailing all the relevant factors that led to that output will not happen, nor is it desirable, for that would miss the point of the account. If our pain system is dynamical in the sense discussed, then we know that it is the sort of system that naturally gives rise to these sorts of organized behavior, and we can explain in a rough-and-ready way the connection between the type of system and its subsequent development for any given piece of its trajectory. But, as Chris Eliasmith notes, "in adopting a purely dynamicist approach. . . , it becomes impossible to identify the underlying mechanisms that affect behavior."[44]

From a feature-detection point of view, this is a dangerous precedent to set. We should not "mistake translation for explanation." "Merely [redescribing] . . . the phenomena" does not mean that we have explained them, as Stephen Robertson and his colleagues remind us.[45] It is difficult to know whether advocates of dynamical systems models for the brain are articulating a fundamental aspect about the way we work, or whether they are merely being empirically and conceptually lazy. Without serious data concerning how our neural networks interact with one another and the basis of that interaction, we cannot decide.

The Pragmatics of Neuroscience

At this stage in neuroscience, the experimental techniques we choose to use in investigating some phenomenon determine the events we highlight for the causal action. From one approach, we cannot measure the effects seen in the other, and without a "middling" approach, we cannot pick which way is superior. Once a train of neuronal spikes has been averaged and the mean determined, then there is no way to see whether the differences between neighboring interspike intervals contain any useful patterns. Once we find the differences between interspike intervals, then we no longer see the general firing trend of the neuron. And, for now, there is no neutral way to compare the success or value of one approach against the other. These facts suggest a strongly pragmatic view of neuroscience and of theory choice within neuroscience.

Whatever contingencies force some to select one approach over the other have nothing to do with the relative merits of the framework, for at the moment, neither has an explanatory advantage over the other. The traditional philosophical and social methods for distinguishing among theories fail in neuroscience. Both approaches are equally parsimonious, consiliant, simple, explanatory, elegant, and well confirmed. Moreover, neither political funding decisions nor the social powers of the agents involved have adjudicated this dispute. Both approaches are well respected in their academic and scientific communities and both are well funded. In sum: we have no deep reason for adopting a feature-detector approach over a dynamical systems one, or vice versa. We must simply pick our framework and dig in.

Simply selecting a theoretical approach for essentially arbitrary reasons does not bode well for any claims that we have a deep understanding of the fundamentals of our brains' machinations. If we cannot decide what the basic unit of computation is (indeed, if there are computations at all), then we cannot begin to make definite claims about how the brain cognizes at all. We are still guessing at this stage (though our guesses are educated and circumscribed), with the hope that someday soon, these guesses will pay off as genuine theoretical advances.

5

The Nature of Pain

Common sense, though all very well for everyday purposes, is easily confused, even by such simple questions as "Where is the rainbow? When you hear a voice on a gramophone record, are you hearing the man who spoke, or a reproduction? When you feel a pain in the leg that has been amputated, where is the pain?" If you say it is in your head, would it be in your head if your leg had not been amputated? If you say yes, then what reason have you for ever thinking you have a leg?

—Bertrand Russell

It is time we ask the central question: what is pain? How should we explain it? Answering these questions should explain how we should conceive of psychogenic pains, among other things. However, true to my warning in the last chapter, the best I can do is present a hodgepodge of perspectives here. I shall outline both feature-detector and dynamical systems views of pain. In some sense, for our purposes, it does not matter which side wins in the end, because my conclusion would be the same either way: philosophers (and others) have misunderstood the fundamental complexity of pain processing and, as a result, often say or write silly things about pain.

Pain as a Sensory System

Philosophers regularly take pain to be an unproblematic and simple example of a phenomenological experience. And philosophy's influence is spreading. Much to my surprise, a recent review article in neuroscience began with the following quotation from Hilary Putnam: "The typical concerns of the Philosopher of Mind might be represented by three questions: (1) How do we know that other people have pains? (2) Are pains brain states? (3) What is the analysis of the concept pain?"[1] Upon reflection, I decided that the quotation was entirely apt after all. Philosophers do take pain as their paradigm case in quite a number of projects, and the fact remains that we do not know exactly how pain processing works in the brain, so there is lots of room for wild and rampant speculation.

A little digging into the philosophical literature uncovered a wide range of opinions and arguments regarding how we think about pain. Indeed, I daresay just about every conceivable position is currently held today by some leading thinker or other. We find some philosophers and neurophysiologists arguing that pain is completely objective; it is either intrinsic to the injured body part, a functional state, a set of behavioral reactions, or a type of perception. We also find some philosophers and psychologists arguing that pain is completely subjective; either it is essentially private and completely mysterious, or it does not correlate with any biological markers but is completely nonmysterious. Finally, we find a few philosophers who disagree with both conceptions and hold that pain is not a state at all; it either does not exist as we commonly conceive of it or it is an attitudinal relation. (See figure 5.1.) Furthermore, each of these positions has become grist for someone's mill in arguing either that pain is a paradigm instance of a conscious state or that pain is a special case and should not be included in any general theory of consciousness.

We are left with several significant questions and puzzles. Among them are Putnam's. In this chapter and the next two, I do try to answer Putnam's three questions, but I also want to do more than merely carve out my niche among the myriad of positions. Here I aim to offer a diagnosis for why we have so little agreement concerning the nature of our pain states. In brief, I believe that there are two reasons. First, for many philosophers, there is a basic failure to appreciate the fundamental complexity of our neuronal processing. This is the less interesting cause. My claim is that philosophers are enamored with dissociation experiments but fail to understand their purpose, which is to individuate the component pieces of our larger systems. I argue that our pain sensory system functions according to the same basic rules of all our sensory systems.

Second, for many psychologists, neurophysiologists, and philosophers alike, there is an explicit or an implicit reliance on some sort of gate-

Eliminativist		Averill Churchland Dennett
Completely Objective	*Intrinsic to Part of Body*	Armstrong Bogen Holly Newton O'Shaughnessy Pritcher Wilkes
	Behaviorist	Malcolm Natsoulas Wittgenstein
	Functional State	Davis Edwards Gillet Lycan Shoemaker Tinnen Walkup Wilson
	Perception	Everitt Hall Handcock Tye Pitcher
Relation		Conee Graham Kaufman Langsam Nelkin Stephens
Purely Subjective	*Mysterious or Agnostic*	Addis Dalrymple Ehlich Harrison Kripke Leder McGinn Ornstein Sharpe
	Nonmysterious	Blum Carasso DeGrazia Gennaro Grahek Leighton Mayberry Trigg

Figure 5.1
Possible philosophical positions regarding the nature of pain, with the names of a few of the more prominent adherents listed. See the references for bibliographic information.

control theory of pain. Though theories of this ilk can account for several "low level" puzzling cases involving pain (why it is that stimulating our nociceptors under certain conditions can alleviate pain instead of causing more, for instance), they are notoriously vague when it comes to discussing the central gating mechanisms. This vagueness, I believe, obscures the fact that we actually have two separate systems involved in our perceptions of pain. One functions as a pain sensory system (PSS), quite analogous to our other sensory systems. The other (PIS), which developed independently of our PSS, actively inhibits its functioning.

Differentiating between the two systems helps explain the remaining controversies surrounding the basic nature of pain. While a PSS supports a perceptual view of pain as a completely objective phenomena, adding in a PIS (without explicitly recognizing that fact) accounts for the strongly subjective aspects of pain. I shall claim that a PSS functions according to the same basic rules of all our sensory systems and insofar as the pain system is a simpler system than, say, vision or audition, it makes sense to take pain perception as a paradigm instance of a conscious experience. But, insofar as we also have a PIS, pain also becomes a special case in our collection of conscious phenomena. Hence, contra Putnam, we should not be using the experience of pain as an intuitive and unproblematic example of conscious experience.

However, as a final conclusion emerging from my understanding of pain, we shall see that the sensation of pain—what most philosophers of mind focus upon as absolutely central to being in pain—is neither a particularly fundamental nor a particularly important component to our pain processing. One current popular research question in philosophy of mind is determining whether some philosophical approach or other (identity theory, functionalism, weak supervenience, etc.) can capture in an appropriate way what sensations feel like. If I am right about how we should understand pain, then the fervor devoted to this project might better be spent elsewhere, for what something is like becomes less important in explaining our mind.

The Complexity of Our Sensory Systems

Let me begin by outlining a few facts regarding our other sensory systems. I do this as a preliminary to discussing pain not because we understand, for example, visual processing, so much better than pain processing—we do not—but because many of the facts of perceptual processing regarded as commonplace (even among philosophers of mind) are the same sort of facts that seem to confuse philosophers and psychiatrists when theorizing about pain.

Our visual system is quite complex, spans many areas in the brain, and is comprised of several subsystems whose interactions remain a mystery. It is widely known that different aspects of visual processing occur in different processing streams, at least from the feature-detection perspective. For example, color is processed in the intralaminar pathway, while motion is processed in the magnocellular. The auditory system works in an analogous fashion (though the interactions of its subsystems are not as mysterious). The medial superior olive of our auditory system probably computes sound location using interaural time differences. The lateral superior olive, on the other hand, computes sound location by using differences in interaural frequency.

What is important to notice is that it is quite all right for there to exist more than one processing stream in each modality. We might be mystified how color gets joined with shape and motion so that we have a unified visual experience of particular objects.[2] But we are not confused about whether the neuronal paths involved in computing an object's color are visual, or whether computing interaural time differences is auditory. We are perfectly happy to have each modality be involved in several, maybe ultimately unrelated, computations. We say (or, at least, I say) the parts of the brain that normally respond to impinging photons are part of the visual system, and the parts of the brain normally sensitive to air compression trains are part of the auditory system.

Naturally, this is a gross oversimplification of how our sensory modalities are actually individuated: without unpacking what is meant by "normal functioning," the definitions are virtually unworkable. By way of partially rectifying this gloss, let me briefly touch upon the top-down and bottom-up investigative methodologies in neuroscience (and in psychology, to some degree), since these analytic tools help disambiguate what counts as normal functioning. More important, they allow us to make claims about which computational algorithms and cell assemblies are and are not included in our brain systems and subsystems.

First, scientists use the method of double dissociation to isolate the processing streams that comprise our subsystems. If we can get X to occur without Y and also Y to occur without X, then scientists take this as grounds to claim that X and Y function as independent units. For example, explicit priming tasks in psychology demonstrate that we can record the meaning of a word or phrase without storing its syntax; implicit priming tasks show that the syntax of a word or phrase can influence later linguistic processing while the meaning remains inert. I call this a top-down strategy because we start with a crude parsing of our system writ large (e.g., linguistic processing) and then divide that system into its component pieces (syntactic processing, semantics). This method of investigation forms the backbone of Daniel Dennett's functional decomposition.[3]

Second, scientists rely on a teleological analysis to unite the various and sundry parts into wholes. Breaking down larger pieces into smaller ones is not enough to get the explanatory job done, especially when several of our systems overlap inside the head. Our brain houses lots of individual processors; knowing all the pieces does not identify the larger puzzles. Why do scientists believe that color and motion processing belong to the same system but that echolocation belongs to something else? This is not a trivial question since each of the subsystems is (mainly) anatomically and physiologically distinct from the other, and since individual neurons do not know the sort of signal to which they are responding. The information contained in an atmospheric compression wave or a photon wave triplet is transmitted as electrical and chemical energy once one moves inside the body.

Scientists use three converging strategies to isolate and construct systems from the component dissociable subsystems. First, they look for correlations between neural firing patterns and events in the external world, very much what Fred Dretske has in mind with his informational semantics.[4] Neurophysiologists take the smallest pieces of the puzzles, usually individual neurons, or the extracellular spaces around small groups of neurons, and record what they do under a variety of circumstances. They conclude that our color and shape detectors belong together because they are active under similar circumstances, namely, when the organism's retinas are bombarded by photons. Auditory cells are active in different contexts. Luckily for the scientists and their correlation project, true polymodal cells are relatively rare.

Second, scientists look at the neural connections fore and aft. Aside from knowing how a cell or an area resonates with the environment, they also need to know what this cell or area is connected to—where the information the cell or area lights up to goes—and what is connected to the cell or area—how it gets the information it does respond to. Determining the processing algorithm of any cell group is not as easy as it might sound; it is not a matter of merely recording all the stimuli it likes and then deciding what all the stimuli have in common. As Lehky and Sejnowski remind us,[5] even cells that we think we know well, such as Hubel and Weisel's simple edge-detectors, might not be involved in the computations we think they are. It is entirely likely, given Lehky and Sejnowski's simulation results, that the so-called "edge-detector" cells actually are involved in computing an object's axes of curvature. Or, given dynamical systems considerations, they might not be involved in computations at all.

For another, more striking example, consider synesthesia, a condition in which one gets a bimodal experience from monomodal inputs—one can see and hear colors or taste and hear words.[6] Although we would probably want to say that someone seeing blue columns when she hears a bell ringing is having a visual experience, we would not want to say that atmospheric compression waves are visual inputs, even for this person. The inputs are still auditory; they come in through the ears and pass through the traditional auditory centers. They just happen also to travel through some of the visual pathways. If we only had access to single-cell recordings of synesthetic cells, we would obviously misidentify what those cells were doing. Knowing how things are connected prevents us from leaping to what would otherwise be an entirely rational (but also entirely false) conclusion.

Finally, scientists consider historical and evolutionary facts whenever possible. We are biological organisms equipped to move through our environment. We evolved that way because (roughly speaking) those who can move most effectively through their environment succeed in reproducing the most. When thinking about our perceptual systems, especially when worrying about various components' purposes, we should keep in mind how the hypothesized system or subsystem is supposed to function with regard to motor assembling. For most, if not all, information processing in the brain is related to the motor system in one way or another. For example, the visual areas all have at least some indirect contact with some motor structure or other, either the basal ganglia, or the motor cortex, or the tectum, or something.[7] Motor information needs to be "siphoned off" the visual pathways at all stages along the ascending route so that the visual input can be used for motor output.[8] Quite often what seems strange or curious from a psychological point of view seems quite natural from an evolutionary standpoint.

If we can group subsystems together into larger systems via their function—which is just what it is about that system that increases the reproductive rate of organisms that house it[9]—then so much the better. The brain puts great emphasis on the priority of motor tasks, and we should pay attention to this emphasis. Whatever purpose we ultimately proposed has to fit with our biological natures. (Often, however, such considerations are not possible or are little better than just-so stories, for the details of the advantages have been lost over evolutionary time. Why do we see in color, for example? What reproductive advantage would it have given our ancestors long ago? The answer is not easy, nor is it clear.)

I call this collection of research strategies "bottom up" because we begin with the smaller units in the brain and then arrange them into nested hierarchies. We group the double-dissociated subsystems, based on gross similarities in response patterns, connections to other systems and organs, and putative selective advantages, into hierarchically arranged classes. The process is not cut-and-dried by any means, but it is the best we have at the moment. Perhaps someday we will be able to identify which system various cell assemblies belong to definitively in virtue of the inherent rhythms of the cells' firing patterns, or something like this.[10] Until then, though, the best we can do is make educated guesses based on converging evidence.

Both approaches are required for a complete explanation of psychobiological phenomena. By breaking cognitive engines into interacting component pieces, the top-down strategy helps explain why organisms behave the way they do, and by categorizing and grouping the isolated parts, the bottom-up strategy helps explain what purpose the analyzed behavior serves. Reminding ourselves that we use both strategies in understanding our neural systems will rid us of the tendency to make our pain system into a cartoon, and reminding ourselves of our biological heritage will aid in justifying a counterintuitive system that prevents pains from occurring. Ultimately, I claim that our system for perceiving pain works in exactly the same fashion as our visual and auditory systems: it is a complex system with dissociable subsystems. Furthermore, it is a system that appears quite natural when considered against an evolutionary backdrop.

A Sketch of Our Pain System

The classic feature-detection view of our basic pain system is of two three-neuron subsystems.[11] (See figure 5.2.)[12] Each subsystem has a set of neurons that resides in the dorsal root ganglion of the spinal column. These neurons extend their axons to whatever tissue they innervate and receive external input there. They also have a second axon that projects across to the dorsal horn. The axon in the dorsal horn connects with a second set of neurons housed in the dorsal horn whose axons run out of the spinal column and up to the thalamus. The third set of neurons projects from the thalamus to the postcentral gyrus in cerebral cortex.

In 1911, Head and Holmes proposed a dual system of afferent projections in our pain sensory system: an epicritic system that processes information regarding intensity and precise location, and a protopathic system that delivers the actual pain sensations. Almost nine decades later, we still believe they were fundamentally correct. We now know that we have a "sensory discriminative" subsystem that computes the location, intensity, duration, and nature (stabbing, burning, prickling) of the stimuli. This subsystem is subserved by the A-∂ fibers. These mechanoreceptive neurons are myelinated, so information can travel quite quickly along them (approximately 5–30 m/sec, as opposed to .5–2 m/sec for information traveling along unmyelinated pathways[13]). Consequently, they transmit what is known as "first pain" or "fast pain." The threshold for activation is constant from person to person, and this subsystem remains active (assuming no other defects in the organism) only as long as the raw nerve endings are stimulated.

We also have a "affective-motivational" subsystem that supports the unpleasant part of painful sensations. This system feeds directly into our

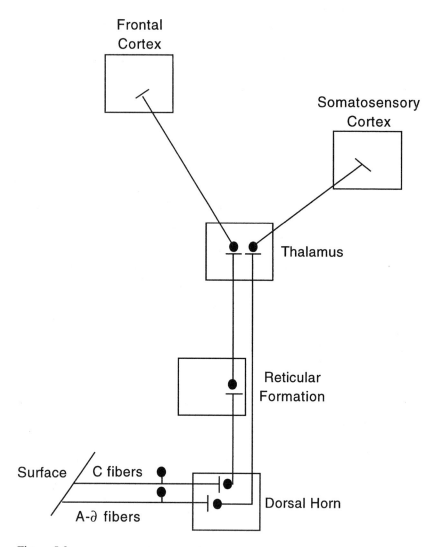

Figure 5.2
Diagram showing our pain sensory system. The first set of neurons take in information from the periphery and then synapse with a second set of neurons in the dorsal horn. These neurons ascend, some terminating in the reticular formation of the brain stem, others traveling to the thalamus. Axons that terminate medially in the thalamus synapse with a third set of neurons that project to the frontal cortex. Those that terminate laterally synapse with neurons that project to the somatosensory cortex.

motor response systems and is considered to by phylogenetically older than other aspects of our multifaceted pain system. This polymodal subsystem begins with the well-known unmyelinated C-fibers. Once they are activated, they will continue to fire for some time, even after the noxious event has ceased. This subsystem gives rise to what is known as "slow pain" or "second pain," so called because this is what we feel second whenever we are injured—a diffuse and persistent burning pain. The traditional view is that when someone has chronic pain, a protracted second pain might be what is being referred to.

Similar to the color and form processors in the visual system, the A-∂ fiber and C-fiber pathways remain largely segregated. For example, generally speaking, they terminate in different layers on the dorsal horn. However, there is more interaction than what we find in either the visual or auditory system. The dorsal horn contains "wide-dynamic range" (WDR) neurons that respond to both A-∂ and C neurons, as well as to other peripheral stimuli. WDR neurons are also sensitive to visceral stimuli. It is possible that referred and sympathetic pains depend upon this sort of visceral-somatic convergence.[14]

Once nociceptive information exits the dorsal horn, it travels either to the reticular formation in the brain stem or to the thalamus. Laminae I and V project to the lateral nuclei in the thalamus,[15] and laminae II, IV, and VI project to the medial nuclei. Each type of nuclei underwrites a different sort of information; the lateral nuclei process discriminative information (fast pain), while the medial nuclei and reticular connections process affective-motivational information (slow pain). The two thalamic streams remain separate on their trip to cortex as well. Nociceptive neurons in the lateral nuclei synapse in somatosensory cortex, which then can compute the location and characteristics of the pain; those in the medial nuclei synapse in the anterior cingulate gyrus in the frontal lobe, which figures in our emotional reactions to pain. The frontal lobe (and its connections) process our actual suffering.

Philosophy's Error

Now we can see how and why several philosophers are mistaken in their conclusions that there are no such things as pains,[16] or that pains are located in our limbs,[17] or that pains are purely subjective[18] or that pains are reactive behaviors.[19] Each of these positions identifies pain with one of the neuronal groups within the classic pain system, while failing to recognize that our pain system is complex and contains at least a duality of subsystems,[20] each of which processes a different sort of information. (See figure 5.3.)

In general, philosophers make these mistakes because they misunderstand the double dissociation methodology. We can, either through purposeful intervention or accidents of Nature, dissociate our discriminative pain processing from our affective-motivational pain processing. Ingestion of morphine (or other opiates), lesions to the medial thalamus, and prefrontal lobotomies all result in sensations of pain without a sense of suffering and without producing characteristic pain behaviors (wincing, moaning, complaining, etc.).[21] In these cases, patients can localize their pains but are not upset by the fact that they are in pain. We can also get reverse effects, to a degree. Fentanyl causes one to react in pain yet inhibits our discriminatory abilities for the pain.[22] Lesion studies and studies using hemispherectomies show that even with cortex completely missing, we can still have a pain sensation; we simply lack fine localization and intensity discrimination.[23] Patients with Parkinson's disease and Huntington's chorea often have pain sensations but are unable to indicate exactly where they feel the pains.[24]

We also find instances of the nociceptive centers in the thalamus and cortex being activated without corresponding activations of A-∂ or C fibers. Fully 80 percent of lower back pain sufferers present no external or internal injury.[25] Phantom limbs and phantom pains in phantom limbs are quite common experiences in new amputees.[26] Stimulating the medial periaqueductal gray region, tectum, or thalamus directly can also result in painful experiences.[27] Finally, as we have seen in chapter 2, our emotional states heavily influence the degree of pain we feel, quite independent of actual injury. Indeed, "psychogenic" pains have been documented since the late 1800s, when D. H. Tuke reported the case of a butcher who got fouled up on a meat hook and appeared to be in agony. However, when examined by the local chemist, it was discovered that the meat hook had only penetrated his jacket sleeve and, even though the butcher was screaming in "excessive pain," he was completely unharmed.[28]

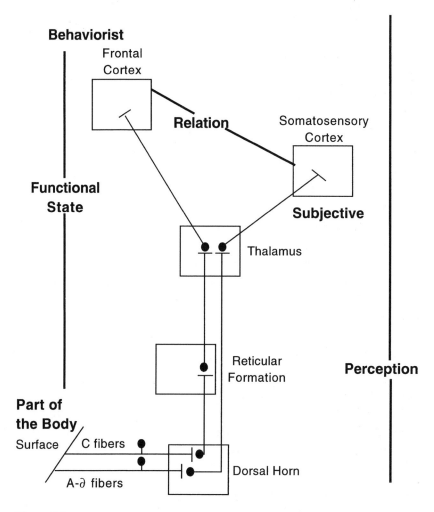

Figure 5.3
Part of the pain system identified with different philosophical views regarding the basic nature of pain. Most views identify pain with one subsystem or with one sort of neural processor. Two exceptions are functional state and perceptual views of pain, though perceptual views of pain often overlook or underestimate the motor component of pain processing.

Correlatively, there are also examples of our peripheral nociceptors being activated without this information being processed as it normally would be in the thalamus or cortex. About 37 percent of emergency room visitors feel no pain at the time of their injury.[29] Athletes and soldiers can continue performing free of pain, even though they have been severely injured.[30] Hypnosis allows some subjects to engage in what would otherwise be painful activities without being in pain.[31] Placebos are notoriously helpful in relieving pain. (Interestingly enough, they relieve pain at half the rate of the real drug, regardless of the supposed strength of the drug.[32]) And of course, some lesions to the thalamus and cortex can result in the cessation of pain experiences, even though the peripheral neurons continue to operate normally.

However, each of these double dissociations only individuates neuronal groups or subsystems within our overarching pain system. I make this claim by analogy with our other perceptual systems. Blindsight patients can discriminate shapes and figures they claim not to be able to see consciously. Sufferers of Anton's syndrome insist that they can see perfectly well, even though they are completely blind and have severe bilateral damage to their visual association areas. However, no one uses these facts to argue that vision does not exist, or that vision is located in our eyeballs, or that vision is purely subjective, or that vision is behavioral. We may not know exactly what to say about blindsight or Anton's syndrome, but no one claims that blindsight is not a disorder of the visual system or that patients with Anton's syndrome are not having a visual experience of some sort.

By misunderstanding what a perceptual system in the brain encompasses, many philosophers miss the boat regarding the basic nature and structure of pain. Double dissociation alone does not individuate our basic systems; that is used to isolate the subsystems that operate within the larger system. We then need to build our different systems out of the component pieces. Teleological considerations help us to do so. To wit: the neurons in our pain system all respond to roughly the same sort of information; they increase their rate of firing in the presence of noxious stimuli on skin or deep organs. Moreover, the connection among the six-neuron tract is a stable, common, and isolable pathway. Connections fore and aft show a stream of information flowing from the nociceptors on the skin up through cortex.[33] Finally, a pain sensory system tied to the somatosensory processors makes good evolutionary sense. As creatures eking out lives in a hostile environment, having a system that could warn us when damage occurred and could force us to protect damaged parts until they healed would be tremendously beneficial. (Indeed, as our discussion of Tanya in chapter 3 indicates, persons who cannot feel any pain at all often live a nasty, brutish, and short life.[34])

Neither our conscious experience of pain, the damaged tissue itself, nor our bodily or emotional reactions are fundamental to pain processing. Each is but one component of a larger processor. Hence, it is a mistake to try to claim one or the other as pain simpliciter. And it is equally erroneous to conclude that since we cannot identify one or the other with pain, there is no such thing. The entire pain sensory system functions largely the same way as any of our sensory systems. Their pieces are united by our best guess of their function, based on the three types of converging evidence discussed above. Hence, we have concluded that the components of our visual system take the information contained in photons bouncing around in the world and use it to compute the location, orientation, texture, color, and movement of objects in the environment. The components of our auditory system take the information contained in atmospheric compression waves and use it to compute the placement of things. And the component of our pain system take pressure, temperature, and chemical readings of our surface (and interior) and use this information to track what is happening to our tissues. The A-∂ cells and the C-fibers do this, as do the spinothalamic tract and its connections to cortex. In sum, it appears that we have a complex but well-defined sensory system that monitors our tissues to promote the welfare of our bodies.[35]

The Awfulness of Pain

Not surprisingly, though, appearances are deceiving. With the classic story of pain processing, we can determine how philosophers and others go astray in their thinking about pain: in assuming that pain is simpler than it is, they end up identifying pain with some component or subset of the entire complicated process. However, the classic feature-detection story of pain qua sensory system only scratches the surface of pain's complexity and, in so doing, gives the illusion that our pain system is well defined. What counts as pain processing as opposed to an emotional reaction to pain or a belief that one is in pain, for example, is difficult to determine, for they all shade into one another. Once we move beyond the spinal column, discrete computational streams become difficult to identify and trace. What counts as the process proper and what counts as merely an influence on the process? What marks the end of one process and the beginning of another? There are no principled answers for pain.

But again, this problem also appears in our other sensory systems as well (though I shall not take the time to do the comparative analysis here), so pain is not special in this regard. Perception, interpretation, judgment, and reaction are all tightly bound up with one another, so much so that separating cognitive "events" from one another becomes an artificial laboratory exercise. Pain is a far cry from the simple sensory event that philosophers assume.

Images of Pain

Knowledge of the higher brain processes involved in pain comes largely from imaging studies, which have only recently become cheap and easy enough to use fairly extensively in basic science research. Unfortunately, imaging studies of pain are still relatively rare, and replication is the exception, not the rule. (I should note, though, that true replication in any imagining study is highly unusual.) Experimental paradigms are not codified across laboratories, so definitive results are hard to come by. Nevertheless, we can see general trends and patterns developing across the different studies. At the least, it is clear that the classic view of pain processing is woefully oversimplified and quite limited.

The first thing we learn from looking at the imaging studies is that blood flow or other measures of cerebral activity often decrease during painful stimulation. (We see deactivations most consistently in contralateral posterior cingulate, contralateral somatosensory cortex, and orbital gyrus; see figure 5.4.) The decrease appeared in the very first imaging study in the mid-seventies and has remained a constant datum since then.[36] Though what the decreases mean is still under discussion, one good explanation is that they indicate neural inhibition. Of course, in-

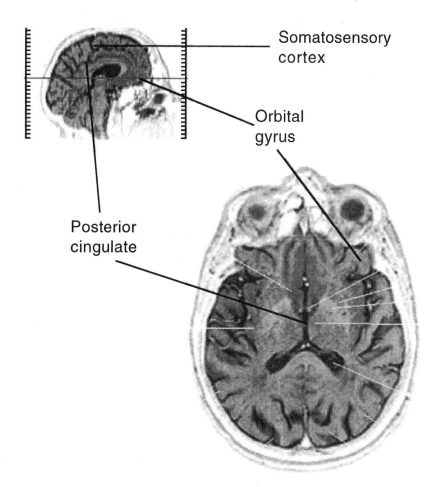

Somatosensory cortex

Orbital gyrus

Posterior cingulate

Figure 5.4
Brain image schematic showing the approximate locations of the areas that consistently indicate decreased blood flow during a painful experience. We assume that decreased blood flow correlates with neural inhibition in the brain.

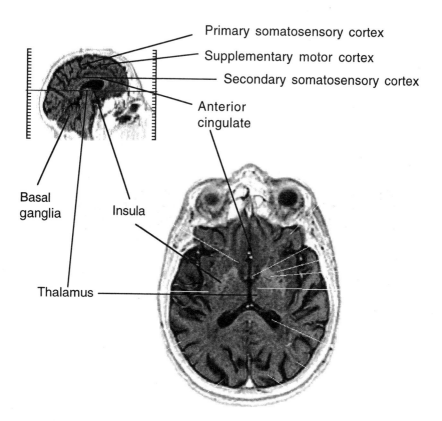

Figure 5.5
Brain image schematic showing the approximate locations of the areas that consistently indicate increased blood flow during an acute painful experience. We assume that increased blood flow correlates with increased neural activity.

terneurons inhibiting the firing of other neurons would consume energy (and so their activity should show in any scan). However, these neurons are quite small relative to excitatory neurons and so their activity relative to excitatory cells might show up as an overall decrease in the area.[37]

In addition to the decreases, brain scans of induced acute pains indicate activity in the anterior cingulate cortex, anterior insula, primary and secondary somatosensory cortex, supplementary motor cortex, thalamus, and basal ganglion.[38] (See figure 5.5.) Excluding the primary somatosensory system, thalamus, and orbital gyrus, the brain regions responding to painful stimuli do not respond to nonnoxious thermal stimuli or to

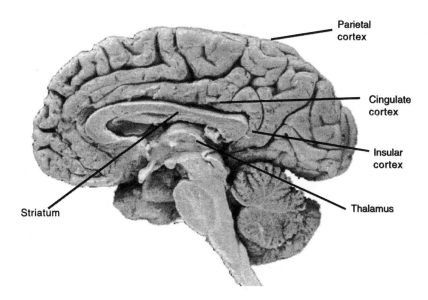

Parietal
cortex

Cingulate
cortex

Insular
cortex

Thalamus

Striatum

Figure 5.6.
Midsagittal section of the brain with the approximate locations of the areas that respond significantly to painful stimuli.

vibrotactile stimuli. That is, the activated areas are devoted specifically to sensing and processing information about pain itself and not to analyzing any inputs that might merely resemble something painful, such as warmth or pressure. In general, parietal, insular, and cingulate cortical regions, plus the thalamus and the striatum, respond significantly to painful stimuli. Figure 5.6 provides a sense of where these areas reside in the brain. Other regions may be involved as well, although they may not show any change in activity relative to baseline (because they are active during the baseline circumstances as well).

However, one danger in leaning too hard on these studies of acute pain is that there is no good way to differentiate between processing the experience of pain, on the one hand, and startle reflexes, anticipatory motor programming to withdraw from the pain, changes in alertness, and so forth, on the other. All the brain scans can tell us is which areas of the brain differentially respond to the task; they cannot tell us what role the activated regions are playing in the cognitive or behavioral economy of the subject. We have many responses to pain; some include the experience of pain itself, but others include our evaluation of the incident, our decisions about how to react, our bodies getting ready to respond, our planning for the next event. Sorting which is which is not trivial.

The Emotion of Pain

Nonetheless, we can infer some things about the functional roles of the activated areas, particularly when we compare acute instances of pain with tonic ones. When the stimuli are repeated continuously over time, ipsilateral insula, thalamus, and the cerebellum also become active.[39] Here we see the first glimpse of a general arousal that might be tied to pain as the brain activity becomes bilateral and more distributed. Indeed, it looks as though tonic and chronic pains show a very different activity pattern than brief acute pains.[40]

In particular, some argue for a biphasic pattern of pain processing in cortex that closely parallels the two sorts of lower-level pain processing assumed in the classic view. Vania Apkarian suggests that the cortical activity seen in the somatosensory regions during acute pain reflects the subjects' decision to remain in the painful situation for the duration of the experiment.[41] This decision requires information concerning where the painful stimuli impinges on the body and how intense or disturbing the phenomenological experience is. This process is a relative of the A-∂ fiber-based sensory discriminative subsystem, now sometimes called the "lateral pain system."[42] The difference between the classic feature-detection perspective and the new view is that Apkarian makes early pain processing to be largely motoric and likely to turn on one's local motivations in behavior. In fact, studies comparing what happens in the brain when a finger is heated beyond the pain threshold versus when the same finger is vibrated or moved show about 90 percent of the activated cortical areas in common. The overlap tells us that what happens in the brain in the early pain processing phase is very similar to what happens during motor programming and execution.

Following these early decisions, though, one can still perceive pain. This aspect of pain processing does not depend upon our somatosensory regions, which is why activity there decreases even though painful stimuli continues to impinge on the nociceptors. Despite the emphasis of the classic view on the centrality of the thalamus as a nociceptive/pain relay station, this later nonmotoric processing probably has extrathalamic sources, for we see a decrease in thalamic activity in conjunction with increases in activity in anterior cingulate, supplementary motor, and anterior insular regions (though decreases in primary and secondary somatosensory regions and in primary motor cortex). This second phase, known as the "medial pain system," corresponds to some sort of central reaction. Pain still persists, even though the immediate behavioral response has been plotted and executed. Something else has to be done, and perhaps what we are seeing is the brain's alternative strategy for dealing with the stimulus.[43]

Similar decreases in brain response are seen when subjects anticipate a painful or unpleasant stimulus, and its magnitude is associated with the level of anxiety the subjects reported experiencing before the input.[44] (This correlation is striking because there is no correlation between the activity of primary somatosensory cortex and pain or intensity ratings.) Though I do not want to argue that the way to cope with stress is to become nervous, it is clear that the brain responds in the same way when we expect a pain to be coming down the pike or when we continue to experience pain after our motor decisions have been made. The brain clearly has some other coping mechanism for pain beyond simple and quick motor responses.

"Coping mechanism" should be understood in quotes, though, for often what our brain decides to do to "cope" is not terribly helpful. We can see this, in particular, in our susceptibility to Pavlovian classical conditioning. We can easily condition sensory processing—including pain processing—to produce concomitant negative emotions, such as fear, depression, or anxiety.[45] This "conditioning" is really a by-product of thalamic activity, and subcortical conditioning strongly resists extinction. Most of us have had some experience with this phenomenon (if not personally, then vicariously through someone we know) in dentists' offices. Fear and loathing of dental procedures, so often the subject of parody, is quite real. One painful experience in a particular setting can induce the same emotions in the same setting later. Patients who have undergone repeated painful diagnostic or treatment procedures exhibit similar effects: they are terribly and disproportionately anxious about their next hospital visit.

Tying fear to pain intensifies the affective dimensions of pain when what is normally considered to be a minor pain is paired with intense negative emotion.[46] It also means that the thalamus no longer needs to be active to continue the emotional response. Once a cognitive or emotive reaction is programmed into a system, it will kick in full-strength with appropriate triggers. And it will continue to run, even if the trigger is brief, even if the trigger is then turned off. Such is the nature of classical conditioning, and unfortunately, we have very little higher-level control over those circuits once they get set up.

Classical conditioning is just one way in which pain can become interwoven with affect. Extrathalamic connections may be even more powerful, as I discuss below. My point here is simply that our pain system is intimately related to our perceptual, cognitive, and affective apparatuses. Except under unusual circumstances, we cannot react to pain without also bringing forth a lot of additional baggage. There is no such thing as a simple pain state, nor a simple pain.

Aristotle considered pain a "passion" of the soul, an affect distinct from our five senses. It is important to understand, though, that Aristotle's "passions" are wider in scope than ours. He meant "passion" (pathe) to refer to anything we perceive or feel that comes to us unbidden. Things we cannot control intellectually are passions. These would include our emotions as well as our perceptions. Consequently, the dividing line between the emotions and our sensory experiences is not as clear for Aristotle as it is for many cognitive scientists. One of my themes in this chapter is that an Aristotlian view is probably right on this score.[47] Distinguishing among emotional, sensory, and cognitive responses is quite difficult to do. They all run together in the brain.

In any event, contemporary scientists are concluding what the ancient Greek philosophers already knew: "Emotion is not simply a consequence of pain sensation that occurs after a noxious sensory message arrives at somatosensory cortex. Rather, it is a fundamental part of the pain experience. . . . [The experience of pain] is above all else a powerful and demanding feeling state."[48] The brain's reaction to pain information is a complicated and multidimensional. It involves large chunks of our cognitive and emotional lives and utilizes processing resources distributed throughout our neural tissue. So far as the brain is concerned, pain is an important and all-encompassing event.

Chronic Pain Possibilities

One might expect that these results would give us important clues about what chronic pain is like, at least for the brain. Unfortunately, however, the small number of imaging studies done on clinical persisting pain give inconsistent results.[49] We find activity in the primary and secondary somatosensory cortex and thalamus either unchanged, inhibited, or increased, depending on the study (though the trend is to see a decrease in thalamic activity and no change or a decrease in primary and secondary somatosensory areas). Hsieh et al. postulate that "the brain may recruit different operational mechanisms in processing a long-lasting pain state with persisting emotional distress versus phasic perceptual challenges with a low tone of affection."[50] It is conceivable that chronic, pathological, or clinical pain is simply different in kind from acute, phasic, or tonic pain, even when the latter last for a long time.

Nevertheless, one fact consistently emerges: the brain activity in chronic pain patients changes radically when they simultaneously experience acute pain but are relieved of their chronic pain through a block or some other similar treatment. Clinical pain patients show one pattern of activity in somatosensory cortex when given a painful thermal stimulus before they are administered a nerve block eliminating their chronic pain. After the block, they show the opposite pattern. Even though the patterns may differ across subjects, within subjects the change in pattern remains the same. We see similar effects with the frontal cortex. It is active under chronic pain and during acute pains; it is not active when chronic pain is blocked.[51]

These facts tell us that our perception of some pain depends upon the ongoing neural activity against which the pain is processed. Apkarian explains: "Although the [acute pain] stimulus is perceived [to be] of similar magnitude both during and in the absence of the chronic pain, during chronic pain the noxious stimulus acts mainly as an extra-exacerbation of the chronic pain. In contradistinction to this, in the absence of chronic pain, the noxious stimulus induces a motor decisional component that increases the activity in the somatosensory areas that feed into the motor system."[52] How we think about our pains depends upon what else is happening in our cognitive economy at the time. Under some circumstances (when we aren't experiencing ongoing pain), pain makes us decide to move in some fashion. Under other circumstances (when we are experiencing ongoing pain), it doesn't.

This backdrop against which we perceive new painful stimuli includes both our perceptual and our affective states. Hsieh et al. point out that the anterior cingulate is active in a majority of chronic pain studies in an area that does not correspond to regions that light up during attentional or motor tasks. (Instead, this area is close to the one that is involved in itch perception.)[53] This part of the frontal lobe developed out of a primitive hippocampus formation; we can think of dorsal frontal cortex, which includes the cingulate regions, as an evolutionary extension of hippocampus.[54] It appears to be devoted to emotionality; most likely, it is part of the loop between cognition and emotion (though which drives which is still a matter of controversy[55]).

We know that the anterior cingulate and the prefrontal cortex are involved in processing chronic pain, while the thalamus is not. Despite assurances from classic pain theory that the thalamus is the major relay station for pain between the spine and cortex, it is clear that other connections have to be involved in chronic pain. One likely possibility for these connections is via striatal areas and the limbic system itself (our emotional headquarters) because the limbic system is strongly interconnected with the cingulate and prefrontal cortex.[56] (A second likely pathway is via the spinoreticular tract.)

There are some single-cell studies showing a response to nociception in the limbic areas under experimental conditions, though nothing is known about chronic pain responses there.[57] The difficulty here, as discussed in the last chapter, is that we are running up against technical limitations. Single-cell animal studies work for short duration acute pains. We have very few, if any, good models for chronic pain in animals. Nevertheless, with the little information we do have, we can draw some tentative conclusions.

The classic three-neuron theory discussed above gives little role to cerebral cortex, including primary and secondary somatosensory cortex, in pain processing. Stimulating these areas does not produce pain, nor does removing them cause pain to decrease.[58] Imaging studies agree with the classic position on clinical pain: the thalamus and somatosensory areas are only minimally involved in chronic, pathological, or psychogenic pains.[59] The thalamic and somatosensory regions seem to be important for fight or flight and other related motor decisions, but not for pains for which behavioral decisions have already been made and executed.

Ronald Melzack suggests that chronic pains are induced in the spine but then sustained centrally through activity in the cingulate, hippocampus, and fornix.[60] He might be right. Radical frontal lobotomies relieve the suffering of intractible pain, though without changing awareness of the pain itself.[61] Patients who have undergone the procedure report that the pain is still there, but that they just don't "worry about it." In fact, it can even be "agonizing," but somehow that fact does not distress them in the least.[62] Frontal lobotomies, among other things, sever projections from hypothalamus to cingulate cortex; in effect, they discombobulate the part of the brain that processes affect. Consequently, lobotomy patients can still perceive everything that they used to; they simply do not have the same (or in some cases, any) emotional reactions to their perceptions.

A recent study adds weight to the proposal that pain's significant affective dimension is connected to the frontal lobes. When PET scans were done in subjects who had received hypnotic suggestions that their pains would not hurt, activity in anterior cingulate cortex decreased, while activity in primary somatosensory cortex remained unchanged.[63] (How and why hypnosis influences pain is a topic examined in chapter 8.) As before, the level of activity in the cingulate cortex is correlated with how bad the pain seems, while the activity in somatosensory cortex is not.

In addition to the limbic system, our brains contain other neural mechanisms (aside from thalamus) by which the affective load of pain could be carried. There are four major extrathalamic afferent pathways that project to neocortex. Of these, the dorsal noradrenergic bundle (DNB) orginating in the locus coeruleus (LC) is most closely tied to negative emotions and projects to what is known as the "limbic brain."[64] The LC consistently increases its activity with nociception[65] and increased activity of the LC is correlated with alarm, fear, defensive postures, startle, and freezing in primates.[66]

One hypothesis is that the LC is a central analog of a sympathetic ganglion.[67] It reacts when the organism is under biological threat—when the organism is in pain, to be sure—but also when the heart beats rapidly or when internal organs are distended. The LC and consequently the DNB are geared to increase vigilance, emotional response, attention, and motor response. In short, they work to increase the general responsiveness of creatures to threats.[68] If this hypothesis is right, then it is no wonder that the LC and DNB respond rapidly as part of pain processing.

Though we really have no idea how chronic pain appears in the brain, we can at least say that chronic pain is a complex that includes negative affect as a significant component. Ample connections exist in the brain to integrate nociception with emotional response very easily. Perhaps, when we think of chronic pain, we should think in terms of a perceptual-emotional mental unit.

The Dynamical Approach

More important than our stabs at explaining chronic pain, though, is the general picture of pain processing that emerges from these data. Even if we do not yet have the details concerning exactly what is active when in the brain, it is clear that lots of areas are involved at more or less the same time. As with our other sensory systems, pain processing is highly distributed and massively parallel. It glosses over much, maybe too much, to rely on the serial, feedforward transmission implicit in a feature-detection approach. The discussion above gives a hint of the complexity involved in processing pain: pain processing involves adjudicating among various motor response patterns; integrating perception with expectation, memory, and affect, as well as perhaps motives, and longer-term goals; and settling on some sort of (more or less) unified whole from the disparate processed bits.

In everyday life, pain occurs in the context of other experiences. We are always receiving a spate of sensory information in some fashion, and pain is just one extra byte in the mix. Everything is integrated together at each instant of time. Nociceptive signals, other sensory perceptions, memories, associations, feelings, goals, and expectations, all combine into some stable pattern of activity.[69]

C. Richard Chapman suggests that we could use schema theory from cognitive psychology to understand pain.[70] In brief, a schema (or frame, as it is sometimes called) is a pattern of concepts, meanings, and associations produced from memory traces, present experiences, and expectations of the future. Our schemata are ever changing and constantly updating, reflecting the ongoing stream of perception and thought in our mental lives. David Rumelhart describes them as follows: "[S]chemata emerge at the moment they are needed from the interaction of large numbers of much simpler elements, all working in concert with one another. [They] . . . are not explicit entities, but rather are implicit in our knowledge and are created by the very environment that they are trying to interpret as it is interpreting them."[71] Just as in the case of classical conditioning discussed above, simple sensory stimuli can trigger a full-blown meaningful schema. Doing so is merely a matter of completing a dynamic pattern. There is no reason why pain, one sort of sensory stimulus, cannot do this, nor why we cannot have schemata for pain that other things might trigger.

Indeed, recent work concerning what triggers phantom limb pain suggests that the latter is exactly what occurs in some cases of chronic pain. (Remember the third case study from chapter 2, the surfer with phantom pain.) Some cognitive or emotional event activates a conscious schema associated with painful experiences.[72] A remembered pain, then, becomes real once again. The brain creates the experience of pain from available cognitive and emotional schemata and other associations. Hence, the experience of chronic pain isn't the culmination of a sequence of processing steps in a circuit; it is an ongoing construction that relates our current experience to past understandings, framings, of the world.

Once the pain schema is activated, it becomes impossible not to pay attention to it, for Nature designed us to focus on our pains and decide some appropriate behavior immediately in order to ensure our survival. Chronic pain then becomes the endlessly repeated construction of a pain experience, constructed perhaps not because of some bodily trauma, but because some other stimulus input has trigged the loop. A dynamical perspective on pain processing sees pain as a reverberating circuit among a diverse set of brain areas, a circuit that is constructed as it is activated, but one that also depends upon which circuits have come before.[73] The various regions of the brain that we see light up during pain do not function independently of one another. Instead, they are tightly integrated. These interactions are felt in the experience of pain itself as a complex perceptual-emotional state as well as seen in the neuroanatomy of the brain.

6

When a Pain Isn't

At the age of 13, I found that self-injury temporarily relieved [my]. . . . unbearable jumble of feelings. I cut myself in the bathroom, where razor blades were handy and I could lock the door. The slicing through flesh never hurt, although it never even occurred to me that it should. . . . The blood brought an odd sense of well-being, of strength. It became all encompassing. Sometimes I rubbed the blood on my face and arms and looked at myself in the mirror. I did not think how sick I must be. I did not think. With a safe sense of detachment, I watched myself play with my own flowing blood. The fireball of tension was gone and I was calm. I learned to soothe myself this way.

During I feel very focused and full of anticipation. I purposely hold my breath as I cut and let it out when I'm through, so I breathe out as the blood runs out. I feel so calm. All the noise and stupidity in my head is gone, I feel like I'm floating . . . I feel stupid because I feel like I don't have a reason to do it. That's why I keep it to myself.

I feel like I'm going out of control. I have so much anger and hurt inside me that I don't know what to do with. During an episode I start to feel relieved from all my tension and stress and it seems like I'm almost in a trance and don't really notice the things around me. It's really strange.

I think I become so fascinated with it that the pain is the last thing on my mind. Truthfully, I enjoy it way too much. . . . A lot of times I don't want to stop and have to make myself.
—Anonymous accounts of self-injurious behavior

If I were to choose between pain and nothing, I would choose pain.
—William Faulkner

Whether we can or should decompose our multifarious states and processes into their component pieces is a question we cannot answer now. We do not know if a feature-detection, stepwise computational description or a higher-level dynamical system's model will better capture the features of pain processing we find most important. Regardless, from either perspective—both still regretfully incomplete—we can see that processing painful stimuli uses large portions of the brain and is tied to our memories, current perceptions, expectations, and feelings. It is a nontrivial operation.

This is the easy and less interesting reason why philosophers are wrong about how to understand pain. More to the point: their way of looking at our pain system does not clear up all the confusions, mysteries, and conflicts in our account of pain. There are several important empirical facts that any theory of pain needs to be able to explain. These are facts that, by and large, do not have analogues in our other perceptual systems. Moreover, they are facts that lead otherwise intelligent people to make prima facie bizarre statements regarding what pain is and is not. Here I only touch upon a few such facts, but it should be enough to motivate the challenge to theories of pain as well as to justify the approach I shall advocate in understanding self-injurious behavior and other pain anomalies.

I aim to show that we really have two independent pain-related systems, a pain processing system (PPS), discussed in the last chapter, and a pain inhibiting system (PIS). Though I shall not spend much time on the details of how the PIS works, it should be enough to establish that we should think of it as a separate system in its own right, with its own processing goals and strategies.

The Strangeness of Pain

Correlations between Nociception and Perception

There is, in fact, a poor correlation between nociception and pain perception.[1] That is, the relationship between stimulating the A-∂ and C fibers and actually feeling or reporting a pain is not at all straightforward. Several tribal rituals give vivid illustrations of the dissociation. In parts of India, for example, men chosen to represent the gods have steel hooks inserted under the muscles of their back. They then swing above the crowds, suspended on these hooks by ropes, blessing children and crops. They exhibit no pain.[2] I mentioned in the last chapter that about 40 percent of all ER patients reported feeling no pain at the time of injury; another 40 percent report greater pain than one would expect, leaving only 20 percent of all ER visitors having pains appropriate to their injuries.[3] It is not the case that we can dissociate nociception from discriminative and affective-motivational reaction; it is that they regularly and frequently dissociate.

Self-injurious behavior (SIB) provides perhaps the most striking and poignant instances of this phenomenon. As the quotations above testify, some people cause themselves physical harm on purpose and without pain. Indeed, the usual accompaniment to SIB is a feeling of relief and calm. Persons describe being "comforted" by their injuries, being "relieved of [a] . . . desperately restless feeling," feeling "cleansed . . . calm, and in control" after they cut, burn, or otherwise abuse their tissues.[4]

We must be careful to distinguish the sort of self-injurious behavior that some autistic, learning disabled, or psychotic patients engage in and what otherwise (or maybe completely) normal people do.[5] I am concerned with the latter. The SIB of the mentally impaired is stereotypic, often rhythmic head-banging or biting, and has been traced to abnormalities in the serotonergic or dopaminergic systems. I do not know whether this sort of self-injurious behavior is painful. Though quite often ritualized, the self-mutilation of normals is not stereotypic. It generally includes cutting, scratching, burning, pulling hair, breaking bones, hitting, self-flagellation, and poisoning. Nor has it been definitively linked to any neurotransmitters in the brain. Indeed, as I shall discuss below, no one quite knows why some people repeatedly injure themselves, though I shall give my hypothesis below.

Persons who engage in SIB rarely intend to kill themselves; they aren't suicidal.[6] Instead, they use it to escape from depression, to relieve tension or anger, to make themselves feel good, or to overcome a sense of unreality, depersonalization, or alienation.[7] Though some self-harmers do feel pain during SIB, the majority do not. For those who do not, their perception of pain intensity is within normal limits for other sorts of pains. Something about the SIB itself prevents them from experiencing the pain. Indeed, something about SIB makes it feel good. With SIB, not only do we find a poor correlation between nociception and pain, but the nociception has exactly the opposite effect than it is supposed to.

Other examples of nociception being associated with the sensations of pain include the case of Mathieu discussed at the beginning of chapter two. By focusing on his writing, Mathieu was able to control or eliminate the sensations of pain caused by his cancer. This activity would not diminish the output of the A-∂ and C fibers in his visceral tissues—they will continue to fire as always. Yet, by paying attention to something personally important, a little boy does not perceive what he would otherwise.

Our other perceptual systems do not work in this fashion. There is a highly reliable correlation between having the rods and cones in our retina being bombarded by light photons and having some visual experience or other.[8] There is also a highly reliable correlation between the vibration of our tympanic membranes at a certain frequency and hearing sounds. And rarely so far as I know, does stimulating the tympanic membrane cause our auditory experiences to blank out or be replaced by some other mode of phenomenology. Any theory of pain is going to have to explain why our peripheral sensors for noxious stimuli are not well connected to our sensations of pain. Indeed, the relation between external events and internal indicators is part of what individuates our systems. Without better correlation between external events and internal activity, we cannot claim that our putative pain system is in fact a pain system.

Illusions of Pain

In addition to the poor correlation between the external event and the internal reaction, several fairly common illusions associated with pain exist. For example, pain is often "referred" to a different part of the body. The pain from deep tissues or the viscera sometimes is felt as a pain on the surface of the body at a point distant from the damaged organ.[9] Heart attacks probably form the most well known example of this phenomenon: Myocardial infarction in males is often recognized by the pain felt in the left arm, shoulder, and hand. These sorts of referral patterns are quite well known among physicians and often aid in making proper diagnoses.

Our best guess about how this works is that it is a sort of hard-wired illusion. The best explanation to date for this is Ruch's Visceral-Somatic Convergence model.[10] Nociception from a damaged internal organ converges onto lamina V of the dorsal horn. Also projecting to the same area are the neurons that synapse on the surface of the skin or some other distal tissue. As a result, the brain misattributes the source of the nocicep-

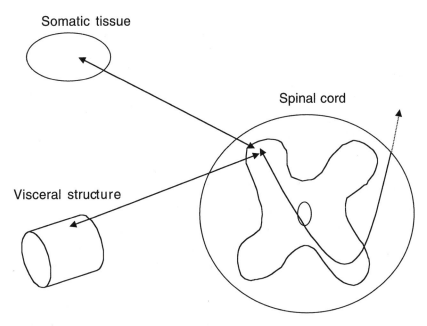

Figure 6.1
The Visceral-Somatic Convergence model for referred pain. Signals from an injured visceral organ project to neurons at the dorsal horn of the spinal column. Input from a healthy distal tissue converges on the same neurons. The signals mix at lamina V of the dorsal horn, which results in the brain attributing the pain to the somatic structure. (Adapted from Fields 1987.)

tor signal to the skin instead of the organ. (See figure 6.1.) Nevertheless, understanding the source of the pain "illusion" does not diminish the fact that pain performs its notification duties poorly, giving us the experience of pain being localized in perfectly healthy tissue while the real culprit feels completely intact to us.

The phantom limb pain discussed in chapters 2 and 5 is another sort of pain illusion. When limbs are surgically removed, it is quite common for the patient to continue to experience the limb being there as part of the body.[11] The further the severed limb is from the torso, the more vivid the phantom experience.[12] These experiences can produce quite odd behavior in people, since their limbs may also seem to be frozen in socially unacceptable positions. Someone who senses that her arm is sticking straight out from her side will enter doorways sideways, for otherwise the "arm" would bang up against the doorjam, and refuse to sleep on the amputated side, for the "arm" would be in the way. Some sense that their phantom limbs can move and so automatically try to use them for daily tasks. Still others find that their phantom limbs are contorted or flexed into uncomfortable positions. Over time, the phantom sensations generally recede. The limb appears to shrivel or telescope in until at last no phantom feelings remain.

In some cases, part of the phantom experience includes sensations of pain. (While there is no agreement about the incidence of phantom pains relative to phantom limbs, we do know that at least a significant majority of the amputee population experiences phantom limb pain for at least a while after surgery.[13]) We really have no idea why people have either phantom limb sensations or phantom limb pains. Further denervation or other tampering with the amputated limb seems only to make the problem worse.[14] One guess about what phantom limb pains are is that it is a central pain caused by hyperactivity in the spinal transmission neurons. Removing peripheral receptors causes the central receptors to go a bit haywire, since they no longer receive the inputs they are designed to. The hyperactivity travels up to cortex and induces a pain sensation that is referred back to the amputated area.[15]

Final illusions concern the cross-talk between our heat sensors and our nociceptors. Low-level stimulation of our thermoreceptors (the larger A-β fibers), which are not supposed to be connected to pain perception, inhibits the experience of pain,[16] while a higher-level stimulus exacerbates pain.[17] Gently pressing a grid with alternating cool and warm bars on the skin often causes the sensation of a strong burning pain.[18]

Here too these sorts of illusions seems to be hard-wired. For the case of altering our sensation of pain by stimulating the larger A-β fibers, we know that the A-∂ and C neurons in the dorsal horn are connected via inhibitory interneurons. These interneurons are stimulated by low-threshold A-β fibers. This means that stimulating A-β cells dampens the activity of the A-∂ and C neurons in the dorsal horn, which in turn means that less nociceptive information would travel up to the brain.[19] (See figure 6.2.) In the thermal grill illusion, neurophysiological recordings now show that there are several ascending neurons sensitive to both pain and temperature. A bit of central disinhibition plus these bimodal neurons explain how this illusion can occur. It can also explain why cold things burn.[20]

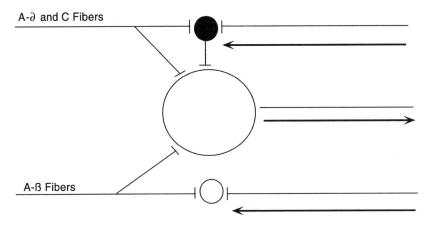

Figure 6.2
Low-level gate control. Cells in the dorsal horn and trigeminal nuclei, which respond to A-∂ and C fiber input, have excitatory (filled circle) and inhibitory (open circle) interneurons associated with them. A-β fibers activate the inhibitory neurons as well as input to the nociceptive cells. Descending controls input to the interneurons.

However, the relationship between tactile stimulation and pain is not completely clear here. Recent evidence indicates that painful stimuli can substantially decrease our sensations of touch.[21] Nevertheless, there are some parallels between pain illusions and our other systems, if we buy that the illusions are hard-wired. In a similar fashion, we see a straight stick as bent when placed halfway in water, and we arrange groups of dots into rows and columns. We make these perceptual errors because, either through learning from experience or by design, our brains develop shortcuts in computing our percepts that inevitably fail us under certain conditions. These heuristics work most of the time well enough for us to survive, even thrive, but they are not fail-safe. Similarly, our pain system may be designed to operate efficiently but inaccurately. One question remaining is whether the incidence of pain illusions outstrips that of other perceptual illusions and, if it does, why that may be.

IASP's Reaction
Recognizing strange facts about pain processing such as these has led the International Association for the Study of Pain (IASP) Subcommittee on Classification to conclude the following:

Pain is always subjective. . . . Many people report pain in the absence of tissue damage or any pathophysiological cause; usually this happens for psychological reasons. There is usually no way to distinguish their experience from that due to tissue damage if we take the subjective report. . . . [Pain] . . . is always a psychological state.[22]

Could they be correct? Are the connections between actual tissue damage, or some other injury, and our sensation of pain so weak that it is better to discount nociception entirely when defining pain? The IASP subcommittee clearly thinks so in their definition of pain: "an unpleasant sensory and emotional experience associated with actual or potential tissue damage, or *described in terms of such damage*"[23] (italics mine).

It is my contention that this sort of subjectification of pain is not preferable, for a variety of reasons. First, if pains are not correlated with actual injury, or the potential for damage, then we lose our intuitive evolutionary story about why we have a pain-sensing system. If our pain system has somehow become detached from the job it is supposed to perform, then its existence and poor performance no longer have clear explanations.

Second, pains become very peculiar phenomena indeed, quite unlike our other qualitative experiences. We can have visual or auditory hallucinations—we can be mistaken about what we think we are perceiving—however, if pain is purely subjective, then there is no way for us to have an illusion of being in pain. Phantom pains become just regular pains instead of some special case demanding special consideration and treatment. Of course, saying something is strange is not a reason for saying that it does not exist, but it is a reason to be cautious in making such metaphysical commitments. And, indeed, I do think that the IASP subcommittee (and people like McGinn and Kripke) are quite wrong in their understanding of what pain is.

Gate Theories of Pain

In general, gate theories of pain argue that the robust feedback loops in our pain system serve to inhibit, enhance, or distort incoming nociceptive information. In addition to the complex structure of our pain system that I outlined in the last chapter, there are further ascending connections from the spinal cord to the brain stem, circular pathways from the spinal cord to other areas in the spinal cord itself, and descending feedback loops from the cortex, hypothalamus, and brain stem back to the spinal cord.[24] Some portions of this theory have been worked out in considerable detail. And some of the mysterious pain phenomena listed above can be explained in terms of well-confirmed portions of Melzack and Wall's gate theory of pain.[25] The accounts of the heat illusions, for example, are gate theory explanations.

Moreover, though more research needs to be done, the alternate routes in the central nervous system might help explain why cutting the primary dorsal horn nociceptive channel, or parts of the spinal cord itself, may not remove chronic pain.[26] However, a Melzack-Wall type of gate-control theory of pain cannot be the entire story, for three reasons. First, we do not have anything approaching a complete theory at this stage in the game. Though the theory does explain low-level phenomena, nothing has been worked out in particular regarding the clearly "psychological" influences.[27] Melzack and Wall themselves simply gesture toward a central gating mechanism that presumably would explain hypnosis effects, any remaining chronic pains, the dismal correlations between ER injuries or back injuries and pain, SIB, phantom limb pain, and so on. But without providing more details—where this central gating mechanism is located in the brain, how it functions to alter our pain perceptions, why we have such a powerful mechanism, for example—they have said little more than ". . . and some other stuff happens in the head that explains everything else." As Wall himself remarks about the many areas implicated in inhibiting our sensations of pain, "Unfortunately we know little of their relative importance and nothing of the actual circumstances in which they come into action."[28]

Second, and more important, even if we could get the details on some sort of central gating mechanism, this would not mean that pains are not largely subjective (which is but a step away from being purely subjective). If top-down cortical processes (which is what I take "purely subjective" to mean here) are mainly responsible for our sensations of pain, then the IASP Subcommittee would be right and pains would be deeply peculiar. They would be the only perceptual experiences we have that are normal (that is, normal functioning creatures have them), natural (that is, not the product of tweaking something in a laboratory, but occurring in the wild, as it were), commonplace (we have them all the time), believed to be giving us information about the external environment (external to the brain, that is [but internal to our bodies]), but in fact not. Dreams might be the only exception, but, unlike with dreams, we do not realize when a pain is over that it really was not about the external world after all.

Most philosophers, psychologists, and neurophysiologists who do not fall prey to the less interesting mistake do hold some version of a gate control theory. Some advocate it explicitly (e.g., Dennett, Melzack, Wall); others maintain it implicitly (Hilgard, Tye). Either way, I believe this commitment to be premature. If there is any way for us not to hold that our pain system is purely, or largely, or even significantly, subjective, then we should not do it. I propose that instead of acquiescing to the IASP Subcommittee's conclusion, we should take the mysterious and unexplained pain phenomena as evidence that at least the traditional views (even with the additional bells and whistles) are wrong. I suggest that we should reexamine the data from a different perspective.

A Pain-Inhibiting System

If standard (higher-level) gate theory approaches are misguided, then we still have a change at understanding pain from a solid neurophysiological and biological perspective without making pain into something peculiar. As will be clear in a moment, I advocate dividing what Melzack and others have lumped into one cortically driven pain system into two separate systems: a nociceptor-driven pain sensory system (PSS) and a largely top-down pain inhibitory system (PIS). First, though, let me sketch some data that I believe are relevant to this perspective, data that the more traditional gate theories either overlook or minimize; I shall then outline some theoretical considerations that point toward a two-system model.

Proponents of gate theories write as though just about any psychological event or any area of the cortex has the potential to influence the perception of pain, what Melzack calls a "neuromatrix."[29] This huge network of neurons extends widely across the brain and is responsible for our sense of physical self. Too broad to be destroyed by any focal lesion, it is responsible for most instances of abnormal or chronic pain, for it produces an abnormal pattern of activity or "neurosignature" when it no longer receives appropriate inputs from the limbs or torso.

However, as I discussed in the last chapter, though there are lots of feedback loops and other sorts of pain connections, not every area in the brain is sensitive to pain information, at least from what the imagining studies tell us. Though lack of activity does not prove conclusively that an area is not sensitive to pain information, these sorts of studies should give advocates of global cortical influences on our perception of pain pause for thought. In addition, as I described in chapter 4, the basic structure of the brain is a vastly underconnected network. About the only area into which everything feeds is the entorhinal cortex of the limbic system. This convergence is probably very important for the emotionality of pain, as well as its sensitivity to context. However, it is not related in any obvious way to a "neuromatrix" or bodily sense.

Moreover, the neuronal areas sensitive to pain information are different from what we originally believed. Apkarian concludes that "the brain imagining studies of pain . . . point to a very different emphasis in research regarding the central processing of pain. . . . [S]ystems outside of the spinothalamic system may control the type of processing taking place in the spinothalamic system. [Chronic pains] . . . seem to activate cortical areas outside the spinothalamic domain, which in turn inhibit the spinothalamic inputs to the cortex."[30] That the thalamus is probably not important in processing our perceptions of pain stands in direct contrast to what many take to be common knowledge regarding how our pain system works.

Because new facts regarding the transmission of pain information in the brain are only slowly emerging, we should be fairly conservative in our conclusions. All I want to claim at the moment is that the traditional views of pain are probably oversimplified to the point of being misleading. Accepting this conclusion opens the possibility of describing our pain system differently than has been in the past. Important for our purposes, it allows the possibility of dividing what we have been calling our pain system into two different and independent processing streams. I believe that doing so helps clear up the remaining puzzles in pain phenomena.

We have known for some time that many of the inhibitory streams are not merely feedback loops in our ascending nociceptive fibers, for they are anatomically distinct from these processors. Three areas are primarily responsible for inhibiting nociceptive information in the spinal column: the cortex, the thalamus, and the brain stem. The dorsal raphe is probably heavily involved as well.[31] In particular, neocortex and hypothalamus project to the periaqueductal gray region (PAG), which then sends projections to the reticular formation (see figure 6.3). The reticular nuclei then work to inhibit activity in the dorsal horn.[32] This processing stream works by preventing a central cortical representation of pain from forming.[33] Endogenous opioids, stimulating the PAG, and morphine all dampen incoming information in the same way in the dorsal horn. That is, this inhibition stream does not merely disrupt the transmission of nociceptive information, but it actively prevents it from occurring.

Moreover, this subsystem is not the only pain inhibitor at work. Stress-induced analgesia can occur without any opioids being released and is not prevented from occurring when opioid-blockers are administered.[34] Moreover, different neural substrates are involved in inhibiting fast pains and slow pains. Stimulating the hypothalamus reduces tonic pain and is not related to stress-related analgesia.[35] Though we only know a little about our pain inhibition in the brain (we do not know, for example, what counts as "normal" function for our opioid analgesics, what environmental circumstances activate them, or how they actually affect pain sensations or behavior), concensus is emerging that we have several distinct inhibitory subsystems.[36]

More important than being anatomically distinct and dissociable from nociception, the inhibitory streams are teleologically distinct from our PSS system as well. The inhibitory streams are not merely general-purpose dampers; they are triggered by a very specific constellation of peripheral and cortical inputs. Otherwise, their removal would drastically increase our sensations of pain or make them all chronic. Such is not the case though. Lesioning the PAG does not appear to be tied to the onset of chronic pains.[37] Moreover, we do know that the inhibitory systems are activated (or inhibited) by nociception plus cortical arousal (stress) on the organism.[38] Fear and learned hopelessness also affect their activity.[39] Hence, the correlates for the firing of these neurons differ in kind from what our ascending nociceptive system is sensitive to.

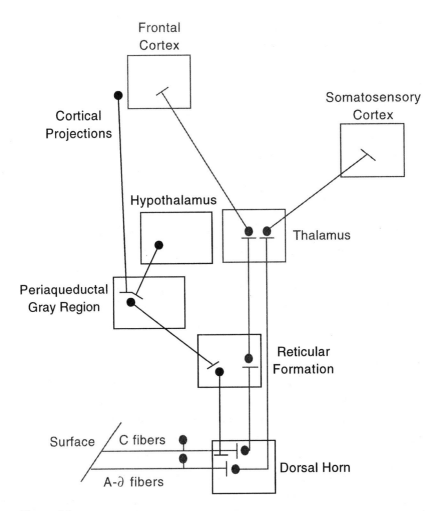

Figure 6.3
Diagram depicting the pain inhibitory system in contrast to the pain sensory system. Projections originating in cortex and hypothalamus descend to the periaqueductal gray of the midbrain, the reticular formation and then finally to the dorsal horn, where they inhibit the ascending nociceptive transmissions.

In addition, if we look at the connections of the inhibitory streams, we can see that they differ substantially from the PSS. It would not be proper to call them sensory systems or subsystems for they have no connections to the periphery. The pain inhibitory streams halt at the dorsal horn. Also, unlike our ascending nociceptive streams, the hypothalamus and dorsal raphe nuclei receive massive inputs from cortical processors, which presumably could carry information about our goals and immediate plans, what else is occurring in the environment, and our larger emotional context.[40] They have immediate access to information that the ascending pathways do not.

Finally, a two-system theory of pain sensation explains the adaptive value of pain. When we are under stress, it is often more adaptive not to feel pain than to be incapacitated by pain.[41] If we are fighting or fleeing from an enemy, it would be preferable to do so unencumbered by the need to nurse or protect our limbs, even if this results in more nursing or protecting later (when we are presumably safe). It is important to know when damage is occurring in our bodies, but it is equally important to be able to shut that information out when circumstances demand. A dual system would allow just such a contingency; we could inhibit our pains as needed, but then feel them again when the danger is gone. A PSS and a PIS then serve two different goals: the PSS keeps us informed regarding the status of our bodies. It monitors our tissues to maintain their intactness whenever possible. In contrast, the PIS shuts down the PSS when flight or fleeing is immanent, and then enhances the PSS response in moments of calm. If our brains are geared for motor control, then the dual pain system makes good biological sense.

In sum: the bottom-up and the top-down investigative strategies support the conclusion that our pain inhibitors form a separate and distinct system. They react to different types of stimuli. They have different points of input and output from the PSS. And their existence is supported by evolutionary considerations.

Self-Injurious Behavior and Other Oddities

But can a PIS explain Matthieu, SIB, and other instances of radical pain malfunctioning? I believe the answer is yes. Here I shall only concentrate on self-injurious behavior, but I think a related story could be told for other cases of "nonpain."

The Demographics of SIB Patients

What do we know about nonstereotypic SIB? The vast majority of self-injurers are women in their mid twenties to early thirties, well educated, middle or upper class, intelligent, and with a history of being physically or sexually abused or having an alcoholic parent.[42] Anorexia and bulimia often coincide with SIB, too. I should point out, though, that many self-injurers were not abused nor neglected, nor do they have eating disorders. Abuse may be a predictor of SIB, but it is not an important causal factor in many cases. Indeed, it turns out that the best indicator for SIB is a previous episode of SIB.[43]

Women who practice SIB generally function well in society, except for their tendency to hurt themselves and the concomitant trouble that can cause with doctors and emergency room visits. Many self-harmers are diagnosed as have Borderline Personality Disorder (BPD). However, it is unclear how seriously we should take this diagnosis. Most patients diagnosed with BPD only meet a subset of the DSM criteria, and self-destructive tendencies are at the core of many BPD patients, so it could be that a diagnosis of BPD is nothing more than a recognition that self-injurious behavior is occurring.[44]

Some SIB patients have Obsessive-Compulsive Disorder (OCD). Their self-injuries usually take the form of hair pulling (also known as trichotillomania) or scratching and picking at their skin. The current view is that OCD is due to a serotonin imbalance, perhaps reflecting unchecked nesting or grooming instincts. However, these patients form only a tiny subset of SIB patients and the etiology of OCD self-injurers differs substantially from the rest.

A minority of practitioners have suggested that SIB should be considered a disorder in itself, as opposed to a symptom of some other disease. Some advocate a Repetitive Self-Harm Syndrome as a new Axis I impulse-control syndrome (similar to OCD).[45] Others propose an Axis II personality disorder, similar to Dissociative Identity Disorder.[46] Perhaps in self-injurious behavior, self-harmers split into three roles: an abuser, a victim, and a disinterested bystander.

How should we understand SIB? Why would some self-inflicted injuries not hurt? Should we even think of it as a disorder? How would we know?

Here is the current state of psychiatric theory. We can find some differences between self-harmers who experience no pain and those who do not routinely harm themselves. For example, sensitivity to heat was measured in female SIB patients diagnosed with BPD who do not experience pain when injuring themselves, those who do experience pain, and BPD patients who do not harm themselves. Those who did not experience pain are worse at distinguishing among noxious thermal stimuli with similar intensity than those who do, BPD patients who do not self-injure, and normal women. The nonpain group was also more matter-of-fact about pain experiences in general, and they discriminated more poorly between imaginary painful and mildly painful situations.[47] Female patients engaging in SIB score higher on the Glover Numbing Scale than do patients with Major Depressive Disorder.[48] They also show an increase in dissociative symptoms during a self-injury episode; after hurting themselves, their dissociation decreases and their mood elevates. The nonpain group dissociates significantly more than the pain group and reinterprets painful sensations as being nonpainful.[49]

There is some evidence that self-injurious behavior—even that not connected with OCD—is associated with a decrease in serotonin function, similar to decreases found associated with suicidal behavior.[50] In these cases, naloxone, an opiate antagonist, can sometimes decrease SIB symptoms.[51] But administering opiate antagonists effectively is a tricky business. They work best when the duration of pain is rather long.[52] Brief experimental pains are not affected very much by naloxone, whereas the intensity of longer pains, such as postoperative pain, do significantly increase.[53] Are SIB pains supposed to be of a long or short duration? The answer to that question has to depend upon the type of injuries used. We would expect different durations for different sorts of injuries. Hence, inconsistent results with naloxone should not be surprising.

Moreover, all the patients in the SIB-naloxone studies were admitted to a psychiatric hospital and were diagnosed as having other disorders as well. Here we find the same difficulties as those I outlined in the second chapter: too many possible confounds. The SIB-naloxone studies did not use normals as controls, so we have no idea whether the psychiatric patients with SIB respond similarly or differently from self-injurers with no clinical diagnosis. Similarly, we do not know whether their psychiatric ailments are the causes or the consequences (or neither) of SIB. Does prolonged, extreme, or repeated self-injury lead to other psychiatric problems, do the other psychiatric problems lead to self-injurious behavior, are they both caused by some other common cause, or are they completely unrelated to each other? Frankly, the paucity of data on this question is disconcerting.

Converging evidence suggests that, not surprisingly, the etiology of SIB follows many paths. SIB has many causes.[54] In one preliminary study, at least seventeen different self-described reasons for why people engage in SIB have been given, with each of the seventeen endorsed by at least one person as fundamental to her practice of self-injury.[55] These reasons range from punishing oneself for being bad in some way to reducing negative feelings that cannot otherwise be controlled, to asserting control, to diminishing feelings of depersonalization and alienation, to providing a sense of excitement and exhilaration, to controlling others, to being done for no reason at all.

In addition, there is extreme variability in how SIB is practiced. In some cases, it is highly ritualized—"there are certain words carved in my stomach and I recarve the words." In others, it is impulsive—"I slam my hands/arms against something cement with corners until I hear something crack and I am convinced I've broken a bone." In some cases, it is done in private and hidden from others even after the fact—"I hide it by wearing pants and long skirts. I do not go swimming, and I never wear shorts. I am very afraid of my cuts being found." In others, it is done quite publicly—"I often want to stand on top of the world and shout 'Look at me. Look at this. I am ugly. Look at this.' I guess that's my equivalent to giving the finger."[56]

The purported causes of SIB are as variable as the symptoms themselves. Some researchers attribute mental causes to SIB: internal tension, disturbed feelings about one's body or others.[57] Others attribute some neurological causes: decreased sensation, abnormal serotonin levels. Still others advocate a combination of mental and physical causes: the lag between physiological and psychological responses. How should we analyze these suggestions?

From chapter 3, we learn that we cannot appeal to facts known outside science to justify one sort of cause over another. We can bring to the table the bias or prejudice that the world is all physical, but the practice of the individual sciences themselves must determine the appropriate levels of explanation for any phenomenon. We cannot decide that matter beforehand through any sort of philosophical analysis. This moral is reinforced in chapter 4, where we discovered that a host of pragmatic factors determine which theoretical approach neuroscientists take. Different explanatory paradigms can produce equally good explanations of the same events. Which paradigm we chose is often not a principled decision.

Without trying to resolve the issue of which level or levels of explanation are appropriate for explaining SIB—we simply do not have enough data yet about its practice or its practitioners to begin to discern the true proximate causes—allow me to sketch a conceptual framework in which SIB makes some sense. If I am correct, then we shall see that self-injurious behavior really is not a disorder at all; it is a useful and predictable strategy for coping with pain.

Understanding SIB

Let me begin by describing anew the first puzzle of pain that opened this chapter. Often we do not feel any pain when we should. I am willing to bet that, at some point in our lives, we all have experienced this phenomenon to some degree or other—ignoring our burgeoning blisters while finishing gardening, forgetting about our headaches as we teach or speak in public, biting our lips to cope with our stubbed toes. Diverting attention to something else is a common and successful strategy for controlling lesser pains.

In addition to these rather mundane instances of pain control, there are also some striking cases of "nonpain" that occur regularly and predictably, though, thankfully, not to all of us. These cases require more than merely changing our focus of attention, for they are instances of what should be extreme pain and suffering being not felt. One of the earliest recorded descriptions of these sorts of nonpains comes from

Michel de Montaigne in his essay, "Use Makes Perfect." He describes being thrown from a galloping horse. Bleeding profusely from the head, he at first thought he had been shot. But instead of suffering, he felt tranquil: "My condition was, in truth, very easy and quiet, I had no affliction on me, either for others or myself; it was an extreme languor and weakness, without any manner of pain." He waited for death, happy to "glide away so sweetly and after so soft and easy a manner." Needless to say, he did not die then, and after a few hours he reports that he was "in terrible pain, having my limbs battered and ground with my fall, and was so ill for two or three nights after, that I thought I was once more dying again."[58]

David Livingstone, the great explorer and medical missionary, recounts a similar experience when an enraged and wounded lion seized him after he had mortally wounded it with his gun:

Growling horribly close to my ear, [the lion] . . . shook me as a terrior dog does a rat. The shock produced a stupor similar to that which seems to be felt by a mouse after the first shake of the cat. It caused a sort of dreaminess, in which there was no sense of pain nor feeling of terror, though quite conscious of all that was happening. It was like what patients partially under the influence of chloroform describe who see all the operation but feel not the knife. This singular condition was not the result of any mental process. The shake annihilated fear, and allowed no sense of horror in looking round at the beast. This peculiar state is probably produced in all animals killed by carnivores; and if so, is a merciful provision by our benevolent Creator for lessening the pain of death.[59]

What both these stories have in common is that the participants believed themselves to be—and very probably were—near death. Something happens to our bodies when it is put under great, life-threatening duress and stress. We no longer react as we used to, or as one would expect us to. Lewis Thomas interprets these sorts of nonpain events as being evolutionarily kind:

Pain is useful for avoidance, for getting away when there's time to get away, but when it is endgame, and no way back, pain is likely to be turned off, and the mechanisms for this are wonderfully precise and quick. If I had to design an ecosystem in which creatures had to live off each other and in which dying was an indispensable part of living, I could not think of a better way to manage.[60]

But there is more than mercy at work here. Remaining calm and detached during conflict or danger instead of panicking or flailing about probably saved the lives of Montaigne and Livingstone. Being aware of your surroundings, but nonplussed by them, is surely more conducive to surviving extreme circumstances than reacting with frenzied terror or horror.

Emergency room physicians are all too aware of this "trick" our bodies perform. As we near unexpected death from violence, we become calm and accepting. Perhaps the most distressing portrait of a near-death experience is Joan Mason's recital of her nine-year-old daughter Katie's final moments after she was savagely and repeatedly stabbed by complete stranger outside of Woolworth's one afternoon in a small town in Connecticut.

> There was no look of pain in her eyes, but instead a look of surprise. . . . Do you know what it looked like? It looked like a release. After seeing him attacking her in that way, it gave me a sense of peace to see that look of release. She must have released herself from this pain, because her face didn't show it. . . . She looked surprised, but not terrified—as terrifying as it was for me, it wasn't that way for her. . . . [Her eyes] were wide but not in a state of terror—it looked almost like an innocence—an innocent release. As her mother, amidst all of that blood and everything else, it was actually soothing to look into her eyes.[61]

Though we do not understand all the mechanisms involved, it is clear that our pain inhibitory system releases endogenous morphinelike chemicals (known by the contraction "endorphins") or other similar hormones that mask or eliminate our pain and suffering. Most likely, it releases an opiate that affects our serotonin levels, but with fourteen different identified serotonin receptors, at least four different opioid analgesics uncovered, and five different PIS pathways charted in the human,[62] even this guess about how stress reduces pain is vague and unhelpful.

Nevertheless, the conceptual framework underlying near-death nonpains is manifest. Under extreme stress, our bodies release something that dampens, gates, or eliminates pain processing. Whether this "something" is triggered by psychological or physiological reactions is unknown, as is what the something is (or, more likely, what the somethings are).

Bearing this framework in mind, it is now easier to understand what SIB amounts to. If some violent external event can trigger our bodies to follow a natural protocol by which they inhibit pain processing, then there is no reason that we could not induce that same protocol by artificial means. I hypothesize that self-injurious behavior is a coping strategy that takes advantage of our bodies' natural method for dealing with pain under pressure. Though we find few commonalities among those who engage in SIB, there are at least two: self-injurers feel psychological distress prior to harming themselves, and they feel better afterward. The phenomenological descriptions of how self-injurers feel after hurting themselves bear an uncanny resemblance to the descriptions printed above regarding near-death experiences. In both cases, the victims feel calmed, removed from the immediate situation, though very aware of what is happening to them and who they are.

SIB is simply a way to force our brains to initiate a pain-inhibiting sequence. As such, I find it difficult to call SIB a disorder or an illness. Certainly self-injurers are unhappy, and they are seeking ways to cope with or resolve their internal tensions. However, their solution is a rational one; it is one that forces evolved neural systems to do what they were designed to do.

Some have suggested that SIB is perhaps an addiction[63] or habit,[64] maintained by its tension-releasing qualities.[65] I am less sure how to react to these analyses than the others. Part of the difficulty concerns the fluidity of what one means by addiction or habit. Biochemically, addiction is tied to the dopaminergic system, which influences the serotonergic system, among other things, so it is conceivable that SIB and addiction are linked. The most recent biochemical data suggest that the brain releases dopamine to "highlight, or draw attention to, certain significant or surprising events."[66] This presumably helps in learning a behavioral response and may explain why we see massive surges of dopamine in the brain with addictive drugs: this is our brains' way of "rewarding" us for producing "correct" behaviors.

However, I quite sure that we would not want to call every behavior that inspires our dopaminergic system to go into overdrive an addiction. Some of the behaviors it rewards are appropriate, nondestructive, and socially acceptable. Moreover, we do not know whether these increases in dopamine are also found with nonchemical "addictions," such as gambling or, perhaps, SIB, nor whether they are found with complex "habitual" behaviors that supposedly are not addictions, such as chalking the cue stick exactly three times before beginning a game of billiards or waiting to pick up the phone until the second ring is completed. The bottom line is that we really do not know what an addiction amounts to in the brain, though important clues have been uncovered.

On the other hand, if we look to our rather nebulous psychological markers for addiction, such as "dependence, tolerance, sensitization, and craving,"[67] which presumably stem from whatever relevant changes occur in our neural circuitry, then it is not obvious that SIB fits the description. There is no evidence that self-injurers become physically dependent, more tolerant, or more sensitized, to harm. Whether self-injurers crave the experience of hurting themselves is difficult to say. In some sense, they feel compelled to do it, and they do use it to seek relief. But whether this drive amounts to a craving I leave for others to decide.

Perhaps self-injurers are analogous to those "addicted" to exercise. There are some who exercise regularly for its health benefits. There are others who exercise seeking the so-called runner's high. This euphoria is (once again) the product of the brain reacting to physical stress; however, this time the stress is from intense physical labor and not bodily injury. There are purportedly some fitness freaks who are "addicted" to this high and will exercise to get it through injury, severe pain, inclement weather, and so forth.[68] I am dubious about whether we should call this strong affinity for exercise a true addiction; nonetheless, the comparison with SIB remains instructive. In both cases, people use (or abuse) their bodies' natural protection systems to improve their mood, soothe uncomfortable feelings, and cope with the stress of their daily lives. The real difference between the two is that exercise is socially much more acceptable than, say, disemboweling oneself with a knitting needle.

The relation to social context in determining what counts as antisocial behavior cannot be overemphasized. Quite often, what counts as an addiction is determined by local norms. Alcoholism provides a good example. In the eighteenth and early nineteenth century, drinking alcohol was considered part of life: "The general pattern for the eighteenth century was for men and women to drink alcohol every day, at all times through out the day, and in large quantities on almost every special occasion."[69] For example, at a New York dinner reception for the ambassador from France, the 120 guests consumed 135 bottles of Mandeira, 36 bottles of port, 60 bottles of beer, and 30 bowls of rum punch.[70] Even the wildest fraternity parties would have trouble matching that level of consumption today. To drink as much as was considered normal one hundred years ago would be considered alcoholic behavior today.

In addition, our current standards for what counts as problem drinking are context sensitive. Undergraduate students are notorious consumers. Rarely, however, are they labeled alcoholics. However, if I drank as much as my freshmen do, then no doubt I would be considered a problem drinker, if not an alcoholic outright. What counts as addictive behavior, as opposed to mere personal preference or lifestyle, depends heavily on the immediately local values and norms.

To some degree, people who engage in SIB are caught in this trap. Self-injury is common in other cultures. Trephination, the practice of drilling holes in one's skull to relieve pain, is probably the best known instance. It was widespread in ancient cultures; instances today warrant mention as case studies in professional journals.[71] Similarly, people who harm themselves are thought to be somehow abnormal, disordered, deranged. However, given what we know about our pain-inhibiting system, it makes immanent sense that troubled individuals would manipulate it to seek psychical relief.

I do not wish to advocate self-injury as a stress-releasing mechanism; at the same time, we are not serving patients well if we focus on the behavior and seek some psychiatric pigeonhole in which to place it. Though we would be wise to see SIB as a plea for help—people harm themselves for a reason, and happy people do not generally hurt themselves deliberately—we make a mistake in focusing on the behavior itself as the problem. SIB occurs because of some underlying ailment or concern. Resolving that should eliminate or decrease the coping behavior.

Our pain-inhibiting system is a marvelously powerful mechanism. Its anatomy and physiology are only beginning to be understood. We know even less about what the sorts of psychological or environment events trigger it. Still, we can understand why organisms evolved such a mechanism and how it might be manipulated to our advantage. We can also see how it, or it in tandem with our pain-processing system, could easily go make us go awry.

7

"But Is It Going to Hurt?"

English, which can express the thoughts of Hamlet and the tragedy of Lear, has no words for the shiver or the headache . . . The merest schoolgirl when she falls in love has Shakespeare or Keats to speak her mind for her, but let a sufferer try to describe a pain in his head to a doctor and language at once runs dry.
—Virginia Woolf

Pain is not equivalent to a phenomenological experience, damaged tissue, or bodily or emotional reactions. Each of these items is a single component within a more complex system. This fact should not be surprising, for all of our sensory systems operate this way. In each case, many individual pieces work in tandem to process information about the world. Our pain system is no different. Its components take pressure, temperature, and chemical readings of our tissues in order to figure out what is happening to our bodies that might be damaging. Just like all our sensory systems, the pain processing system is a complex but well-honed system evolved to monitor some aspect of the world in order to promote our welfare.

But, we must issue an important caveat: Pains are the product of a complex sensory system that has to struggle to get itself heard. Our conscious sensations are the product of both nociception and activity of a pain inhibitory system (PIS). Even though nothing about painful experiences is deeply mysterious—they are neither random, nor inexplicable, nor tied to our psychological whims—they still are poorly correlated with actual tissue damage. What is interesting and different about our pains is the PIS. It is geared to suppress or enhance the activity of a single sensory system, and there is no other system quite like it in our nervous system. We do have general inhibitory and excitatory systems in the brain, but none of these are specific to a particular neural tract. The PIS entails that our sensations of pain are almost independent of nociception.

This perspective on pain might be disturbing, for it greatly diminishes the importance our conscious experiences have to whether we are, in fact, in pain. This is counterintuitive at least, oxymoronic at most. Nevertheless, if chapters 5 and 6 are correct, then, contrary to how things seem to us, the sensation of pain is not what is most important in pain processing. It is but one minor aspect of our entire pain and pain-inhibitory systems, which themselves are geared to help us flee, fight, or nurse ourselves, depending upon the circumstances. Just like the rest of our perceptual systems, they help us get around in our environment as effectively as possible. From an evolutionary perspective, visual sensations are not the raison d'être of our visual system, and auditory sensations are not the ultimate goal for our auditory system. Sensations of pain are no different.

However, regardless of how I analyze pain scientifically or philosophically, how it feels is of great importance to us in our everyday lives. I too am a qualiaphile, so I too want to know when something is going to hurt and by how much. This chapter is aimed at explaining why, even if we just focus on our sensations of pain, asking whether something is going to hurt is an ill-formed query. Part of the answer is that our seemingly simple sensations of pain are actually quite complex; part of the answer is that there is something right about the philosophical arguments for an eliminativism about our pain language, especially if we take the IASP recommendation that we define pain as a purely subjective state seriously.

The Complexity of Pain Sensations

My main point is that the story of pain is yet more complicated. Even if we restrict our purview to one tiny aspect of pain processing—subjective experience—we find several independent dimensions to pain phenomenology, including the sensory-discriminative and the affective aspects of our pain sensations, as well as our judgments of suffering, memories of previous pain experiences, and our beliefs about the causes and prognosis of the current pain.

Just as we can dissociate the various subsystems of pain processing in the body, so too can we dissociate the various dimensions of our pain sensations. For example, we can distinguish discriminative pain processing from affective-motivational pain processing phenomenologically as well as physically. We can have sensations of pain without them feeling awful and without acting as though we are in pain. In these cases, we can localize our pains but are not upset by the fact that we have them. As Barber concluded: "Apparently, the 'sensation of pain', in itself, is not necessarily 'painful'."[1]

We can also get reverse effects. Certain drugs can cause us to wince in pain, yet if pressed, we would be unable to locate where the alleged pain is. Lesion studies and studies using hemispherectomies show that even with cortex completely missing, we can still have pain sensations; we just can't articulate exactly where or how bad they are. Various degenerative diseases can also provoke nonspecific pain sensations.

As alluded to in the previous chapters, important interactions exist among these dimensions, too. The sensorium fades into the emotive and the cognitive. This blending is not specific to pain processing, though. We see connections between affect and experience in our other perceptual systems, especially our systems involved in processing taste, temperature, and smell.[2] Even vision shows this effect, for we perceive objects we value to be bigger than neutral objects of the same size.[3]

Nevertheless, we need to distinguish the different dimensions of our pain sensations conceptually. How we treat pain clinically depends on which aspect of the pain sensation we want to affect. In only rare cases (and in cases of only a little pain) can we simply eliminate the entire phenomenological experience. More typical are instances in which only one or a few dimensions are affected. For example, if a doctor administers diazepam, then one's affective discomfort is reduced, while the sensory qualities of the pain remains the same. In contrast, fentanyl diminishes sensory intensity but increases the unpleasantness of pain.[4]

However, basic experimental research on pain often overlooks the complexity of pain sensations and assumes that feeling pain refers to some unique or simple experience. Experimental scientists require quantifiable stimuli and simple, repeatable, behavioral responses in order to produce analyzable data. They, like all other scientists, simplify and abstract from the phenomena they study. Their task protocols assume that they can control nociception and that (contrary to fact) there is a tight correlation between a stimulus and subsequent behavior. Consequently, if they recognize the affective or cognitive dimensions of pain at all, they treat them as contaminants or as sources of experimental error.[5]

Happily, in distinction to most basic research on pain, clinical pain assessment techniques make none of these simplifying assumptions. As Melzack remarks: "To describe pain solely in terms of intensity is like specifying the visual world only in terms of light flux without regard to pattern, color, texture, and the many other dimensions of visual experience."[6] Typically, modern psychiatrists look at four major components when evaluating a pain patient: nociception, sensation, suffering, and behavior.[7] The best clinicians attend to historical, environmental, and interpersonal influences on pain perception, as well as the more standard cognitive, emotional, and behavioral dimensions.[8] They believe that understanding the total experience of pain necessitates understanding the physiology, subjective experiences, behavioral responses, and psychosocial environment of the subject.[9]

Clinicians have devised pain rating scales that reflect the affective, intensity, and reactive dimensions of our pain experiences. These scales have been validated using cross-modality matching, which verifies that the magnitude of the descriptors remains (relatively) constant across tests and situations. Figure 7.1 gives one example of this sort of scale.[10] Perhaps the best of the lot is the McGill Pain Questionnaire, one of the most common diagnostics used for pain and reproduced as figure 7.2. This survey charts seventy-eight adjectives for pain along twenty different dimensions. A self-report instrument, it lists numerous words that patients can use or rank to describe the intensity of their sensory, affective, and evaluative experiences.

Though these scales are quite robust across subjects and across time within individuals, their difficulty is that they only measure the intensity and not the qualitative character of pain itself, which is what those suffering from chronic and other pains care most about. (On the other hand, focusing only on intensity does give scientists a way to compare experimental and clinical results.) Nevertheless, despite the limitations of our diagnostics, we can understand pain sensations in terms of locations, affective and somatic qualities, and the intensity of these feelings. Each

Intensity	Reaction	Sensation
Excruciating	Agonizing	Piercing
Intolerable	Intolerable	Stabbing
Very intense	Unbearable	Shooting
Extremely	Awful	Burning
strong	Miserable	Grinding
Severe	Distressing	Throbbing
Very strong	Unpleasant	Cramping
Intense	Distracting	Aching
Strong	Uncomfortable	Stinging
Uncomfortable	Tolerable	Squeezing
Moderate	Bearable	Numbing
Mild		Itching
Weak		Tingling
Very weak		
Just		
noticeable		
Extremely		
weak		

Figure 7.1
Adjective scales derived from the McGill Pain Questionnaire and validated by cross-modality matching. (From Tursky 1976.)

can act independently of the others, or each could affect the others, depending on circumstances.

Quite trivially, we can see that if we merely ask how much something hurts, then it is not clear what we are talking about. Does an intense pain that doesn't bother you hurt more than a mild pain that troubles you greatly? Does a well-localized stabbing pain hurt more than a diffuse aching? A multidimensional perspective on our complex sensory experiences of pain is clearly called for. However, at the moment, our folk and research notions of pain bundle together the bodily location of the

McGill Pain Questionnaire

Patient's Name ____________ Date ________ Time ______ am/pm

PRI: S ______ (1-10) A ______ (11-15) E ______ (16) M ______ (17-20) PRI(T) ______ (1-20) PPI ______

1 FLICKERING, QUIVERING, PULSING, THROBBING, BEATING, POUNDING	11 TIRING, EXHAUSTING
2 JUMPING, FLASHING, SHOOTING	12 SICKENING, SUFFOCATING
3 PRICKING, BORING, DRILLING, STABBING, LANCINATING	13 FEARFUL, FRIGHTFUL, TERRIFYING
4 SHARP, CUTTING, LACERATING	14 PUNISHING, GRUELLING, CRUEL, VICIOUS, KILLING
5 PINCHING, PRESSING, GNAWING, CRAMPING, CRUSHING	15 WRETCHED, BLINDING
6 TUGGING, PULLING, WRENCHING	16 ANNOYING, TROUBLESOME, MISERABLE, INTENSE, UNBEARABLE
7 HOT, BURNING, SCALDING, SEARING	17 SPREADING, RADIATING, PENETRATING, PIERCING
8 TINGLING, ITCHY, SMARTING, STINGING	18 TIGHT, NUMB, DRAWING, SQUEEZING, TEARING
9 DULL, SORE, HURTING, ACHING, HEAVY	19 COOL, COLD, FREEZING
10 TENDER, TAUT, RASPING, SPLITTING	20 NAGGING, NAUSEATING, AGONIZING, DREADFUL, TORTURING
	PPI: 0 NO PAIN, 1 MILD, 2 DISCOMFORTING, 3 DISTRESSING, 4 HORRIBLE, 5 EXCRUCIATING

BRIEF	RHYTHMIC	CONTINUOUS
MOMENTARY	PERIODIC	STEADY
TRANSIENT	INTERMITTENT	CONSTANT

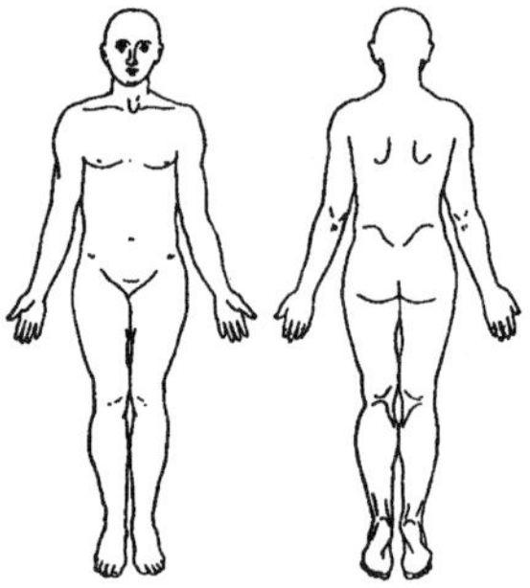

E = EXTERNAL
I = INTERNAL

COMMENTS:

Figure 7.2
The McGill Pain Questionnaire.

sensation, its somatic quality, the feeling of suffering, and negative reaction to the feeling of suffering under the single heading of "pain."

Some may argue that pain then is just a simple term for a complex sensation. That is, we have just uncovered different aspects to a single perception, instead of entirely different experiences. Hence, it would make good folk and scientific sense to keep one name for the complex percept.

I disagree. The four dimensions of our pain sensations should be kept distinct. They are not like the color and shape of an object or the pitch and loudness of a sound. Our perceptions of objects and sounds are comprised of complex units. We cannot see a shape without also seeing that shape as some color. We cannot hear a loud noise without also hearing that noise at some pitch. If a brain is not given some of the information regarding the structure of an object or a sound, then it simply fills in what it is missing.

In distinction, pain sensations function quite differently. We quite often get one aspect of pain without the others. Moreover, if we are lacking an aspect—say, we have the somatic quality without the suffering or negative reaction—then our brains feel no obligation to fill in the missing pieces. Though our commonsense views tie the different aspects of pain sensations into single complex percepts, our brains don't.

There is a second reason for redesigning our ways of understanding our experiences of pain. The language we have for expressing our propositions concerning pain sensations is very crude. Unlike words for hue or pitch, we have few words that speak directly about the qualitative aspects of pain itself. Instead, pain is "described by illustration."[11] The adjectives we do use (e.g., cutting, dull, hot) are metaphorical.[12] In addition, we give short shrift to the emotional side of pain. Ronald Melzack comments that "the affective dimension [of pain] is difficult to express—words such as exhausting, sickening, terrifying, cruel, vicious, and killing come close but are often inadequate descriptions."[13] We simply cannot express in a clear and unambiguous fashion how pain, in all its complexity, feels.

Eliminating Pain

But there is more at issue here than simply cleaning up our workaday language. I hold that adopting a biological perspective on pain entails an eliminativism regarding pain talk. Eliminative materialism espouses the view that our commonsense way of understanding the mind is false and that, as a result, the mental events referred to explaining our everyday behavior and psychological states do not exist. Hence, the language of our "folk" psychology should be expunged—eliminated—from future scientific discourse. Though I do not wish to eliminate most folk expressions concerning our mental life, I do believe that our ways of discussing pain are broken beyond repair. They do not reflect what we know to be true about pain processing; they do not reflect the complexity of our experiences. Moreover, they assume a tacit dualism. Our best strategy is simply to scrap them and start over.

Defending Eliminative Materialism

Traditionally, there have been two routes taken to get to the eliminativist's position. The better developed and more popular approach to eliminativism comes out of philosophies of science developed by David Lewis, Willard van Orman Quine, and Wilfred Sellars. That argument runs as follows:

1. There is no fundamental distinction between observations (and our observation language) and theory (and our theoretical language), for previously accepted conceptual frameworks shape all observations and all expressions of those observations. Our observations are "theory-laden." These include observations we make of ourselves—in particular, observations we make about our internal states. In other words, there are no incorrigible phenomenological "givens."

2. The meaning of our theoretical terms (which includes our observational vocabulary) depends on how the terms are embedded in the conceptual scheme. Meaning holism of this variety entails that if the theory in which the theoretical terms are embedded is false, then the entities that the theory posits do not exist. The terms would not refer.

3. Describing ourselves in our everyday interactions comprises a rough-and-ready theory, composed of the platitudes of our commonsense understanding. The terms used in this folk theory are defined by the platitudes.

4. Folk psychology is a false theory.

Paul Churchland has put the eliminativist position in its starkest terms: "Our common-sense conception of psychological phenomenon constitutes a radically false theory, a theory so fundamentally defective that both the principles and the ontology of that theory will eventually be displaced, rather than smoothly reduced, by completed neuroscience."[14] Discussion of beliefs, desires, perceptions, and the like should go the way of all discussions using wrongheaded ideas. Just as we no longer talk about dephlogistonating wood or luminiferous ether, so too should we no longer bother talking about our minds and what is happening in them.

This essentially recapitulates the earlier argument about the complexity of pain sensations: our folk ways of talking about pain comprise a rough-and-ready theory of pain. This theory assumes that pains are identical to the sensations of pain and that the word "pain" can capture the essence of that sensation. Both assumptions are false.[15] Pain processing is enormously complicated, and our sensations of pain form only a tiny subset of what these processors do. But even if we focus exclusively on our sensations, since these are most important to our folk ways of being, our folk theory is still inadequate. We simply do not have the language to express all the dimensions of our pain experiences. The descriptors are either metaphorical or nonexistent. Our folk theory of pain needs to be replaced by something commensurate with the phenomenology.

The Referents of Pain Terms   Attacks on this version of eliminative materialism generally have come from three fronts, either on premise two, premise three, or premise four. Premise two asserts meaning holism and a particular theory of reference. If that theory were false, then the eliminativist's second argument would be undermined.[16] There are alternative approaches to reference that do not assume holism; for example, causal-historical accounts do not.[17] If meaning is not holistic, then even if folk psychology were incorrect, the terms used in that theory could still refer, and elimination of folk psychological terms would not be warranted.

Though an interesting and important rebuttal, deciding here whether meaning holism is true would take us too far afield. However, even if it were to turn out that a causal-historical account of meaning is correct, this would not change the basic substance of the eliminativist's charge: the alleged referents of folk psychology do not exist as assumed. Of course, one might prefer to keep the folk language with new referents, but this is only a semantic patch for a deeper metaphysical problem.

Consider: not only can we distinguish between the sensory, affective, and cognitive dimensions of pain phenomenologically, we can also manipulate them independently of one another. We can feel a shooting pain in our leg but not suffer in the least from it; we can be in agony from pain, without feeling any particular sensation localized to any part of our body. We could just decide by fiat that "pain" is going to refer to the localized sensations, or we could just decide that "pain" is going to refer to the suffering. But either way, we do violence to our folk notion of pain, which requires that a single simple sense datum seems to both occur in some place and be unpleasant.

Similarly, we could decide that "being possessed" means "having epilepsy." As with our revised definition of pain, we would still capture some of the surface features of the phenomenon. However, to claim that "being possessed" is a neurological condition is to replace our theory of demons with something else. Likewise, to say that "pain" only refers to a sensation without awfulness or to awfulness without sensation is to rend the folk theory of pain. Meaning holism or not, if what we refer to as pain turns out to be neither a conscious experience nor a perceptual simple, then what we are trying to point to in the world with the word does not exist, for these are the two defining features of our folk notion of pain.

Direct Knowledge   Arguments that our folk psychology is not really a theory deny premise three.[18] These arguments have an old and venerable position in the history of philosophy. Descartes was the first to espouse direct knowledge of mental life: "I can see clearly that there is nothing which is easier for me to know than my mind."[19] Ludwig Wittgenstein also captures some of the sentiments behind this objection when he writes, "I am not of the opinion that someone has a soul; my attitude towards him is as towards a soul."[20] Expanding on this idea, he points out:

We do not see facial contortions and make inferences from them (like a doctor framing a diagnosis) to joy, grief, boredom. We describe a face immediately as sad, radiant, bored, even when we are unable to give any other description of the features. —Grief, one would like to say, is personified in the face.[21]

Even if my point regarding premise two is taken and some ideas concerning our mental states are both theoretical and off base—there may not be any particular thing that is identical to being hornswoggled, for example—still there are some things we are surely right about.[22] Pain is touted as one of these items. Georges Rey notes that "clearly there are some first-person states—for example, sensory ones, like pain—about which people do seem to have some special first-person apprehension."[23] We just know when we are in pain, no inference or judgment required. Churchland himself comes dangerously close to this line, arguing that there is something correct about our beliefs about sensations; when all is said and done, they will only be reduced to their neurophysiological underpinnings, not eliminated altogether.[24]

This "special knowledge" argument reminds me of those who claim to know God directly; they simply experience Him in the fabric of the universe. Alvin Plantinga, for example, argues that he can take his belief in God as basic.[25] Given the way he was raised and the social community in which he is embedded, it is reasonable for him to start with a belief in God. No justification for this belief is required, for the belief arises from Plantinga's interaction with his environment.

I don't find Plantinga's argument persuasive, nor am I convinced by Descartes, Wittgenstein, or Rey. Plantinga might be right that we take some of our beliefs as basic because we have been raised in a certain way or because we live in a certain environment. These facts might explain why we believe the way we do, but they cannot justify our beliefs. Growing up as part of the white supremacist movement might explain one's beliefs about African Americans, but it would not justify the proposition that people with lighter colored skin are superior to those with darker colored skin, despite the fact that white supremacists assert that they can simply sense the truth of this claim by looking at the people around them.

Some believe that we know certain introspective facts indubitably. Saying that they can sense the truth of their experience directly does not show the claim to be true, however, for what they introspect about their conscious experience is a statement about their psychology and nothing more. We need some independent reason to believe that sensory experiences or introspective reflections or whatever are, in fact, infallible. We can say that they seem infallible to some people, but that isn't going to help.

Indeed, it is quite easy to demonstrate that our introspective knowledge of pain can be mistaken. If we burn our hand by touching something hot, we jerk our hand away from the heat source. This is a reflex action; the nociceptive information travels up our arm to the spinal column and then back down again. It takes about 20–40 msec from stimulus to behavior. The information also travels up the spinal column to the brain. We feel the burn as well. Unlike the reflex movement, this processing is more complicated, and it takes about 200–500 msec from stimulus to percept, a full order of magnitude longer.

Nevertheless, if we introspectively report on what the incident feels like, we would say that we moved our hand away after we felt the pain; feeling pain initiated the motor sequence. For whatever reason, our brains backdate our pain sensations so that they seem causally relevant to our reflex behavior. But clearly we can't cause the effect after it occurs, so our introspective report has to be wrong. We don't have complete first-person knowledge of our pains. Whatever knowledge we do have is embedded and informed by a conceptual framework of our brains' devising. Despite Rey's protests to the contrary, our pain experiences have all the earmarks of being theoretical in nature.

Other detractors point out that even if a completed psychology does not rely on the propositional attitudes or consciousness or some other defining characteristic of our folk theories, that would not entail that those sorts of mental states do not exist; they just would not be referred to in scientific discourse.[26] Our notion of pain would be analogous to our ideas about tables and chairs, germs and gems, and birthday presents and birthday cake. These are perfectly legitimate terms. We use them all the time, and we use them correctly and unproblematically. We just don't use them in science. Being cultural artifacts of one stripe or another, they do not refer to things about which we would have laws. Plantinga could go on talking about God, and the white supremacists could continue to talk about white supremacy; we just should not expect a science of God or human superiority. Notions of pain might work in a similar fashion. We might not have a mental science or laws about pains, but our folk psychology could still be used as it is now, in our everyday explanations of our behavior. It works well enough, in our specific cultural contexts, to get the job done. Hence, there is no need for elimination or replacement.

There is something undoubtedly right about this charge. In many ways, pain experiences are environmentally determined. Puppies raised without ever experiencing pain and without ever seeing any other dog in pain will exhibit no pain behavior. They will repeatedly sniff a lighted match without fear and then show no reaction when burned. Children learn both pain behaviors and the emotional concomitants to pain from the reactions of others around them.[27] Expressions of pain and reports of sensation and experience are significantly different across cultures.[28] Much of our experience of pain and how we react to and express these experiences is socially relative, a cultural artifact of sorts.

However, social relativity is not enough to show that our folk ways of understanding pain are adequate. Different cultures have different experiences; they also have different ways of understanding these experiences. But varied expressions for varied phenomenology does not guarantee that the descriptors are sufficient within their contexts. I argue that ours, anyway, are not, for at least two reasons. First, people with pain experiences that do not fit under our folk theories are assumed to have some psychiatric problem. Chronic pain without a diagnosed physical cause is deemed a mental disorder. Nonpainful self-injuries are considered a mark of Borderline Personality Disorder. Second, the fact that different chemicals affect the qualitative experience of pain differently cannot be expressed using our folk measure of pain intensity, namely, how much it hurts. This has and has had serious consequences for patients trying to relieve their pain or suffering with drugs. I claim that there is a fundamental inadequacy to our folk theories. The burden is now on the folk psychologist to demonstrate how—despite appearances—our folk theories of pain are actually successful.

The Necessity of Pain Talk Others charge that premise four is false; folk psychology might be a rudimentary theory, but it is not radically false.[29] While agreeing that our everyday explanations might not be entirely empirically adequate or complete, champions of folk psychology argue that no other theory is either. In addition, our folk psychology has developed over time, is coherent, and its status with respect to neuroscience is immaterial. These arguments are generally coupled with the claim that no other alternative, either real or imagined, could fulfill the explanatory role that folk psychology plays in our understanding of ourselves.

So, until the eliminativist's promise of a better conceptual scheme is fulfilled, folk psychology is here to stay. At least, some properly revised version of folk psychology would remain.

In addition, there is something radically incoherent about the elimination of various mental states. Barbara Hannan puts the complaint thus: "Concepts referred to as part of 'folk' semantic and psychological theories, such as meaning and belief, are arguably necessary . . . for the experience of the person or self as rational agent."[30] The only way to appreciate another human being as a human being is by assuming that she is a reasonably rational creature. We posit internal states, which makes our interlocutor appear, as Donald Davidson puts it, "consistent, a believer of truths, and a lover of the good."[31] The only way to understand ourselves is by using a particular mentalistic theory—rationalistic folk psychology. Anything else would give us something less than full human-ness. Hence, folk psychology is not a "theory" we can do away with and still enjoy our richly intentional lives. (Indeed, given its normative elements, it is not a theory in the traditional sense at all. Moreover, it presupposes what it allegedly is designed to explain.)

Others agree.[32] Let us take the example of the folk notion of belief. Eliminativism tells us that there is no such thing as belief. Presumably, then, we would be forced to say that Paul Churchland believes that there is no such thing as belief. How else are we to capture the gist of Churchland's view? There doesn't seem to be any way of expressing an eliminativist's position other than by using mentalistic language. This strikes some as an incoherent position, a semantic contradiction. Eliminative materialism collapses onto itself and reduces to absurdity.

We can devise a similar argument for the elimination of pain talk. We have all experienced pain; therefore, it would be impossible for us to claim that pain doesn't exist. We might claim that we don't understand pain, or that we are mistaken about particular aspects of our sensations of pain, but we cannot accept a theory that claims pains don't exist. Certainly, we could not accept a theory that claims that the sensations of pain don't exist.[33] That claim would be a simple reductio of the theory. Any theory that denies pain also denies an important aspect of our conscious lives; it doesn't capture a fundamental element about us that it should.

In answering this argument, eliminative materialists have generally held that something else will replace "pain," or some instances or aspects of "pain."[34] They don't want to deny the sensations themselves, only the way we describe them. We are making mistakes in language, not mistakes about what is actually in the world. As Wittgenstein explains, pain "is not a something, but not a nothing either! . . . If I speak of a fiction, then it is of a grammatical fiction."[35] The facts of the world remain, regardless of the theories (folk or otherwise) we use to capture them.

But this move has a simple response. Defenders of a revised folk psychology answer that, as used in this context, the new term and concomitant theory would be a mere revision of "pain." Without better exposition of what the replacement for our folk psychology term will be (and how it will be radically different), we simply cannot tell what the future holds for our commonsense theory of pain: simple revision, peaceful coexistence, or outright replacement.

My reply to this claim should be obvious by now. The solution for the eliminativist, of course, is to offer a serious replacement for our folk terms.[36] Chapters 5 and 6 outline a substantive, biologically based theory of pain processing. The combination of a PSS and a PIS account for the appearance of pain sensations being disconnected from physiology. Moreover, the clinical scales for assessing pain give us ways to describe at least one dimension of the complex nature of our pain sensations.

Though other aspects of our folk psychology may not be wrong, our folk theory of pain is woefully inadequate. We might play at revising this theory, but any change that remains faithful to what we know about pain processing is going to entail that pain no longer refers to a simple conscious percept. This sort of change crosses the line from mere revision to outright replacement.

Eliminating Our Scientific Theories

There is a second, less popular (and underappreciated) argument in support of eliminative materialism. It stems from a linguistic analysis of pain language. Paul Feyerabend and Richard Rorty argued that the commonsense terms for mental states tacitly assume some version of dualism.[37] Mentalism, by its very nature, assumes at least a dualism of properties—those that earmark the mind and its processes and those that

indicate the brain and its processes. According to Feyerabend, "physiologically inclined . . . empiricists" assert that the relationship between
the two sorts of features is a bridge law:

X is a mental process of kind A if X is a central process of kind *alpha*.[38]

But this "law" only shows the inadequacy of mentalistic theories, for it
"not only implies, as it is intended to imply, that mental events have
physical features; it also seems to imply (if read from the right to the left)
that some physical events . . . have non-physical features." This is a
difficulty with the very way in which the materialist "has formulated his
thesis."[39] Insofar as materialism is true, mentalistic terms cannot refer
to anything in the physical world. Thus they should not be used in
discussing ourselves or our psychologies, for we are purely physical
beings.

Even though this approach is not used much today, it does have
considerable application to our scientific pain discourse. If we take the
IASP recommendations seriously (and prima facie we should, since they
are the formal body charged with defining pain), then we have to accept
that (1) pain is equated with the sensation of pain (whatever that is), and
(2) this sensation is not correlated with any particular physiological cause
in the body (e.g., tissue damage, nociception, activation patterns in the
brain). Taken together, these two planks give us a dualism. If the IASP
is correct and "only through [private experience] is pain defined,"[40] then
the relevance of the body fades away.

This fact has not escaped the notice of some health professionals,
especially with respect to alleged psychogenic pain.[41] They point out that
the psychosocial dimensions of pain have been misconstrued; doctors
often talk about pains for which they can find no somatic cause as being
imaginary or mental in a pejorative sense. Douglas DeGood laments that
"all too often" psychogenesis "connotes a dualistic view of mind *versus*
body" (italics added).[42] Psychogenic pains become mental states with no
physiological underpinnings or mechanisms.

Empirically minded philosophers are used to retreating to token-token
identity or supervenience as a way of getting around the main thrust of
Feyerabend's argument. They deny the bridge law. Each individual instance of some mental event—my current perception of the blue sky—is
identical to some brain event or other; however, the mental event type—

perceiving blue in general—does not correspond to any identifiable brain type. Percepts of blue supervene on the brain (or they supervene on the brain plus environment). There are many different brain configurations that might give rise to a blue experience. The brain determines each individual case of perceiving blue, to be sure, but we cannot make interesting generalizations about these events unless we move up to a higher (or different) level of abstraction, namely, the mind.

Nevertheless, no philosopher comfortable with or committed to this approach to explaining mental events wants to disconnect our mind from the brain completely. Quite the opposite, in fact. Though perceiving blue may supervene on the brain, we can still identify our visual areas. We still believe that visual experiences, for the most part, originate with the rods and cones in our retinas. Visual information flows along particular tracts in the head, whether one be a dynamist or a feature-detectionist. Our individual experiences might not be type-identical to any brain state, but our sensory systems certainly are. Vision happens in the visual areas, and my visual areas are importantly similar to yours.

But no one holds that visual processing is the same as a visual experience. With the failure of type-type identity for our visual experiences, making this claim would effectively disconnect vision from anything physical. When I experience this blue sky, many things are happening in my brain. Only a few constitute the experience itself. The rest reflect the remainder of my cognitive life, my efforts at homeostasis, underlying moods and emotions, the behavioral programs I am initiating, and so forth. We all know this. How could we pick out which firing patterns are connected to the percept? Knowing that visual experiences occur in the visual areas helps narrow the search space considerably. Knowing something about the general anatomy and physiology of our visual system helps even more. But if we just claim supervenience and deny any interesting generalizations across brains, then we are stuck. If we are limited to having only a snapshot of the brain's activity coincident with the blue percept, then we cannot identify which subset of the activity is the percept and which concerns other processes. Indeed, we would not be able to tell that any of the activity was relevant to the experience at all.

From only one instance, we can generalize to anything. Uncovering nomic relations requires repeatable examples. Multiple instantiability tout court denies the prospect for discovering any mind-brain connections. We might still want to say that token-token identity between individual experiences and particular tweaks of the brain holds, but that would only be an expression of faith, for we would no longer have any way of justifying the correlations. If we cannot identify even roughly the areas in which vision occurs in the head, then we have no basis for claiming that this visual experience is occurring there as opposed to somewhere else, or nowhere.

In contrast to this perspective, the IASP is claiming that pain is the same as the experience of pain. It is denying that pain itself, not our individual experiences of certain sorts of pains, is correlated with anything in the brain. This is the equivalent of denying that vision itself corresponds to some brain areas. Hence we lose one good reason to believe that pain is physical. For we would have no way of connecting brain activity with a particular phenomenal experience nor generalizing from sets of neural firing patterns to types of qualia. If the IASP is correct, then, as a materialist, I can no longer even ask the question "Does it hurt?" in good conscience.

Or, better, if one is antecedently committed to materialism, then there cannot be any such thing as this sort of pain. Materialism claims that all mental causes are physical. This tells us that pain, whatever it is, has to be correlated with something in the body. The mistake is identifying pain with the experience of pain. This we should eliminate. Given the poor correlation between nociception and sensation, given the existence of the pain inhibitory system, given the psychosocial dimensions to our pains, we should see pain, like vision, as a complex sensory system. The sensations may not correlate with events in the external world, but the activity of the system certainly does.

What forces the elimination of the IASP definition of pain is the claim that it is not connected to any particular physical cause or event. To my knowledge, there is no other sensory process about which the scientific community makes that charge. And, as Feyerabend, Rorty, and others have shown, there is a good philosophical reason why.

The Irony of Pain Elimination

There is an irony in my arguments for the elimination of pain: I am claiming that we need to eliminate all our pain talk because we need the propositional attitudes for a full appreciation of pain processing. Our beliefs, judgments, and desires regarding our present sensations of pain are important components of our pain experiences. However, beliefs, judgments, and desires are exactly the items that traditional eliminative materialists wish to rid themselves of.

As my discussion in chapter 3 should have made clear, I do not believe that we philosophers can antecedently decide exactly what our contentful mental states are like and how to individuate them precisely. Those sorts of details lie in the hands of the relevant sciences. We can critique, cajole, and nag, but we cannot define. At the moment, psychology, psychiatry, and neuroscience all refer to content states in their explanations of thought, behavior, and internal circuitry. Consequently, we should accept this explanatory move as legitimate and do what we can to make it work, if at all possible.

Connectionism and the Mind

Nevertheless, I should address a final argument, concerning the appropriate level of organization in explaining mental events or intelligible behaviors. An ongoing debate in philosophy exists over whether understanding the connections between stimuli and outputs in "lower level" terms might mitigate the need for truly contentful states. If we can reduce the complexity of our minds to interacting sets of feature detectors and other relatively simple processors, then the notion of beliefs causing actions could be redescribed in lower-level neurobiological terms, perhaps in the language of action potentials and locally distributed neuronal connections.

This argument most recently has been presented in terms of connectionist or parallel distributed models in artificial intelligence, though the basic premises date back at least to Quine and his claim that we should look to neurophysiology to connect stimuli with behavior. The connectionist version adds a few wrinkles, since the debate becomes one of whether we can find any interesting contentful states among the nodes or neurons themselves. Some believe that we can;[43] others that we cannot.[44] If we can, then connectionist models pose no threat regarding eliminating the mind. The mind could just be the appropriately designed parallel distributed processor. If we cannot and if connectionism presents the best way to understand stimuli-behavior interactions, then either we should eliminate the mind from our scientific discussions, or we should have two completely autonomous ways of explaining ourselves—connectionism for the brain and contentful psychology for the mind.

This debate parallels those I sketched in chapter 3 over what it means to be a naturalist in many important ways. In both cases, philosophers and scientists suggest that redescribing the phenomena in question makes the mental go away. And, in both cases, there are those who believe that important generalizations and patterns are missed when content is described away. Though, as my discussion in chapters 3 and 4 should have made clear, I believe that it is much too early in our explorations of mind and brain to draw any definitive conclusions about how we should account for psychological or neurobiological events, I do want to note that one increasingly popular way of viewing this debate is in error.

Marr's Levels
Among those who wish to defend the viability of contentful explanations of behavior, there is an increasing tendency to hold that connectionism, even if it is a true description of our brains, it is not the best way to understand our minds at all. A connectionist network might give us the details for how to implement a mind in a brain, but it won't tell us about the mind itself. Arguments to this end generally rely heavily on a particular way of parsing explanations in cognitive science. More recent arguments to this end have also relied on attractor dynamics as a way to get interesting contentful states to be both physical but also separate from the underlying neural details. Both bits of the argumentative scaffolding need work. In particular, the explanatory distinctions do not allow the autonomy presumed, and the move to use one sort of model to describe one level of organization and another model to describe another level just does not work.

Fifteen years ago, a young scientist named David Marr offered us a complex view of theorizing in artificial intelligence. His tripartite division among levels of explanation still remains an important touchstone in philosophy of psychology. Among other things, Marr suggested that "the top level [of explanation] is the abstract computational theory of the device, in which the performance of the device is characterized as a mapping from one kind of information to another, the abstract properties of this mapping are defined precisely, and its appropriateness and adequacy for the task are demonstrated."[45] Terry Horgan and John Tienson have called this the level of cognitive function.[46] At the center level, what Horgan and Tienson call the algorithmic level, we find "the choice of representation for the input and output and algorithm to transform one into the other." Finally, at the bottom, there are "the details of how the algorithm and representation are realized physically—the detailed computer architecture, so to speak."[47] This is the level of implementation.

Horgan and Tienson adopt Marr's starting position and then expand the Marrian conception of the explanatory levels to reflect the recent emphasis in cognitive science on system dynamics and nonlinear modeling of information processing. The functions of level one and the algorithms of level two presume tractable and computable relations among variables. However, as mentioned in chapter 4, neither of these assumptions are warranted (yet) with respect to the mind. Hence, we need to generalize Marr's original typology. We should now think of the three levels as (1) the level of cognitive-state transitions, instead of cognitive functions; (2) the level of mathematical-state transitions, instead of algorithms; and (3) the level of (again) implementation.[48] Cognitive functions are a subset of all possible cognitive-state transitions, for some cognitive-state transitions will be NP-incomplete; similarly, algorithms form a subset of all possible mathematical-state transitions, for some mathematical-state transitions are not computable. Nevertheless, as in Marr's system, each level remains a functional decomposition of the one above and is multiply realizable by the level below.

In generalizing Marr, though, Horgan and Tienson still keep his basic conception of explanation in cognitive science. They claim, along with many in AI, that what we care about with respect to the brain and understanding cognition are not the brain-ish properties of our nervous system. Instead, the "abstract functional/organizational properties" sensitive to or reflective of the intentional aspects of mental phenomena are where our focus should lie, for it is these "physical state transitions" that underlie our information processing.[49] However, the physical state transitions are not, properly speaking, either physical or mental. We should think of them as being purely mathematical descriptions of the processes our brains (or some other machines) go through in dealing with contentful thought. This middle level then "mediates between the other two: cognitive states are realized by mathematical states, which in turn are realized by physical states of the cognizer's hardware or wetware."[50] There are three levels: the lowest one an implementation of the processes the middle level describes; and the middle level a mathematical working out of the general higher-level account of what the processing is. According to Horgan and Tienson, explanation in cognitive science consists of describing a cognitive system in three different ways, at three different levels of organization or analysis.

However, I am not confident that these distinctions are viable. Consider first the distinction between the so-called neurobiological properties and the functional/organizational properties of the brain. Of course, there are going to be neurobiological properties that are not relevant to determining or defining content. Nevertheless, any abstract organizational property of the brain that is "systematically appropriate" to content will also be a neurobiological property, by definition.[51] For example, certain patterns of activation appear over rabbit olfactory bulb whenever the animal is presented with an odorant that has previously been paired with some stimuli (food, say, or an electric shock).[52] Electrodes placed around the relevant olfactory neurons can record these patterns. The resultant EEG waveforms index a neurobiological property, since they indicate summed electrical discharges from groups of cells. At the same time, these patterns are deeply connected to content, since they appear when and only when the rabbit receives meaningful olfactory inputs, and they vary as the meaningful stimuli do.

Despite the assumption to the contrary, outlining the general functional organization of our wetware is just another way to describe our brain. Whenever we discuss a particular cognitive system, for example, our brain, the level of implementation and of mathematical-state transitions amount to the same thing. Even if the mathematical state-transitions can describe more than one physical system—brains and some computers, say—they will still remain an abstract account of the brains (and the computers). In other words, the mathematical descriptions seen as filling the second level of explanation are also one way to describe the level of implementation."[53]

What about the level of cognitive-state transitions? Here I think we run into a parallel situation, given how the higher levels are described.

Horgan and Tienson claim that "there might be many different mathematical ways of delineating a certain dynamical system or class of dynamical systems."[54] In other words, there might be many mathematical realizations of a dynamical system corresponding to one class of trajectories. Here is how I believe we should unpack this idea: Every physical or mathematical dynamical system has a set of trajectories that correspond to it. Some of the sets of trajectories define various sorts of invariant attractors; some of them do not. Horgan and Tienson believe that we can sort dynamical systems by the topologies, or structure, of their attractors.

For example, a Lorenz attractor, also known as a butterfly attractor, can be represented by a system of differential equations in a three-dimensional space. These equations generate trajectories, some of which lie on the attractor. (See figure 7.3.) Another completely different mathematical system could be described by a set of discrete transformations in 3-space. This new set of equations, which is unrelated to the equations for the Lorenz attractor, also defines trajectories, some of which also lie in the butterfly-shaped region. These two systems, then, have invariant attractors with the same topology. We could say that they belong to the same topological class. The conjecture—though there is no proof at all of this idea, mathematical or otherwise—is that we can uniquely characterize any dynamical system by its dimensionality and the topology of its attractors.

If this hypothesis is true, and I think it is, then we are well justified in claiming that the mathematical state-transitions of a system are multiply realized by the cognitive state-transitions. However, if this hypothesis is true, then it is also the case that the higher level description of "cognitive-state transitions" is just another description of the "mathematical-state transitions," albeit perhaps more general. To see what I mean, let us return to the trajectories that correspond to the Lorenz attractor. We can define this attractor, the trajectories, by any number of different sets of equations. These would all describe the mathematical-state transitions that comprise a butterfly-shaped region in 3-space. Presumably, we can also characterize this very same region by describing its topology. This sort of topological description should capture what Horgan and Tienson mean by a cognitive-state transition, for it would articulate the fundamental shape of the relevant "landscape." (A cognitive-state transition

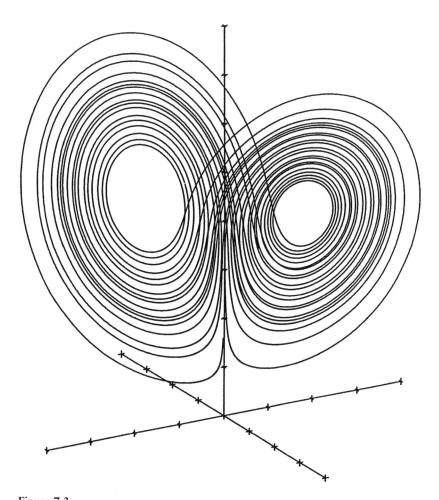

Figure 7.3
The Lorenz attractor or butterfly attractor. At any instant in time, the equations
that describe this attractor fix the location of a point in three-dimensional space;
as the system evolves over time, the motion of the point represents the changing
variables. This system never repeats itself exactly; instead, the trajectory loops
around and around forever, confined to a rather small attractor region in 3-space.
(Adapted from Gleick 1987.)

would then be a qualitative topological description of the manipulations that could occur in dynamic information processing.) But regardless of whether you use a set of equations or the topology to describe a Lorenz attractor—or any other sort of attractor—you would still be describing the same set of trajectories, namely, the set that defines the attractor region in multidimensional space.

I conclude that there really is not an interesting explanatory or mathematical distinction between the three levels of analysis that Horgan and Tienson articulate. They are all different ways of characterizing exactly the same interaction. The underlying hope was that the cognitive-state transitions would somehow give us the transitions we normally find between contentful mental states, while the mathematical-state transitions would be a more fine-grained analysis of the evolution of contentful states from states without content. However, demonstrating an isomorphism between the folk content of beliefs, say, and a description of a dynamical system (at any level) requires careful argument. It is not obvious; it certainly cannot be presumed. But unfortunately, Horgan and Tienson, at least, stop short of explicating any systematic connections between either their mathematical-state transitions or their cognitive-state transitions and what we normally mean by content.

However, even if we could spell out what exactly is contentful about the various state transitions, I am dubious we would find much of significance to distinguish among their three types of description, for each presents us with different ways of accounting for the very same set of trajectories that, in turn, describes (probably) a set of neural firing patterns. Marr's three levels, as generalized to be applicable to dynamical systems descriptions of information processing, give us distinctions without a difference.

If Horgan and Tienson, and others, are correct in emphasizing the centrality of dynamical systems in psychology, then the traditional distinctions between descriptions of function and descriptions of implementation disappear, for they would both amount to the same thing. As a consequence, the need to distinguish higher-level contentful interactions from lower-level mathematical descriptions in explanations of cognitive activity also disappears, for all a dynamical systems analysis gives us are informationally sensitive trajectories in multidimensional spaces under different descriptions. A dynamical systems analysis is more radical than even its proponents envision.

Back to Pain
In arguing that Horgan and Tienson's take on Marr does not give them the autonomy of psychological descriptions that they would like, I cannot conclude that talk of beliefs and desires is on its way out, to be replaced by descriptions of mathematical trajectories, or that dynamical systems will give us a new way to talk about our old friend content. Either alternative seems likely, or equally unlikely, from our position of almost complete ignorance about the fundamental level of organization of a minded brain.

But regardless of how we end up understanding our contentful mental states, they will be important in explaining pain sensations. In chapter 5, I suggested that we should understand at least some of our psychological responses to pain in terms of schema theory. It is now well documented that people selectively look for evidence to confirm their active schemas or current beliefs about the world.[55] This is true for pain experiences as well. If we believe that pain is eminent, then we are more likely to feel pain and report stimuli as painful.[56] If we are expecting something pleasurable, then we are more likely to experience pleasure.

Work by James Pennebaker[57] gives a robust illustration of this phenomenon. He gave subjects one of three consent forms: they either agreed to partake in an experiment that might result in a brief but intense (and harmless) pain, or one that would produce a pleasurable experience, or one in which the sort of experience they would have was not mentioned. In each case, however, the experiments proceeded in exactly the same way: subjects worked a series of mathematical problems and then placed their finger in a machine that contained a vibrating emery board. They were then asked to rank the sensation on their finger along a sixteen-point pleasure-to-pain scale. The only indication that subjects ever had about what sort of experience they might have came from the consent form; the experimenters said nothing. Remarkably, subjects who signed the forms that suggested they might feel pain reported the vibration as "stinging" or "burning" and indicated that the sensation fell on the pain end of the scale. Many believed that they had been shocked electrically.

Subjects who signed the forms intimating pleasure reported a "tingling" feeling and ranked their sensations on the pleasure end of the scale. Subjects who received no indication of what the experience might be like reported the sensation as "vibrating" and ranked the experience as neutral. Even though the subjects, in this case, undergraduates, all received the same input, their responses differed significantly, varying as their expectations did.

There are also some brain data that support the notion that beliefs and expectations play a large role in how sensations are experienced. PET scans were done on irritable bowl syndrome patients who, after just having a rectal balloon inflated, were told that the balloon was being inflated again, even though it wasn't. These patients claimed to feel pain in their rectal area, and these felt pains correlated with activations in prefrontal cortex.[58]

Unlike most eliminativists, I maintain that we need our contentful mental states to be able to account for pain processing, pain sensations, and pain behavior. Though we should eliminate our current pain talk and replace it with something more psychologically and biologically accurate, we cannot do without important aspects of folk psychology. In particular, we cannot do without some notion of belief (or one of its sisters).

That belief and expectation play an important role in how we experience pain has not been lost on those trying to find cures for chronic pain. One popular approach to controlling chronic and unremitting pain is to use therapies designed to get patients to change their minds about whether they are in fact experiencing pain. The assumption is that if they believe that they are not in pain, then they will not be, and, consequently, their pain will be gone. Whether this or other therapies actually work and why is topic of the next chapter.

8

What We Do Know about Treating Pain

I see it through the windows in my mind. . . . That jagged rock beneath my brow—where is it now? . . . There is that tiny finger pressure against my nose, under my eyebrows, just back of my ears. . . . The fire back of my eye is dying of its own accord. I am floating, floating. Aware. The pain? Oh, yes, the pain. It's there. Somewhere.

—The forty-two-year-old woman's description of her headaches after intensive therapy at UCLA Pain Control Unit (as quoted in Bresler and Trubo, *Free Yourself from Pain*)

Illness is the doctor to whom we pay most heed: to kindness, to knowledge we make promises only: pain we obey.

—Marcel Proust

Treating psychological or biological malfunctions does not require knowing the cause or the exact etiology of the disease, nor does it require understanding exactly how the therapy works. Using diuretics to manage edema did not depend upon knowing the glomerular permeability of the kidney. Using electroconvulsive therapy and drugs that influence amine metabolism to alleviate depression continue to be successful, even though we only have a murky idea about why they work. Similarly, we have many techniques for treating pains that we do not understand—we do not understand the pains, and we do not understand the treatments. Indeed, the best therapies for treating chronic pains are the least understood, and the most obvious and best understood "solutions" fare the poorest.

The Traditional "Cures"

It is important to recognize that "treatment" of chronic pain usually means a behavioral or psychological change, not the elimination of pain nor a cure in any traditional sense.[1] The goal for most therapy is to give patients "the most effective opportunity to manage their . . . chronic disease syndrome . . . [and] the skills and knowledge needed to increase their sense of control over pain."[2] Other popular buzzwords in pain management are "optimal functioning," "active participation," "self-efficacy."[3] In sum, improving a patient's functioning takes priority over relieving the pain itself.[4]

I leave it for the reader to decide whether this is the optimal strategy for dealing with chronic, intractable pain. Regardless, the unfortunate truth is that chronic pain is not controlled effectively, even when the goal is just to manage the sensation and not to eliminate the processing itself.[5]

The list of accepted methods to control pain is incredibly long and diverse. Figure 8.1 categorizes some of the more common techniques. No technique works obviously better than any of the others.[6] In fact, there is little experimental data to support the efficacy of any traditional therapy.[7] For chronic pain, some combination of methods is generally used, for no one method works alone. Combinations of methods rarely work either, however.

We have many fancy new drugs and our operating techniques may be greatly improved, but translating this knowledge into everyday clinical practice is problematic. Many current treatments for pain are based on an overly simple view of how pain works, the view that pain originates with some noxious stimuli and then is transmitted to and later interpreted by the brain. Hence, interventions and analysis of those interventions have focused on either removing the offending stimuli, altering conscious awareness of the painful sensation, or changing the resultant pain behavior.[8] Either that, or the person is labeled psychologically disordered with psychogenic pain and a round of psychiatric therapy is in order.

Surgery

The most obvious route to curing pain is to cut out the offending area. If we could lesion the parts of the brain active during chronic pain, then it seems that the pain should disappear. However, ablative surgery, which tries to block or interfere with the transmission of pain along the pain processing pathways, often provides only temporary relief. In a large

Drugs	spinal opioids nonsteroidal antiinflammatory drugs tramadol tricyclic antidepressants anticonvulsants cyroanalgesia analgesics transdermal drugs implanted intraspinal drug-delivery systems patient controlled analgesia
Non-invasive therapies	superficial heating agents cryotheraphy ultrasound transcutaneous electrical nerve stimulation radiofrequency thermocoagulation intrapleural bupivacaine
Denervation procedures and invasive therapies	spinal cord stimulation deep brain stimulation ablation
Palliative procedures	patient education distraction psychological counseling behavior modification

Figure 8.1
Accepted medical interventions for pain.

percentage of cases, the pain recurs in about a year. This fact prompts Leriche's famous dictum: "Le résultat est bon pourvue que les malades meurent vite." (The result is good if only the patients die soon.) In addition, ablative surgery can leave permanent neurological deficits. It should be used as a measure of last resort, and indeed, its prevalence has been steadily decreasing. It is, in fact, now mainly used for patients with a short life expectancy.[9]

Working to improve surgical techniques is difficult since there are few animal models of human pain. The spinothalamic tract is a relatively young system, appearing in higher primates but not in the lower primates. Animal incisions in similar areas give different results. Consequently, all tests and trials for the surgical correction of pain are performed on humans and are still being perfected by trial and error.

Nevertheless, one reason why surgery provides such a poor long-term outcome is fairly clear: creatures lacking the spinothalamic tract still have pain; hence, they must have alternative paths. In most cases of evolution, when something new comes on the scene, it overlays what was there previously; it does not replace it. Therefore, it stands to reason that we too have some phylogenetically older pain signaling systems. Oblating all these systems in the correct place is difficult to do, especially since we don't know exactly where they are. Surgery is supposed to prevent pain by removing some of the nociceptive inputs in the PSS. Theoretically, this would allow the PIS to prevent the remaining nociceptive signals from being fully processed. However, our central nervous system is plastic, and as long as some of the older pain system is intact, it will work to reroute the nociceptive signals through that system. The PIS might also stop inhibiting nociception for a variety of reasons. Ultimately and unfortunately, the pain returns full force.

Drugs

Perhaps, some have thought, the best way to control chronic pain—since we do not understand it—is to focus on the PIS. In particular, opioids or other chemical mediators inhibit the spinal cord by decreasing the amount of endogenous chemical activity associated with tissue damage.[10] (Nociception releases such chemicals as bradykinin, histamine, prostaglandin, serotonin, norepinephrine, and substance P [which also stimulates prostaglandin and collagenase production].[11]) These sorts of drugs are often used in managing chronic cancer pain. Morphine, oxycodone, fentanyl, methadone, and levorphanol are all accepted interventions with cancer pain.

However, their use in controlling noncancer pain is fiercely debated, for all these substances are highly addictive and quite often they induce depression, change one's personality, or impair cognitive function.[12] Many with chronic pain require detoxification from opioids, sedative-hypnotics, and muscle relaxants. Becoming addicted to one type of pain reliever or another is quite common with chronic pain patients, as they search in vain for relief, if not a cure.

On the other hand, that these patients experience physical dependence and drug tolerance may not be problematic, as long as those outcomes are not terribly maladaptive and their pain relief is significant.[13] Indeed, some cannot function at all without low doses of opioids.[14] The professional literature draws a distinction between being physically dependent on a drug required for a normal life and being addicted to recreational drugs for pseudosocial reasons. The former can be acceptable, as long as the benefits outweigh the costs; the latter isn't, regardless of the cost-benefit analysis. I am dubious that a principled distinction can be drawn between the two; many "recreational" addicts claim that they require their drug of choice for important life-enhancing reasons. Still, we cannot say with authority that all addiction is bad; it all depends on who is totting up the cost-benefit balance.

But regardless of whether we find addiction to pain medication socially acceptable, the opioid family does not give us a panacea. Most nerve pain patients do not respond to opioids, and others receive only modest amounts of relief. Still others get relief at the cost of cognitive function and psychological health.

Pain Clinics

Pain clinics are multidisciplinary and multifaceted; they seek to treat the entire person and all aspects of pain. However, they specialize in pain management; hence, they do not focus on curing pains at all. These clinics are proliferating quite rapidly. Recent estimates put over 2,000 such clinics in the United States alone. However, there is little comprehensive research done on their efficacy.[15] Most are centered around either the cognitive-behavioral approach developed by Dennis Turk[16] or the operant conditioning approach developed by W. E. Fordyce (though few today use either technique exclusively). I should also stress that most clinics use these techniques in combination with physical treatments as well.[17] The cognitive-behavioral perspective is founded on the following five propositions:

1. Individuals actively process information instead of passively receiving it.
2. Beliefs and judgments can affect mood, physiology, environment, and behavior. Conversely, mood, physiology, environment, and behavior can affect beliefs and judgments.

3. The individual and the environment jointly determine behavior.
4. Individuals can change the way they think for the better.
5. Individuals can and should actively work to change their own maladaptive thoughts, feelings, and behaviors.[18]

Cognitive therapy holds that psychological dysfunction is at least partially responsible for chronic pain. If errors in cognitive appraisal or other beliefs are at the heart of psychological dysfunction—as cognitive therapists assume—then treating chronic pain is a matter of replacing pain-promoting beliefs with ones that minimize the emphasis on pain processing. Cognitive therapists believe that "all the symptoms of chronic pain, except for those arising from on-going nociception, can and should be explained in purely cognitive terms."[19] Their goal is to replace active pain schemas with ones that do not interpret current experiences as painful or negative. The assumption is that the pain schemas are somehow wrong or irrational while the replacement beliefs are correct or rational. The message that the therapists try to instill in patients is that they are not helpless; instead, they have inner resources that will allow them to cope with their lives successfully, if only they can develop their cognitive skills appropriately.

The difficulty with this approach is that the pain processing, the root of the problem, is not treated at all; only one's beliefs and judgments concerning the subjective experience change. Of course, altering one's cognitive schema can and does alter the subject experience. It can diminish the intensity of the pain as it also reduces the negative value one places on it. But it isn't a cure, of course, the PSS (up to the higher cortical areas) is still being activated as it was before, and the cortex is still responding to the inputs. It just isn't responding in the same ways as it did.

Operant conditioning, the other favored method of pain clinics, is often criticized for denying the experience of the patient. The therapy promotes nonpain behavior, despite (presumably) the remaining sensations of pain. Those who champion pain clinics and operant conditioning therapy claim that pain is learned via some sort of environmental reinforcers, and it can be unlearned in the same way. They claim that if the behaviors change, then the subjective experience will follow.[20] (This contrasts with the cognitive-behavioral approach, which claims that if we change the experience, then the behaviors will follow.) This is nowadays described in terms of cognitive dissonance; if a person's beliefs are at odds with her behavior, then she will switch her beliefs to match her actions.

Success of this method is measured in purely behavioral terms. If, after treatment, patients are able to live in a manner indistinguishable from pain-free subjects, then the treatment is deemed a success.[21] Of course, acting as though one is not in pain is not the same thing as not being in pain.[22] Reviews of treatment programs have borne this out. Behavioral therapy changes pain behavior significantly; however, no decrease in pain sensation can be traced to the behavioral modifications themselves. Instead, they are connected to relaxation techniques often taught alongside the behavioral reprogramming.[23]

Perhaps a better description of what operant conditioning is doing with chronic pain patients concerns our negative judgments about suffering, which are learned. As I shall discuss in the final section in this chapter, plenty of evidence exists that our PSS and PIS systems are innate and fully functioning early in life, prior to most learned behaviors or abilities. As argued in chapter 7, how we react to our sensations of pain and suffering is largely social. If this analysis is correct, then pain clinics do not alleviate the somatic quality of pain sensations nor do they alleviate suffering. Instead, they just teach us to accept these feelings and to live with them. Certainly, as with cognitive-behavioral therapy, this is better than no treatment, but it is less then ideal.

In our brief review of the most popular ways of treating pain, we can see that none of the approaches really addresses the full complexity of our pain processing system (or systems, as the case may be). Curing a pain has to be more than merely removing a piece of the processing system, enhancing the pain inhibitory system, changing the conscious experience, or altering behavior, for each of these only touches a tiny part of the PSS. Even taken together, they cannot fully remove pain, which would require quiesence of the entire pain processing tracts. At their best, they are only damping down part of pain processing. And, in many cases, it is not even the most important part. The long and the short of it is that there is little theoretical reason to believe in the efficacy of any of these approaches.

Nontraditional Approaches

As mentioned several times now, emotional factors heavily influence one's perception of pain and suffering. In cases in which stress, distress, abuse, or genuine mental disorders exacerbate the intensity of the suffering, traditional analgesics do not work. Often some sort of psychiatric treatment is used. But what is most successful in treating chronic, intractable pains are the "nontraditional" methods, including hypnosis, biofeedback, relaxation therapy, acupuncture, and psychotropic drugs.

Hypnotism, in particular, is a highly effective pain-relieving technique.[24] Studies have shown that it is more effective in removing pain than acupuncture, psychotherapy, biofeedback, drug placebos, and relaxation therapies, and, most interestingly, it is more effective than morphine, aspirin, or valium.[25] In fact, it seems to work better than any waking analgesic.[26] Hypnosis has been shown to work with repetitive strain injury,[27] childbirth,[28] burns,[29] chronic back pain,[30] cancer pain,[31] oral pain,[32] and fibromyalgia,[33] as well as in children[34] (though it is not clear how long the effects last[35]). In addition, success with hypnotism is not related to demographics, medical status, psychological distress, personality traits, coping strategies, or pain appraisals.[36]

Questions we need to address include why hypnosis is so successful, how it works, and whether we can generalize what we learn about hypnotism to treating or curing pain in general. Let us start, though, with a brief tour through the history of hypnosis, which will clear up one mystery: why hypnosis is not a popular method of treatment, even though it works as well as it does.

A Brief History of Hypnosis[37]

Using hypnotic techniques to control pain is probably one of the oldest therapies around—ancient Greek priests apparently induced trances in their Aesculapian temples to effect "miraculous cures"[38]—however, it was not until the late 1700s that significant scientific attention was devoted to the phenomena. The Austrian physician Franz Anton Mesmer popularized what he called "animal magnetism" as a treatment for healing all sorts of diseases and established two very popular clinics in Paris devoted to magnetic treatments. He theorized that doctors have healing powers similar to those attributed to magnets. Certain diseases, he believed, were caused by an imbalance in magnetic fluid in the human body. An appropriately trained physician could channel this ubiquitous but subtle fluid—which also links and connects all objects in the world—into patients, thereby restoring their imbalances and healing them.

The French medical community was less receptive, even though at the time their healing repertoire was limited to leeches, potions, bleeding, and purges. Part of the difficulty was Mesmer's great drama in effecting his cures. Patients awaited his arrival in a darkened room, arranged in benches around an oak tub filled with iron filings and iron rods. The walls were mirrored and curtained; the floor thickly carpeted; the air perfumed. Those closest to the tub or "baquet" held the iron rods to their bodies; those further out touched those holding the rods. Some patients responded immediately to the animal fluid's movements through the rods and human bodies. Finally, Mesmer arrived, dressed in light purple robes and carrying a long magnetized pole. Patients would shake, convulse, moan, or scream as the magnetic fluid filled their bodies. Mesmer attended personally to those who had trouble sensing the fluid's movement; he would pass his pole over them as he glared at them, almost daring them not to feel the changes in the magnetic fluid. Most did. Despite the flamboyance and unorthodox approach—or maybe because of it—most of his patients claimed to be cured.

Ultimately, the King of France appointed two commissions to investigate the efficacy of animal magnetism. The first, in 1784, included members of the Royal Academy of Sciences and the Faculty of Medicine and was headed by no less than Benjamin Franklin (who was then the Ambassador to France); the second was comprised of members of the Royal Society of Medicine. Both distinguished groups concluded that there is no scientific evidence for animal magnetism of the sort Mesmer proposed. Neither, however, maintained that Mesmer's cures did not work, nor that his patients did not recover. But they believed that the patients' improvements were due to the psyche somehow overcoming the physical and not to any sort of subtle fluid.

Though Mesmer wrote rebuttals to the charges, his reputation was damaged beyond repair and his clinics fell into disrepute. His student, Marquis de Puységur, continued pressing the possibility of magnetic cures. (Actually, Puyégur came to believe that what was most important in effecting a cure was the "rapport" shared between doctor and patient and not the channeling of fluids.) Puységur identified the deep trance that his patients entered into and considered it necessary for the healing process, calling it "magnetic somnambulism," after the resemblance between the trance and sleepwalking.

Under hypnosis, patients superficially appear to be asleep; however, they can respond to commands, answer questions, and move intentionally. They tend to discuss themselves as though the waking states belonged to another person, being remarkably indifferent to and objective about whatever problems they have when awake. Puységur and later his follower Deleuze carefully investigated the metaphysical properties of magnetic somnambulism. They both came to the conclusion that it uncovered a separate person within the body. Still, despite a split between Puységur and his teacher, and the attempts at "scientizing" mesmerism, it remained out of favor as a therapeutic technique, mainly for moral reasons. There was a fear that an inappropriate relationship could or would exist between a young suggestible female patient and the "magnetizer." As a result, mesmerism was condemned outright by the Congrégation du Saint-Office in 1851.

We are not sure how long hypnosis has been used as an anesthetic during surgery; the first official published case occurred in 1826 in Paris in which Hippolyte Cloquet, a well-known surgeon, performed a mastectomy on a young woman using no other method of pain control. A commission was appointed to investigate these extraordinary results and, after five years of inquiry, concluded that the results were authentic.

Nevertheless, even though hundreds of operations were performed during the early 1800s using hypnosis as an anesthetic, the procedure was still openly viewed with suspicion and outright hostility by most professionals. Pierre Martin Roux, speaking for the French Academy of Medicine, counseled that "quackery will find enough voices outside these walls to defend it; it must find none amongst us."[39] In an editorial in the *Boston Medical and Surgical Journal* (now the *New England Journal of Medicine*), J. V. C. Smith fussed that "whole scores of silly girls were exhibited in public on platforms, pricked with needles, had their toes crushed and teeth extracted, all which they (the mesmerists) represented to be wholly unconscious." He continues, "The country is swarmed with traveling mesmerizers who lectured in every town and hamlet . . . and made such high pretensions, that gentlemen who presumed to question the honesty of the vagabonds made themselves quite unpopular with the multitudes."[40]

At about the same time, the English doctor James Braid renamed mesmerism "hypnosis" in an attempt to sever its connection with Mesmer's disastrous introduction of hypnotism as a genuine cure. Braid saw hypnotism as a genuine and nonmysterious phenomenon and strove to remove the atmosphere of ceremony and occult that surrounded it. In particular, he devised a simple technique by which to induce it:

Take any shiny object . . . between the thumb, index and middle finger of the left hand; hold it at a distance of between 25 and 45 centimeters from the eyes, in such a position above the forehead as to induce the greatest necessary effort on the part of the eyes and eyelids of the subject to stare at the object. The patient must be made to understand that he must keep his eyes continually on the object and his mind must remain totally attached to the idea of this sole object. One will observe that because of the synergistic action of the eyes, the pupils will firstly contract; shortly afterwards they will begin to dilate, and after having become thus considerably dilated and after having made an oscillating movement, if the pointing and middle finger of the right hand, extended and slightly separated, are taken from the object towards the eyes, it is highly probable that the eyelids will close. . . . After an interval of about ten to fifteen seconds, by gently lifting the arms and legs, one will find that the patient, if he is strongly affected, is disposed to keep them in the position in which they have been placed.[41]

The pendulum of scientific acceptance of hypnotism should have begun to swing in the other direction. Hypnotists were having too many successes and were becoming more closely affiliated with the medical establishment for it to keep its connection with charlantansim much longer. Nevertheless, even though hypnosis had been recommended as a standard procedure for surgery, its popularity on that front plummeted due to the advent of chloroform around the same time. Ether anesthesia was seen not only as a triumph over pain but also as one over mesmerism. That many died from inhaling ether during operations, and that chloroform still won out over hypnotism as the anesthesia of choice, tells something of the nature of the dispute among methods at the time.

Still, enough operations had been performed using hypnosis that doctors had begun to document hypnotism's singular effects. In particular, they had noticed the selective quality of hypnotic anesthesia. Patients could be unaware of any pain during a major surgical procedure, yet still complain of the cool temperature of the operating theater. Or they could lose sensation in their right arm, but not their left.

Nevertheless, even as hypnotism once again waned in popularity, the notion of a secondary self persisted under scientific scrutiny, for scientists believed that there was no other way to explain the selectivity of hypnotic anesthesia. Patients would have to recognize, in some sense, the very objects or sensations they are supposed to ignore or suppress, in order to be oblivious to just those items and not everything else. As William James notes, "A subject must distinguish the object from others like it in order to be blind to it. Make him blind to one person in the room, set all the persons in a row, and tell him to count them. He will count all but that one. But how can he tell which one not to count without recognizing who he is?"[42] Binet agrees: "There is always an unconscious judgment that precedes, prepares, and guides the phenomenon of anesthesia. The perception of the forbidden object continues to operate, but it becomes unconscious."[43] He hypothesizes that "the perception forbidden by suggestion undergoes the same fate as the sensations arising from anesthetic regions. It is relegated to a second consciousness, where it determines ideas, judgments, and actions, which are all equally unconscious to the principal personality."[44]

This notion of a second self persists in explaining consciousness today—what Hilgard calls the "hidden observer"—for exactly the same reasons it was hypothesized then.[45] Now, there is a bit more experimental data to support this idea. Hypnotized subjects will claim to be feeling no pain, even though they will also admit indirectly via automatic writing that part of them hurts or, when pressed, they will confess that something is experiencing the pain ("My arm hurts, but I don't hurt."). (One question that needs investigating is whether these hypnotic subjects resemble the patients with frontal lobe lesions who report pain but are not bothered by it.)

In any event, by the mid-1800s, the general consensus was that hypnotism involved the power of suggestion, which Hippolyte Bernheim, a professor of medicine at Nancy at the time, called "the aptitude to transform an idea into an act."[46] Jean Martin Charcot, one of the nineteenth century's foremost neurologists, presented data regarding the structure of the hypnotic trance to the Academy of Sciences in 1882. This time, the reaction of the Academy was quite different: Charcot's paper was greeted enthusiastically. Hypnosis became a legitimate item for scientific inquiry after all; however, its application to pain control was still rather limited.

In the late nineteenth century, there was again a brief flurry of interest in hypnosis in psychiatry as a way to uncover the unconscious beliefs and desires of hysterical patients and as a way to treat people with multiple personality disorder. But as Freud abandoned hypnotism for his own talking therapy, so did the rest of the psychiatric community. World War I and World War II renewed interest in hypnosis as a way to cure soldiers of shell shock and battle fatigue. After the Second World War, professional societies centered around the study of hypnosis emerged, and two research centers for hypnosis were established at Stanford and Harvard.

By the 1970s, interest in hypnotism as a way to control pain became melded with the behavior modification literature both from an operant conditioning perspective and from a cognitive perspective (though the behavior modification studies rarely availed themselves of the relevant data from hypnosis). However, it is only recently that the connections between the cognitive control of pain and hypnosis have become clearer. And it is only very recently that we have begun to get any idea of what hypnotism does to the brain. Until then, we have been stuck back in the 1800s with our theories, believing in homunculi and other mysterious entities (though these things go under more respectable sounding labels like "dissociated control"[47]) in our quest to explain this very odd effect.

What We Do Know about Hypnotism

People differ in their abilities to distort their perceptions and experiences on the basis of suggestion. Though how hypnotizable one is can be altered a bit through training and experience, the degree to which one can be hypnotized is remarkably constant throughout one's life.[48] We can now evaluate one's level of hypnotizability clinically using standard tests;[49] however, we have no clear idea what it is we are measuring when we determine that someone is a "low hypnotizable" or a "high hypnotizable." We know it is not compliance, conformity, gullibility, or persuasibility,[50] but beyond that it is not clear what psychological prop-erties are important for hypnotic suggestion.

We do know that whatever hypnotism is, it is mainly a central effect. When highly hypnotizable subjects are told to feel no pain and they report that they are indeed feeling no pain, their involuntary autonomic responses to pain still continue.[51] Their hearts beat faster, their blood pressure increases, they sweat, their bodies release stress hormones. (This fact actually has been known since at least the early 1800s, when B. H. West noticed that during a molar extraction, the hypnotized patient had "a flush over the whole face and a slight quivering of the lip, with a countenance indicative of considerable pain."[52]) A natural guess is that hypnotism is tapping into endogenous firing of our PIS. Yet, studies designed to test whether opioid production is associated with hypnosis produce largely negative results.[53] Given the rapidity by which suggestion can reverse hypnoananesthia, it is doubtful that peptides or hormones are inhibiting nociception or pain sensation.[54]

Part of the difficulty in studying hypnosis scientifically has been that both the hypnotic trance and the verbal pain report depend upon subjec-tive, first-person data. We cannot control or measure them in the way we might when delivering a drug or determining a heart rate. Even today some claim that hypnosis only involves the subject relabeling a pain sensation instead of eliminating or attenuating it.[55] Nevertheless, neuro-psychologists and neurophysiologists have recently turned their attention to hypnosis and have begun to look at what happens inside the brain and nervous system under hypnoanalgesia. For example, high hypnotizables show lower EEG amplitudes globally over both hemispheres during hypnotic analgesia; they also show a significant reduction in the spectral midfrequency peak of heart period variability, which indicates that sym-pathetic activity is decreasing. In contrast, low hypnotizables show lower EEG amplitudes only in some frequencies in the posterior regions and no change in heart rhythms.[56]

It is now clear that hypnosis involves striking changes in the excitatory and inhibitory patterns in cortex.[57] We get stereotypical evoked potential (EP) waveforms with hypnosis. When subjects were hypnotized and told not to perceive some visual stimulus, the beginning of the EP waveforms remained unchanged from the unhypnotized control waveforms, but later recorded event-related potentials inside the head to painful stimuli under conditions of attention and hypnotically suggested analgesia.[86] Their subjects were two patients with obsessive-compulsive disorder who had electrodes implanted in anterior cingulate cortex, the amygdala, the temporal cortex, and parietal cortex for diagnostic reasons. It turned out that one was hypnotizable, and one wasn't. The hypnotizable and hypnotized patient showed reduced positive EP components in left anterior cingulate cortex followed by an enhanced negative component in left anterior temporal cortex when she was instructed not to feel pain. She also reported very little pain under those conditions. The nonhypnotizable patient showed no changes in brain waves and reported feeling significant pain.

These findings dovetail with the imaging studies in chapter 5 that tied the anterior cingulate to pain processing. It makes sense that under hypnotic analgesia, the activity there would diminish. However, it is also very important to underscore the increase in activity in the anterior temporal cortex. This tells us that this area is working harder at doing something during the task. Perhaps it is actively seeking to control and suppress the pain response elsewhere in the brain. The assumption is that, as James and Binet noted almost a century ago, in order to ignore a particular experience or stimulus, you have to notice it first and then work to eliminate awareness of it. In other words, not feeling pain during hypnosis (and a noxious stimulus) requires more labor on the part of the brain than just going ahead and feeling the pain that is already there.

What Counts as a Cure

What does this parade of data tell us about hypnosis, treating pain, and "mental" cures of physical ailments in general? We can draw a few tentative conclusions. First, as with the other, more traditional methods of treatment, hypnosis does not cure the pain in any normal sense. Instead, under hypnosis, the frontal lobe actively seeks to shut down activity in the anterior cingulate, somatosensory cortex, and perhaps other places as well (the sympathetic nervous system, for example). This means that, instead of there being less activity in the brain associated with pain processing, there is actually more.

Perhaps the mechanism of hypnosis is related or analogous to our attentional system. If it is, then that would explain why distraction tasks work with high hypnotizables as an analgesic as well as why similar areas of the brain light up during focused attention and hypnosis. On the other hand, this hypothesis does not explain why being hypnotized per se adds anything to the treatment. Why doesn't distraction alone work just as well? It also does not explain why hypnotism is so effective at altering physiological function (digestion, blood flow, and so forth). At best, an attentional component to hypnotism is part of the full story.

Why does hypnotism work as well as or better than other available treatments? Insofar as we don't understand exactly what hypnotism is or how it works, I cannot give a good answer to that question. However, I can say that data suggest that hypnotism can affect many different aspects of pain processing. Unlike the more traditional therapies, each of which alters only one or two components of pain, hypnosis appears to be able to influence neural activity on a global scale so that not only are the sensations of pain and our judgments of suffering changed, but our pain behavior, the autonomic concomitants to pain processing, and nociception can change as well. Even though hypnosis does not cure pain in the sense of removing it, it can modify many dimensions of our complex pain processing system. As I have argued in previous chapters, being able to do this is key to treating pain effectively and appropriately.

Finally, understanding hypnosis neurophysiologically is fundamental to explaining how it is that merely talking to a person could produce such low-level physiological changes, how "mental" therapies can affect "physical" difficulties. I hope that the brief description of the neurophysiology of hypnosis helps to demystify the phenomenon a bit. Hypnosis is weird—I will be the first to admit that—but if we can see that it is really nothing more than one identifiable brain circuit influencing others in ways that we already understand and can document, then, appearances aside, hypnosis becomes much more mundane. It is just more of the same, from the brain's point of view.

There are, of course, many fundamental gaps in our understanding. In particular, we have no idea why it is that talking can induce the changes in the brain that it does. Why should telling someone to relax and focus on a shiny object change the inhibitory patterns over cortex? Nevertheless, knowing that it does clarifies a bit the relation between the "mental" and the "physical," in the manner chapter 3 requires. In this case, the "mental" event—being hypnotized—is an activated brain circuit that changes the pattern of activity in other brain areas and circuits via its connections to them, and those patterns of activity ultimately produce the "physical" effects—whether they be changes in behavior via neuromuscular connections, changes in heart rate via the parasympathetic nervous system, or what have you. It is a complex, but purely mechanical and unproblematic, interaction. One would assume that other talking therapies work in an analogous manner.

I have now told you my story about pain. A pain by any other name—chronic pain, psychogenic pain, hysterical pain, psychosomatic pain—is still a pain, and it can be understood best as a complex biological phenomenon. I would like to close this tale by briefly examining what my theory and my approach have to say about another treatment issue, the treatment of pain in infants and children. (As an epilogue, the final chapter looks at the larger implications my approach has for analyzing psychopathologies in general.) The current dispute within pain literature over whether and how much children have pain is disconcerting and rife with moral overtones. Frankly, as a parent with small children of my own, I believe that I would be remiss in not addressing it. From a less personal perspective though, we can see that if my analysis of pain is approximately correct, then the controversy is misanalyzed and misargued on both sides of the fence. If my story is correct, then whether and how to treat pain in infants and children has a very simple, straightforward, and noncontroversial answer.

Pain in Children and Infants

A common yet naive assumption is that pain and pain behavior in children are similar to those of adults. A second common and also naive assumption is that infants do not feel pain. Both are questionable.

I have argued that pain is actually a complicated sensory process and that pain sensations, one tiny component of the entire process, are complex as well. Pain sensations contain at least a sensory component, a sense of localization, a negative reaction to the sensation, and a negative judgment about the reaction. And all of these aspects of pain sensations are informed to some extent by memories of previous experiences with pain. Certainly as children grow and mature, their sense of what feeling pain is will change and become more precise as their mnemonic, cognitive, and emotive capacities grow and mature as well. Children experience pain,[87] but as their life experiences differ, so too their pains will differ from those of adults.[88]

Actually we know quite little about pain processing in children or infants, and what we do know is limited to how they react in largely artificial and clinical situations in which the sensation of pain itself cannot easily be distinguished from any general distress at being in pain.[89] Some experimental data do bear out my conjecture that children experience pain differently from adults. Most studies show that younger infants have diffuse and less well modulated reactions to painful stimuli than do older infants or children.[90] Pricking a young infant with a pin provokes an unlocalized reaction with only an occasional withdrawal reflex; doing the same thing to a twelve-month-old infant elicits a more focused, defensive movement.[91] Anticipatory fear develops at about six months, though in younger infants, previous experience with a noxious stimulus is correlated with less crying to the same stimulus a second time around.[92] Even the youngest infants are affected by painful experiences, though how those effects are expressed changes over time.

Studies of infant reactions to inoculations provide some of the best evidence of diachronic changes in pain response. Over time, the pain reaction itself decreases and anger becomes the more prevalent emotion. The duration of the negative emotion also decreases with the age of the infant, as does the rigidity of the infant's body.[93] These results support the idea that the older we are, the better able we are to anticipate and modulate our pain responses.

There are fewer data concerning pain perception in children. Studies indicate that pain thresholds decrease with age but the ability to localize pain increases.[94] Distress-related behaviors also change: younger children tend to resist an offending procedure and to cry generically; older children are more specific in what they say (not surprisingly) but also flinch, components were reduced in size.[58] We get similar effects with pain. Hypnotic analgesia attenuated later EP amplitudes; hypnotic suggestions of increased sensitivity to pain increased later EP amplitudes.[59]

The later changes in the pain EP might turn out to be a brain response to anxiety, though. When we decrease anxiety but leave pain sensation unchanged (with benzodiazepine), then the later wave component disappears altogether. Consequently, the later EP waveforms might reflect part of the emotional aspects of pain, not part of the sensory discrimination, as once thought (though this point is still being debated).[60]

Hence, some have argued that both hypnoanalgesia and hypnoanasthesia only reduce the suffering component of the pain experience without actually removing the pain sensation itself. Hypnotized patients are very relaxed and so any anxiety they might normally feel about an upcoming painful procedure or current painful situation is greatly attenuated. In addition, the rapport between patient and practitioner that Puyégur believed so important might also prevent patients from owning up to the pain they really experience.[61]

Experimental data do not support this contention. Though hypnotized subjects are indeed relaxed and not anxious, when we compare the pain felt with anti-anxiety drugs to pain under hypnotism without any suggestions of analgesia and to pain experienced by highly hypnotizable subjects using hypnoanesthesia, we find that hypnotism can affect both the affective and perceptual dimensions of pain experiences; it is more than a mere tranquilizer.[62] Indeed, to get a true hypnoanasthetic effect, the subject has to be specifically told not to feel the pain; merely focusing the subject's attention on something else or mentioning pleasant experiences are not enough[63] (though high hypnotizables can decrease their pain experiences with both direct and indirect suggestions[64]).

In addition, when looking at the amplitudes of EP waveforms, high hypnotizables show a significant reduction under conditions of relaxation, dissociation, and focused analgesia, and the EP waveform amplitude decreases for low hypnotizables under relaxation and dissociation. It appears that hypnotic analgesia reduces reports of pain intensity more than reports of pain unpleasantness; hypnotic relaxation reduces pain unpleasantness more than intensity,[65] though this issue is not settled.[66] In any event, high hypnotizables can reduce their pain experiences with things like analgesia suggestion, guided imagery, word memory, and pursuit-motor tasks, none of which work as well with low hypnotizables. However, when the data are reanalyzed and controlled for habituation, conditioning, and neural receptor fatigue, there is only a significant difference between the baseline and the focused analgesia condition with the high hypnotizable group and none for the low hypnotizables.[67]

Nevertheless, the tranquilizing effects of hypnotism should not be underestimated. Even low hypnotizables experience some diminution of pain under hypnotic suggestions of anesthesia or analgesia, even though this reduction does not show in their EP waves.[68] This decrease in pain has been traced to the relaxing effects of attempted hypnosis and is comparable to what one gets with a placebo drug.[69] Interestingly and inexplicably, high hypnotizables show up to four times greater reductions in pain than do low hypnotizables with relaxation alone.[70]

We also know that hypnosis does indeed attenuate the R-III nociceptive spinal reflex.[71] Some of what the hypnotic suggestion for analgesia must tap into are the descending antinociceptive mechanisms that exert control at the spinal cord. (I should note, however, that this effect is very small and that we still have no idea how this could be happening, if it actually is.) But this is not all that hypnotism is doing, since the reduction in the reflex does not match the reduction in pain intensity, as described by the subjects. In addition, the reduction in pain intensity does not match the reduction in unpleasantness that subjects also report. This tells us that hypnotism acts along at least three dimensions: it reduces the input from the spinal column to the brain, it prevents what nociceptive and pain information does make it to the higher cortical centers from reaching consciousness, and it keeps us from judging what sensations we do experience as awful.[72]

Converging evidence suggests that the frontal lobes, perhaps as part of a frontal lobe-limbic system circuit, are involved in hypnotic dissociation.[73] When the EPs are measured over the frontal areas during hypnotic analgesia, the amplitude of the negative components increases relative to waking measurements. If the noxious stimuli are repeated regularly, then there is a left hemisphere positivity that occurs prior to each stimulus occurrence as the frontal lobes anticipate and prepare for what is about to come.[74]

One hypothesis is that highly hypnotizable people are better than low hypnotizables at filtering out information using a frontolimbic attentional system. Data indicate that the frontolimbic system underlies effortful, directed attention (as opposed to selective attention, thought to be housed in the posterior cerebral cortex).[75] Perhaps this system works by modulating "lower-level systems (other parts of the brain) by activating or inhibiting particular schemata."[76] It could then function to decrease pain sensations by inhibiting our pain schemata. Since dissociation and distraction techniques also work to decrease pain reports in high hypnotizables, this suggests that the hypnotized are diverting attention from their painful experiences in order to control them.[77]

If this were the case, though, it should fare no better than cognitive-behavioral therapy, which is explicitly designed to reform internal schemas. Clearly, hypnotism is doing more than this. In particular, hypnosis can alter physiological responses as well. It can reduce the number of migraine attacks, as well as reduce the pain felt.[78] It can also change gastric acid secretions and activities in the bowels for persons suffering irritable bowel syndrome.[79] It can reduce the amount of bleeding during surgery and for hemophiliacs[80] as well as decrease inflammation with burns.[81] See figure 8.2 for a summary of demonstrated nonpain medical applications for hypnosis. In sum, hypnosis can effect partial cures as well as actively inhibiting pain. (I wonder what would happen with the concomitant physiological responses to pain that normally do not change under hypnosis—the increased heart rate, etc.—if hypnotized subjects were told to control those in addition to not feeling the pain.)

Though we have no idea how these changes could be occurring, the autonomic nervous system is somehow probably involved. The hypothalamus regulates the autonomic function via its connections to relay stations in the lower brain stem, which in turn are connected to the sympathetic and parasympathetic nervous systems.[82] The hypothalamus is also a major output pathway for the limbic system, which is part of the frontolimbic circuit, of course.

Using regional cerebral blood flow imaging, Helen Crawford and her colleagues discovered that highly hypnotizable people have increased blood flow over the orbitofrontal cortex and over the somatosensory cortex during hypnotic suggestions of analgesia. Interestingly, low

Cardiovascular system	Decease in hypertension Control of bleeding and vascular flow Control of hemophilia Control of Raynaud's disease
Dermatological	Healing burns and wounds Healing psoriasis and eczema Healing warts
Immune system	Controlling allergic reactions Controlling asthma attacks
Central nervous system/muscles	Decreasing frequency of migraines Controlling firbromyalgia Reducing tinnitus Rehabilitating nerve damage
Gastrointestinal	Altering gastric acid secretion Controlling irritable bowel syndrome
Gynacological	Controlling hyperemesis gradivarum Reducing premenstrual tension Altering menstrual cycles
Genitourinary	Controlling enuresis Controlling detrusor instability
Cancer care	Decreasing nausea and vomiting from therapy

Figure 8.2
Documented nonpain medical applications for hypnosis. (From Gonsalkorale 1996.)

hypnotizables' blood flow decreases over somatosensory cortex during hypnotic suggestion.[83] Crawford et al. believe that "the mental effort involved in inhibiting somatosensory information during successful hypnotic analgesia accompanies increased cerebral blood flow in the fronto-orbital cortex." In addition, "the increased CBF of the somatosensory cortex may be reflective of this mental effort as well."[84] People under hypnoanalgesia are actively working with the pain processing itself; they are not simply changing their judgments and reactions to the outputs of the PSS.

The anterior cingulate cortex is connected to both prefrontal cortex and the limbic system.[85] Juri Kropotov and his lab in St. Petersburg have recorded event-related potentials inside the head to painful stimuli under conditions of attention and hypnotically suggested analgesia.[86] Their subjects were two patients with obsessive-compulsive disorder who had electrodes implanted in anterior cingulate cortex, the amygdala, the temporal cortex, and parietal cortex for diagnostic reasons. It turned out that one was hypnotizable, and one wasn't. The hypnotizable and hypnotized patient showed reduced positive EP components in left anterior cingulate cortex followed by an enhanced negative component in left anterior temporal cortex when she was instructed not to feel pain. She also reported very little pain under those conditions. The nonhypnotizable patient showed no changes in brain waves and reported feeling significant pain.

These findings dovetail with the imaging studies in chapter 5 that tied the anterior cingulate to pain processing. It makes sense that under hypnotic analgesia, the activity there would diminish. However, it is also very important to underscore the increase in activity in the anterior temporal cortex. This tells us that this area is working harder at doing something during the task. Perhaps it is actively seeking to control and suppress the pain response elsewhere in the brain. The assumption is that, as James and Binet noted almost a century ago, in order to ignore a particular experience or stimulus, you have to notice it first and then work to eliminate awareness of it. In other words, not feeling pain during hypnosis (and a noxious stimulus) requires more labor on the part of the brain than just going ahead and feeling the pain that is already there.

What Counts as a Cure

What does this parade of data tell us about hypnosis, treating pain, and "mental" cures of physical ailments in general? We can draw a few tentative conclusions. First, as with the other, more traditional methods of treatment, hypnosis does not cure the pain in any normal sense. Instead, under hypnosis, the frontal lobe actively seeks to shut down activity in the anterior cingulate, somatosensory cortex, and perhaps other places as well (the sympathetic nervous system, for example). This means that, instead of there being less activity in the brain associated with pain processing, there is actually more.

Perhaps the mechanism of hypnosis is related or analogous to our attentional system. If it is, then that would explain why distraction tasks work with high hypnotizables as an analgesic as well as why similar areas of the brain light up during focused attention and hypnosis. On the other hand, this hypothesis does not explain why being hypnotized per se adds anything to the treatment. Why doesn't distraction alone work just as well? It also does not explain why hypnotism is so effective at altering physiological function (digestion, blood flow, and so forth). At best, an attentional component to hypnotism is part of the full story.

Why does hypnotism work as well as or better than other available treatments? Insofar as we don't understand exactly what hypnotism is or how it works, I cannot give a good answer to that question. However, I can say that data suggest that hypnotism can affect many different aspects of pain processing. Unlike the more traditional therapies, each of which alters only one or two components of pain, hypnosis appears to be able to influence neural activity on a global scale so that not only are the sensations of pain and our judgments of suffering changed, but our pain behavior, the autonomic concomitants to pain processing, and nociception can change as well. Even though hypnosis does not cure pain in the sense of removing it, it can modify many dimensions of our complex pain processing system. As I have argued in previous chapters, being able to do this is key to treating pain effectively and appropriately.

Finally, understanding hypnosis neurophysiologically is fundamental to explaining how it is that merely talking to a person could produce such low-level physiological changes, how "mental" therapies can affect "physical" difficulties. I hope that the brief description of the neurophysiology of hypnosis helps to demystify the phenomenon a bit. Hypnosis is weird—I will be the first to admit that—but if we can see that it is really nothing more than one identifiable brain circuit influencing others in ways that we already understand and can document, then, appearances aside, hypnosis becomes much more mundane. It is just more of the same, from the brain's point of view.

There are, of course, many fundamental gaps in our understanding. In particular, we have no idea why it is that talking can induce the changes in the brain that it does. Why should telling someone to relax and focus on a shiny object change the inhibitory patterns over cortex? Nevertheless, knowing that it does clarifies a bit the relation between the "mental" and the "physical," in the manner chapter 3 requires. In this case, the "mental" event—being hypnotized—is an activated brain circuit that changes the pattern of activity in other brain areas and circuits via its connections to them, and those patterns of activity ultimately produce the "physical" effects—whether they be changes in behavior via neuromuscular connections, changes in heart rate via the parasympathetic nervous system, or what have you. It is a complex, but purely mechanical and unproblematic, interaction. One would assume that other talking therapies work in an analogous manner.

I have now told you my story about pain. A pain by any other name—chronic pain, psychogenic pain, hysterical pain, psychosomatic pain—is still a pain, and it can be understood best as a complex biological phenomenon. I would like to close this tale by briefly examining what my theory and my approach have to say about another treatment issue, the treatment of pain in infants and children. (As an epilogue, the final chapter looks at the larger implications my approach has for analyzing psychopathologies in general.) The current dispute within pain literature over whether and how much children have pain is disconcerting and rife with moral overtones. Frankly, as a parent with small children of my own, I believe that I would be remiss in not addressing it. From a less personal perspective though, we can see that if my analysis of pain is approximately correct, then the controversy is misanalyzed and misargued on both sides of the fence. If my story is correct, then whether and how to treat pain in infants and children has a very simple, straightforward, and noncontroversial answer.

Pain in Children and Infants

A common yet naive assumption is that pain and pain behavior in children are similar to those of adults. A second common and also naive assumption is that infants do not feel pain. Both are questionable.

I have argued that pain is actually a complicated sensory process and that pain sensations, one tiny component of the entire process, are complex as well. Pain sensations contain at least a sensory component, a sense of localization, a negative reaction to the sensation, and a negative judgment about the reaction. And all of these aspects of pain sensations are informed to some extent by memories of previous experiences with pain. Certainly as children grow and mature, their sense of what feeling pain is will change and become more precise as their mnemonic, cognitive, and emotive capacities grow and mature as well. Children experience pain,[87] but as their life experiences differ, so too their pains will differ from those of adults.[88]

Actually we know quite little about pain processing in children or infants, and what we do know is limited to how they react in largely artificial and clinical situations in which the sensation of pain itself cannot easily be distinguished from any general distress at being in pain.[89] Some experimental data do bear out my conjecture that children experience pain differently from adults. Most studies show that younger infants have diffuse and less well modulated reactions to painful stimuli than do older infants or children.[90] Pricking a young infant with a pin provokes an unlocalized reaction with only an occasional withdrawal reflex; doing the same thing to a twelve-month-old infant elicits a more focused, defensive movement.[91] Anticipatory fear develops at about six months, though in younger infants, previous experience with a noxious stimulus is correlated with less crying to the same stimulus a second time around.[92] Even the youngest infants are affected by painful experiences, though how those effects are expressed changes over time.

Studies of infant reactions to inoculations provide some of the best evidence of diachronic changes in pain response. Over time, the pain reaction itself decreases and anger becomes the more prevalent emotion. The duration of the negative emotion also decreases with the age of the infant, as does the rigidity of the infant's body.[93] These results support the idea that the older we are, the better able we are to anticipate and modulate our pain responses.

There are fewer data concerning pain perception in children. Studies indicate that pain thresholds decrease with age but the ability to localize pain increases.[94] Distress-related behaviors also change: younger children tend to resist an offending procedure and to cry generically; older children are more specific in what they say (not surprisingly) but also flinch, groan, and become rigid.[95] In addition, children with chronic pain often report having pain, but show no typical pain behavior. In contrast to adults, they do not act as though they are in pain.[96] On the other hand, the affective and cognitive dimensions of repeated acute pain in children often resembles those of chronic pain in adults.[97]

These differences are important for how children's pain is treated, for unless we know that, for example, flinching and groaning are uncommon in young children, then, in comparing children's reaction to adults', we would consistently underestimate the amount of pain young children experience. Indeed, nurses do this regularly.[98] Or, unless we know that children with chronic pain often exhibit no pain behavior at all, then we might accuse them of malingering, being hypochondriacal, or worse.

Moreover, because children in general lack the simple coping skills that adults have, they are often more anxious, believe that pain will continue unabated, are more depressed, more frustrated, and more worried, and, consequently, feel more pain than adults do under similar circum-stances.[99] In fact, it is likely that younger children feel more pain and distress than older children do for the same stimuli since the number of available coping strategies for dealing with pain increases with age, as does their use.[100]

In contrast to this conclusion, though, children are consistently treated as experiencing less pain that adults. A recent survey found that only 30 percent of all cancer centers in the United States for children regularly premedicated children undergoing bone marrow aspiration. Other coun-tries often use a general anesthetic with this procedure because it is so painful.[101] Studies of the differences in treatment in the 1970s and 1980s found that less than 50 percent of children aged four to eight who had undergone surgery had received any analgesia during their hospital stay. Those who did get any medication received roughly two doses of anal-gesia. In contrast, virtually all adults receive some sort of pain medication following surgery, and, on average, it amounts to about 21 narcotic and 17 non-narcotic doses per person per hospital stay.[102] In the past, it was common to paralyze children without sedating them in intensive care because of a widespread (but erroneous) belief that children cannot tolerate analgesic and amnesic drugs.[103] Even though the doctors and nurses believe that children and adults suffer similar sorts of pain during burn debridement, a survey showed that only 20 percent of all burn units use analgesics when they debride children's burns.[104]

I believe that I can safely assert without further argument that we can and should do better for our children. We certainly know better.

From the perspective of some, though, this is not the most grievous injustice done to our children in pain. One of the most hotly debated subjects in pediatric care concerns whether infants are insensitive to pain. The presumption has been that young infants, especially premature new-borns, cannot sense pain. As a result, no anesthesia or analgesics are used with heel lances, venipuncture, inoculations, or lumbar punctures. Rarely is medication used with more invasive procedures, such as circumcision, bone marrow aspirations, or ligation of a patent ductus arteriosus.

Jill Lawson, a parent, is responsible for initiating the controversy. Her few words, written in editorial letters to academic journals, speak volumes about the anguish a mother experiences striving to understand what counts as superior medical care for her own gravely ill infant.

Imagine that your baby needs major surgery. You admit him to a major teaching facility with a solid reputation. Feeling foolish for even asking, you question several doctors about anesthesia. The surgical resident who brings you consent forms promises your baby will be put to sleep, and you sign. Imagine finding out later that your son was cut open with no anesthesia at all.

This is not a cut-and-slice horror movie. This is my life. . . . My son . . . was a very tiny, very sick premature baby . . . at a gestational age of 25–26 weeks. During the almost two months of his life, he was on a respirator, with several lung diseases, a heart problem, kidney problems, and a brain bleed. . . . In the United States each year, thousands of preemies with identical medical profiles are born and kept alive, and many of them have the same surgery.

[He] . . . had holes cut on both sides of his neck, another hole cut in his right chest, an incision from his breastbone around to his backbone, his ribs pried apart, and an extra artery near his heart tied off. This was topped off with another hole cut in his left side for a chest tube. The operation lasted 1 1/2 hours. [My son] . . . was awake through it all. The anesthesiologist paralyzed him with Pavulon, a curare drug that left him unable to move, but totally conscious.

When I questioned the anesthesiologist later about her use of Pavulon, . . . she said, it had never been demonstrated to her than premature babies feel pain. She seemed sincerely puzzled . . . why I was concerned. It turns out that such care, or lack thereof, is possible because, as a neonatologist explained, babies, unlike adults, don't go into shock no matter how much agony they suffer. Anesthesiologists take advantage of this, coupled with the patient's inability to complain.[105]

This presumption of insensitivity is curious because it is well documented that infants have a stress response to tissue damage, including sweating, increased heart and respiratory rates, the release of adrenaline, and increased transcutaneous oxygen pressure, as well as the standard crying, facial expressions, and motor behaviors.[106] These responses are easily modified by comforting the infant or administering analgesics. Perhaps the cleanest demonstration of this fact was a randomized study of premature infants undergoing ligation of a patent ductus arteriosus.[107] One group received fentanyl, curare, and nitrous oxide, while the other received nothing. The medicated group showed less of a hormonal response during surgery (as measured by the release of catecholamines, growth hormone, glucagon and corticosteriods, and insulin release) and had fewer metabolic and circulatory complications after the operation. Certainly this shows that infants, even premature ones, are sensitive to pain in some sense or other.

Moreover, we know that newborn rat pups react strongly to painful stimuli, even before their visual or auditory systems are completely on line. The behavioral reflexes are correlated with patterns of neuronal activation in areas tied to pain processing in adult rats.[108] Though similar studies have not been performed on human infants or fetuses (for obvious ethical reasons), it has been shown that human fetuses, extremely premature neonates, and term newborns all show the same hormonal response to noxious stimuli that older children do.[109]

In fact, though the afferent nociceptive system is completely developed by twenty-nine weeks gestation, it is the pain inhibitory system that does not come on line until later. The possibility of suppressing or inhibiting pain processing top-down comes with the final development of the somatosensory system. This is why infants have a more difficult time moderating their pain processing and why they have enhanced acute pain responses as compared to adults.[110] It also explains why they have poorer localization.

K. J. S. Anand, one of the foremost authorities on infant pain processing, believes that there is a good evolutionary explanation for why pain responses are in place very early.[111] Signaling hunger and tissue damage are the most important facts newborns need to communicate; their very survival depends upon these capacities. Therefore, selection pressures should ensure that they will appear—in largely complete form—earlier than any other adaptive behavior. Perhaps this argument is correct, for certainly pain and hunger behaviors occur extremely early in newborns across the entire mammalian kingdom.

It is a separate question whether infants are conscious of pain experiences or whether they can consciously remember them later. It is a different question still whether (if they are conscious) their experiences are like ours. They probably are not, for they simply have not had the life experiences that would allow them to construct complex schemas for painful episodes. If you believe, as I have argued elsewhere,[112] that such schemas are necessary for consciousness, then young infants cannot consciously experience pain, for they cannot consciously experience anything. If you do not believe that schemas are necessary for consciousness, then, at the least, infant pain experiences are quite different than adult pain experiences. Infant experiences would lack the complexity that we have since they lack the ability to interpret, judge, and relate their current experience to past experiences or to expectations of the future.

Neurophysiological considerations bear this out. In human brain development, thalamocortical fibers do not reach the cortex until twenty-six weeks gestation. Before that, we cannot say that the cortex functions as it should since it is essentially not attached to the rest of the brain.[113] PET scans show that the neural activity of somatosensory cortex, prefrontal cortex, and anterior cingulate cortex increases substantially from birth to eighteen months and does not reach mature form until well after a year.[114]

The question is what to make of these facts. Stuart Derbyshire argues to "unless there is the possibility that the neonate has a conscious appreciation of pain, then any responses to noxious stimulation are essentially reflex responses."[115] This is much too strong a position. There is much that goes on in our brains that is neither conscious nor a reflex. Not all cognition passes through consciousness, nor do all evaluative or emotional reactions, as subliminal priming data show. Moreover, insofar as the experience of pain is but one minor component of pain processing itself, these queries are less interesting. We can say with certitude that all infants react to pain, both behaviorally and physiologically, that these reactions can be modified with relatively simple treatments, and that treating pain has an impact on recovery.

In addition, we know that early exposure to pain, whether remembered or not, affects later experiences of and reactions to pain by altering the developmental course of the nervous system. Infants, like other newborn animals, learn to attach particular meanings or emotions or importance to particular experiences in virtue of what is associated with those experiences. This sort of behavioral malleability is very important if an organism is going to survive in a complex environment. Consequently, manipulating early experiences can have drastic effects later on, as animal studies show. Merely by changing the smells associated with suckling, scientists can alter adult sexual behavior in male rats, for example.[116]

Similar changes occur with pain processing in young infants. It makes a difference to how they are later. In both animals, we find that nociceptive stimuli increases the size of the somatic receptive fields for neurons sensitive to pain and helps maintain dendritic connections that would otherwise be eliminated over time.[117] It looks as though chronic pain and hypersensitivity can result from early acute pain episodes, given how the neural receptors change.[118] Early pain experiences can also influence later personality and temperament.[119] Something as common as circumcision has lasting effects on pain sensitivity if done without anesthesia.[120]

In sum, we have every reason to prevent infant pain, even if it is nothing like our own, even if it is like nothing at all for the infant. In fact, we have reason to use preemptive analgesia[121] with infants, given the impact early pain processing can have on later development. Whether infants or children consciously experience pain—and the degree to which they may or may not be aware of noxious stimuli or suffering—is a red herring. All available evidence leads us to the conclusion that both infants and children process pain, though perhaps not as complex a manner as adults. This processing affects their current behavior and later development in negative ways. Insofar as we have the power to prevent or alleviate some of the pain, then we should.[122]

Understanding pain as a biologically based processing system, with the sensation of pain being only one component among many relevant to whether an organism is in pain, sheds light on how we should approach discussing pain in infants, children, and other nonlinguistic creatures. If we do not worry so much about what a creature might be feeling but concern ourselves more with the larger effects of tissue damage and pain processing, then we can see that treating pain should depend on alleviating activity in several areas of the nervous system and not just on eliminating aspects of sensation.

9

Epilogue: Pain as a Paradigm for Philosophical Psychopathology

Pain—has an element of Blank—
It cannot recollect
When it begun—or if there were
A time when it was not—.
—Emily Dickenson

Although the world is full of suffering, it is full also of the overcoming of it.
—Helen Keller

I have argued that the best way to understand pain processing is using a biological model. This stands in direct opposition to the recommendation of the IASP, most psychiatrists, and many psychologists. Nevertheless, understanding what is happening in the brain dissolves most of the mysteries surrounding pain phenomena.

Pain processing, as compared to many mind and brain processes, is relatively straightforward. This is not to say that we understand exactly why we are in pain, especially in the cases of chronic pain. However, because we do know some things about what pain is, how we approach explaining and treating pain phenomena should provide us with a good paradigm for how to explain and treat other pathologies. We can draw several lessons from my discussion in previous chapters that should be applicable to psychopathologies in general. Here are a few.

• *Understanding the neurophysiology of a disorder is tremendously useful in defining the illness.* Given my view of pain processing, "psychogenic" pain is not a mental disorder at all. It is entirely likely that these sorts of "mental" pains have a traditional "physical" cause that we are as of yet unable to detect. Many of the same areas of the brain are affected by psychogenic pain as they are by regular acute pain. In both cases, our multidimensional pain processing system is activated, with the concomitant psychological reactions, interpretations, memories, expectations, and experiences. Our view of what pain is, how it works, and when it is disordered changes radically with biological information.

Autism might present a similar case in point. Autism was first identified by Leo Kanner in 1943, and he described the symptoms of a male child in vivid detail:

[The child] seems almost to . . . live within himself. . . . He did not respond to being called, and did not look at his mother when she spoke to him. . . . He never looked up at people's faces. When he had any dealings with persons at all, he treated them, or rather parts of them, as if they were objects. . . . On a crowded beach, he would walk straight toward his goal irrespective of whether this involved walking over newspapers, hands, feet, or torsos.[1]

Though well over a half-century has passed since that description, most current clinical accounts do little better. For example, Simon Baron-Cohen writes:

[The patient] never really seemed to look at anyone directly. Rather, he would look fleetingly or else not at all. . . . He would also do things that his parents found embarrassing, like grabbing and eating sandwiches from a stranger's plate at restaurants. . . . Most of the time [he] . . . was to be found on his own, busying himself with one of his special interests, more absorbed in counting lamp posts than playing with other children.[2]

The key features of . . . autism . . . include lack of normal eye contact, lack of normal social awareness or appropriate social behavior, "aloneness," one-sidedness in interaction, and inability to join a social group.[3]

As long as descriptions have remained on the level of the behavioral or the cognitive, autism has remained a syndrome of bizarre and inexplicable symptoms. However, instead of thinking of autism as a cluster of features (and rather poorly described ones at that), we might instead start thinking about autism as something like an atrophied vermis of the cerebellum.[4] This underlying neurobiological structure provides a good peg on which to hang the diverse symptomotology; hence, we need not consider autism any longer to be a syndrome of relatively disconnected attributes. Indeed, knowing how the brain is affected by autism expands our view of the role of the cerebellum in cognitive processing (it is affiliated with attentional shifts as well as motor processing),[5] gives us an approximate gestational time of onset (five weeks),[6] and unites the features of autism under a larger cognitive umbrella (attentional deficits).[7]

As Eric Courchesne notes in an abstract for a recent commentary:

Although remediation-oriented research aims at alleviation of symptoms for today's patients, . . . a basic science perspective seeks insights into the triggering causes and pathogenesis of the disorder from which better diagnosis and remediation may be devised for patients in the future. . . . Research in autism can progress beyond the impasse of disagreement and competition toward information integration and insight by means of dialogue, data exchange, discussion, collaboration, and cooperation.[8]

I have shown that the same is true for pain research, and, I believe, it is also true for research in any other psychological or behavioral disorder.

• *Focusing on neurobiology prevents clinicians and others from covertly adopting some form of dualism to explain various pathologies.* I hold that, however intuitive, the IASP definition of pain is unworkable because it forces one to divide the mental from the physical in unnatural ways. To be more precise: it implies that pain sensations correspond to no particular underlying neurological activity. Materialists must reject this position outright. We need to understand how our neural circuits instantiate psychological disorders, and what exactly has gone awry in the brain to cause such difficulties. This is what a full explanation must contain.

Though I believe the dualism inherent in pain research reaches further than in other clinical areas, the tendency is still there to define and explain psychopathologies solely in terms of mental phenomena, mental phenomena largely divorced from underlying neuronal activity. Hysteria, malingering, dissociative disorders, various sexual dysfunctions, and some addictions are good examples of psychopathologies for which the brain is generally not assumed to be relevant. Nevertheless, adopting a multilevel perspective helps explain why interfering with, for example, neurotransmitters affects higher-level cognitive states, and why using a talking therapy helps those with "lower-level" disorders cope. It also helps forge appropriate treatments and social policies.

Research in addiction provides a clear case in point. We know now that initial exposure to an "addictive" drug, like opium or cocaine, inhibits the cAMP (adenosin 3′,5′-monophosphate) pathway in many neuronal systems in the brain. With repeated exposure, the brain compensates by up-regulating the cAMP pathways in at least some of the neural systems. When the drug is no longer consumed, the pathways remain up-regulated. One hypothesis about how the up-regulation leads to the addictive behaviors and symptoms of withdrawal is that some of the cAMP pathways contain GABAergic neurons, which in turn innervate dopaminergic and serotonergic neurons. Up-regulation would increase the release of GABA, which would then decrease the activity of the dopaminergic and serotonergic neurons.[9] Decreases in dopamine and serotonin is associated with depression, aversion, attentional disorders, dysphoria, anxiety, irritability, and inhibited motivation, all symptoms of withdrawal.

To put these data in a broader context, we can say that drugs like cocaine, ethanol, opium, and THC (to a moderate degree) affect our internal reward system. Consuming the drugs elicits positive reinforcement responses in our brain, and ceasing the drugs causes negative reinforcement responses. The negative-affective state we see with withdrawal may be permanent to an extent, increasing the probability of relapse in former users, especially when they are under stress (which also affects the dopaminergic system).[10]

All the research points to "addiction" being a problem with regulating (or dysregulating) our brain's innate reward system. Once that system is thrown enough out of whack, subjects will compulsively seek the drugs that alleviate their distress and for which they have been internally rewarded for consuming in the past. Though the chemistry of the brain is far from simple, its connection to addiction is becoming clearer and easier to understand. At bottom, addiction is the product of the brain's attempt to maintain its equilibrium under abnormal conditions.

However, these facts have had little impact on professional treatments for drug abuse or public policy for handling abusers, and even less on popular culture's view of users. Most see addiction as a social problem, in which the addict is morally responsible for her unhappy fate. Alan Lesher of the National Institute of Drug Abuse points out that "one major barrier [to connecting science to the public] is the tremendous stigma attached to being a drug user or, worse, an addict. . . . [T]he more common view is that drug addicts are weak or bad people, unwilling to lead moral lives and to control their behavior and gratifications. . . . As just one example, there are many people who believe that addicted individuals do not even deserve treatment."[11]

Similar to the IASP definition of pain, our lay understanding of addicts detaches the symptomology from the physical world. Being "weak" or "bad" or "uncontrolled" can only make sense as a higher-level description of some brain configuration or other. However, from a purely materialist perspective, attaching moral worth to the homeostatic drives of an internal organ is odd to say the least. Our everyday view of drug abuse and what we know to be happening in the brain do not jibe, for the former contains attributes that are (prima facie, anyway) irreducible to the latter.

Lesher concludes that "it is time to replace ideology with science."[12] I agree. I go further: we should replace mentalistic ideology with philosophically sound science.

• *Being aware of the complexity of brain processing, especially processing done outside awareness, decreases the dependence of clinical diagnoses on (notoriously unreliable) subjective reports.* How things seem to us is only the tip of the cognitive iceberg and really only gives us the barest of hints about what is occurring in the brain. Focusing on the malfunctions of entire brain systems, as opposed to a cluster of subjective phenomena, should force clinicians to hone their diagnostic tools and prevent them from lumping different pathologies into the same categories. It should also prevent subject experience from being the sole defining criteria for various disorders.

In addition to my other reasons for why relying almost exclusively on subject experience for cognitive or brain disorders is a bad idea, making experience or reports of experience as a significant (or sole) criterion for psychiatry gives rise to odd facts, facts that might be very important, diagnostically or otherwise, but facts for which we have no idea what they mean when considered from a "mental" perspective alone. For example, pain is the most common complaint in psychiatric patients presenting for the first time.[13] In particular, schizophrenics and persons suffering from depression report feeling pain as the reason for visiting the hospital or clinic and report no other significant symptoms. Why is this? What connection is there between the sensations of pain and suffering and schizophrenia or depression?

None of the usual clinical diagnostics even address this issue. However, if we could understand what these mental disorders are in the brain and how they interfere with our PSS and our PIS, then we would understand the connection. This might let us refine our measuring instruments so that we could diagnose the disorders more swiftly and with greater accuracy. This might force a change in how we understand the "disorder," as a biological appreciation of drug use does. It might also lead us to reformulate basic brain functions, as a biological explanation of autism does.

Obsessive-Compulsive Disorder presents us with another strange puzzle if only considered from a phenomenological point of view. Here is one man's description of what it is like to have lived with OCD:

I cannot really describe the torturous pain of the anxiety brought on by an Obsessive-Compusive Disorder attack. . . . My symptoms were typical of obsessive-compulsives. I would check the gas oven and door locks, sometimes 20 times before I could go to bed at night. I would worry about poisoning myself and others with insecticides or cleaning fluids I may have touched. I would drive home from work, thinking that I left the light on in my office and drive all the way back to see if it was off: "It could start a fire." Sometimes I did this more than once in a day. . . . Each obsessive incident was accompanied by the fantasy that if I *didn't* act on it, something terrible would happen to me or someone else. . . . Making *sure* these outcomes would not occur drives my compulsive behaviors.[14]

From this description, it is clear that he believes that his need to control his anxiety causes his bizarre behaviors. He acts voluntarily. His anxiety might be abnormal, but his responses are rational, all things considered.

But compare this description with his own advice to parents with OCD children:

Your child has absolutely *no control* over what he or she is doing . . . NONE. . . . You cannot intellectually understand why your child does what he or she does. Don't try to understand in this way because . . . normal human reasoning and logic do not exist with this disease. The only logic is your child's relentless pain, his enormous need to stop this pain and his involuntary behavior geared to this end.[15]

Even though he holds that his behavior is of his own devising, at the same time he also believes that it is completely involuntary. He feels as though he is acting freely, yet he believes that he is not. How can this be?

If we expand our view of OCD to include interactions between conscious thoughts and feelings and unconsciously generated drives, then the patient's descriptions and advice seem less paradoxical. He is stuck engaging in his ritual behaviors for biological reasons still unclear (the best theories to date suggest that OCD is a perversion of our innate nesting capacities)—think of a needle stuck in a groove in a record—however, part of what is "stuck" is the experience of freely choosing his behavior.

Still, all of these lessons—that neurophysiology helps us define psychiatric disorders, that it prevents covert dualism, and that it decreases dependence on subject reports—should be tempered by the knowledge that there is quite a lot that we don't know about the brain. I expect that our theories of various psychopathologies will be radically overthrown in short order. We really are flying by the seat of our pants here, and we can only be better researchers and clinicians if we acknowledge that fact up front.

Pain is a very commonplace and relatively simple phenomenon, yet we have difficulty describing it completely, much less treating it successfully. Other pathologies are only more complex and less well understood. Remaining humble is our best intellectual strategy.

Notes

Chapter 1 The Myths of Pain

1. This section owes much to Caton 1985, Chaves and Dworkin 1997, and R. Rey 1993.
2. Galen [1821] 1997, 512.
3. Petit [1499] 1502, 90–91.
4. Rey 1993, 350.

Chapter 2 Pathological Pains

1. Lempert et al. 1990.
2. Frymoyer and Cats-Baril 1991, Report of the Panel on Pain 1979.
3. Meade et al. 1990, 1995, Rowe 1969.
4. Deyo and Tsui-Wu 1987, Murtagh 1994.
5. Merskey and Spear 1967, D. C. Turk 1994.
6. Stephenson and Leroux 1994.
7. Ziegler and Schlemmer 1994.
8. While familial patterns of inexplicable pains are not completely unheard of, they are quite rare. The only other case I could find in recent literature concerns a middle-aged woman in New Zealand who has complained of abdominal pain for over twenty years, resulting in more than thirty-six hospitalizations. Her five children have also had twenty-five hospitalizations for abdominal pain. No physical cause for their distress has ever been found (Joyce and Walshe 1980).
9. Sthalekar 1993.
10. Hausotter 1996.
11. Liniger and Molineus 1930.
12. Engel 1959, as discussed in Gamsa and Vikis-Freibergs 1991, 271.

13. American Psychiatric Association 1968.

14. American Psychiatric Association 1980.

15. American Psychiatric Association 1987.

16. Cf. Blackwell, Mersky, and Kellner 1989, Dworkin and Burgess 1987.

17. King and Strain 1996.

18. Faravelli et al. 1997.

19. Francis, First, and Pincus 1995.

20. American Psychiatric Association 1994.

21. Francis, First, and Pincus 1995, 94.

22. King 1995, Martin 1995.

23. Fishbain 1996.

24. King and Strain 1996.

25. This claim is made on the basis of a computer search for all journal articles published in 1994 through June 1997 on Medline and PsychLit using the subject term "pain" and each of the following second subject terms: "DSM-IV," "somatoform," "psychogenic," and "disorder."

26. Rogers et al. 1996; see also Ghia et al. 1979, Gomez and Dally 1977, Haegerstam and Allerbring 1995, Pillay and Lalloo 1989, and Potts and Bass 1995 for similar failures to secure proper controls.

27. Cf. Drossman 1982, Gustafson and Kallmen 1990, Peyrot, Moody, and Wiese 1993.

28. Cf. Dworkin 1994, Lucas et al. 1995.

29. Allodi and Goldstein 1995; see also Blumer et al. 1982, and Valdes et al. 1988 for equally ambiguous results.

30. Reiter et al. 1991; see also Adler et al. 1989.

31. Walling et al. 1994.

32. Naidoo and Patel 1993.

33. Van Houdenhove and Joostens 1995.

34. Almay, Haggendal, von Knorring, and Oreland 1987, Valdes et al. 1989; see also Almay, von Knorring, and Wetterberg 1987 and von Knorring and Ekselius 1994 for similar arguments concerning melatonin levels in pain and depression patients.

35. Similarly, patients under the age of forty seeking emergency care at a hospital for chest pains without obvious organic cause are more anxious and neurotic than healthy controls (Roll and Theorell 1987). Researchers conclude that anxiety and other personality disorders increase likelihood of psychogenic chest pain, but could also be that more anxious people are more likely to seek emergency care for their pains.

36. Cobishley et al. 1990.

37. Davidson et al. 1985; see also Magni, Schifano, and de Leo 1985.

38. Valdes et al. 1989, Lee, Giles, and Drummond 1993; see also Gatchel, Polatin, and Kinney 1995 and Magni, de Bertoli, Dodi, and Infantino 1986.

39. Blumer and Heilbronn 1982, Lesse 1974.

40. Gamsa 1994b, Wittchen et al. 1993, though see Polatin et al. 1993.

41. Katon, Egan, and Miller 1985, Sullivan et al. 1992.

42. Ciccone, Just, and Bandilla 1996.

43. Chaney et al. 1984, Schmidt and Wallace 1982.

44. Love and Peck 1987, Naliboff, Cohen, and Yellen 1982, Smyth 1984, Watson 1982.

45. Leavitt and Katz 1989, Rook, Pesch, and Keeler 1981.

46. Wade et al. 1992.

47. Cox, Chapman, and Black 1978, Leavitt 1985, Rook, Pesch, and Keeler 1981, Sivik 1991, and Trief et al. 1987, though see Etscheidt et al. 1995.

48. Levitan et al. 1985; see also Magni, Andreoli, de Leo, Martinotti, and Rossi 1986, and Walker et al. 1995.

49. The value of other large-scale diagnostic tools, such as the epidural administration of fentanyl and placebos, is equally unclear; see Cherry et al. 1985 vs. Stanley et al. 1993.

50. Cf. Giles and Crawford 1997.

51. Hendler, Zinreich, and Kozikowski 1993.

52. Mavromichalis et al. 1992; see also Alfven 1993.

53. Grushka, Sessle, and Miller 1987.

54. Benjamin et al. 1988, Freeman 1993, Grushka, Sessle, and Miller 1987, Hendler, Zinreich, and Kozilowski 1993, Kupers et al. 1991, Merskey 1984, 1989b, Ochoa and Verdugo 1995, Sanchez-Villasenor et al. 1995, Sherman, Sherman, and Bruno 1987, Simpson and Gjerkingen 1989, Ziegler and Schlemmer 1994.

55. Hendler, Zeinrich, and Kozikowski 1993.

56. Hendler, Bergson, and Morrison 1996.

57. Hendler, Zeinrich, and Kozikowski 1993.

58. Phillips and Grant 1991.

59. Keel 1984.

60. Barker and Mayou 1992, Lindal and Uden 1988, Trief et al. 1987; see also Joukamaa 1987.

61. Arntz and Peters 1995.

62. Asmundson and Norton 1995, Carlsson 1986, Gamsa 1990, Joukamaa 1991, Kohler and Kosanic 1992, Lesser and Lesser 1983, Sherman, Sherman, and Bruno 1987, Watson 1982.

63. Cox et al. 1994, Sriram et al. 1987; see also Bayer et al. 1993, Lindal 1990.

64. Ahles et al. 1991.

65. Asmundson and Norton 1995.

66. Jensen 1988.

67. Chaturvedi and Michael 1986.

68. Ghia et al. 1981; see also Johansson et al. 1979.

69. G. R. Smith 1992.

70. Ekselius et al. 1996.

71. Kisely, Creed, and Cotter 1992.

72. Apley 1975, Collins and Stone 1966, Cooper et al. 1987, Gamsa and Vikis-Freibergs 1991, Grzesiak and Ciccone 1994, Merskey 1965a, b, Merskey and Spear 1967, Merskey et al. 1985, Muhs and Schepank 1995, Rossi, Cortinovus, and Bellettini 1992, Roy 1982, Salter et al. 1983, Singer 1977, Zeisat 1978.

73. Ciccone, Just, and Bandilla 1996, Linton and Gotestam 1985.

74. Cf. Gamsa 1994b.

75. Gamsa 1994b.

76. Hendler and Kozikowski 1993, 94, 90.

77. Sternbach 1977; see also Lipowski 1990.

78. Baum and Defidio 1995; see also Dworkin 1994.

79. Lim 1994, Sanchez-Villasenor et al. 1995.

80. Ochoa and Verdugo 1995.

81. Shorter 1997.

82. Chibnall, Duckro, and Richardson et al. 1995, Taylor, Skeleton, and Butcher 1984; see also Ryden et al. 1985.

83. Cf. Unruh 1996.

84. Anzai and Merkin 1996, Asnes, Santulli, and Bemporad 1981, Milov and Kantor 1990.

85. Benjamin, Mawer, and Lennon 1992.

86. Garber, Zemon, and Walker 1990, McGrath et al. 1983, Walker and Greene 1989, Walker, Garber, and Greene 1993, though see Robinson, Alverez, and Dodge 1990.

87. Walker, Garber, and Greene 1991.

88. Adelman and Shank 1988.

89. Reiter et al. 1991, Rosenthal 1993, Walker et al. 1992, Walker et al. 1995; see also Walker et al. 1988.

90. Wood, Weisner, and Reiter 1990.

91. Levitan et al. 1985, Rosenthal 1993.

92. Peveler et al. 1996.

93. Fry, Crisp, and Beard 1997; see also Slocumb et al. 1989.

94. Cf. Keel 1984, Menges 1983.

95. Devinsky 1996, Payrot, Moody, and Wiese 1993, Wigley 1994.

Chapter 3 Mind over Matter?

1. American Psychiatric Association 1994.

2. Francis, First, and Pincus 1995, 87.

3. I am going to set aside for the moment whether this belief is part of the pain itself or whether it accompanies my other mental state, the sensation of pain. For our purposes here, it doesn't matter whether you consider the belief that damage is occurring now there part of being in pain as long as you can agree that these mental states sometimes accompany painful events.

4. Quine 1960.

5. Fodor 1987, 97.

6. Some find this claim quite disconcerting and expend a great deal of energy in articulating visions of noncontentful mental states or of psychologies that don't refer to this view of the mind. I am choosing to ignore this cottage industry here, and, instead, I focus my attention on the general issue of how we should understand the mind as a completely natural and nonmysterious phenomenon, given that it has all (or most) of the attributes we normally think of it having.

7. Here I am just stating this as fact. It has been argued extensively in Hardcastle 1996. See also Crane and Mellor 1990 for more discussion along these lines.

8. Fodor 1987, 1990a, b, Block 1986, Devitt 1990a, b, Dretske 1981, 1988, Field 1978, Loar 1981, Lycan 1988, Millikan 1984, Papineau 1987, Schiffer 1982, Stalnaker 1984.

9. Fodor 1990a, 156.

10. Fodor 1987, xii.

11. Fodor 1990c, 202–203.

12. Dretske 1988, 1.

13. Stich 1993, Stich and Laurence 1994; see also Stich 1996.

14. Tye 1994a, b presents a similar view to mine.

15. Fodor 1990a, 156.

16. Stich and Laurence 1994, 160.

17. Stich 1993; see also Stich and Laurence 1994, 178.

18. Schiffer 1982, 119, as quoted in Stich and Laurence 1994.

19. See discussion in chapter 1 for references.

20. See also Fodor's 1974 discussion on "token physicalism."

21. Crane and Mellor 1990 take my position to be so unproblematic and trivial that for them it really isn't a serious position at all.

22. Stich 1993.

23. Lest one think that irreducibility is a hallmark of the psychological sciences, let me hasten to note that the connection between theories in physics exhibits quite a range of specific ontological relations. (I take these examples from Bickle 1997). The reduction between physical optics and Maxwell's equations is relatively smooth; we only need minor corrections to the laws of physical optics to reduce physical optics to electromagnetism. On the other hand, the connection between thermodynamics and statistical mechanics is less smooth; we generally understand thermodynamical theories to picture the limiting conditions on statistical mechanics. But no one uses these facts to argue that physics isn't physical (thank goodness!).

24. Much discussion of the point can be found in Bechtel 1982, 1983, Fodor 1974, Hardcastle 1992, Mayr 1982, Wimsatt 1976.

25. Reiter et al. 1991; see also Adler et al. 1989.

26. I also depart from what the Churchlands argue. They contend that we have to understand reductive relations as relations among *theories* in which objects and properties are defined. Though I do believe that our observations and just about everything else are theory-laden, I do not think that claiming that I am a field in Hilbert space requires biology or psychology (it does require physics, of course). Though there is a coevolution of our ontological commitments and our scientific theories, there are also ontological commitments made prior to any well-developed theory, especially to the midsized objects. However, the Churchlands are focused on answering the second question and explicating the appropriate relationship that holds between mind and body. My project is much less ambitious; I only want to define the minimal requirements for materialism.

27. Rosch 1973, 1978, 1981, Rosch and Mervis 1975.

28. See P. S. Churchland 1986, Rumelhart and McClelland 1986.

29. P. M. Churchland 1989 attempts such an argument.

30. Stich and Laurence 1994.

31. My thanks to R. Hugh Walker for supplying these definitions.

32. See especially Stich 1993.

33. Stich 1993.

34. Burge 1979, 1986, Putnam 1979.

35. Brown 1992, Burge 1979, 1986, Godfrey-Smith 1989, Putnam 1979.

36. Cf. Hardcastle 1997.

37. Brand and Yancey 1993, 3–5.

Chapter 4   What We Don't Know about Brains: Two Competing Perspectives

1. Most of the facts provided in this section come from Cytowic 1996. He provides a very readable introduction to the brain.

2. Brodmann 1909.

3. Lorente de Nó 1943.

4. McCulloch and Pitt 1943.

5. Mountcastle 1957.

6. Hubel and Weisel 1972.

7. Dennett 1971, Bechtel and Richardson 1993.

8. Churchland and Sejnowski 1992, 1–2.

9. Carstens and Watkins 1986; see also Carstens and Douglass 1995.

10. Carstens and Campbell 1992.

11. Coderre and Katz 1998, Torebjörk, Lamotte, and Robinson 1992.

12. Chung et al. 1979, Dougherty and Willis 1992, Kenshalo et al. 1979, Kenshalo et al. 1982, Perl 1976, Price et al. 1978, Simone et al. 1991.

13. Schouenbourg and Dickenson 1985.

14. Cervero, Handwerker, and Laird 1988, Cook et al. 1987, Hoheisel and Mense 1989, Hylden et al. 1989, McMahan and Wall 1984, Woolf and King 1990; see also discussion in Coderre and Katz 1998.

15. Coderre and Katz 1997, 416.

16. Carstens 1996, 24.

17. Cf. Seltzer et al. 1990, Takaishi, Eisele, and Carstens 1996.

18. Other measures did show a decrease in withdrawal latency, so at best, the results are unclear.

19. Cf. Behbehani and Dollberg-Stolik 1994; see also Carstens 1997.

20. Carstens 1996, Takaishi, Eisele, and Carstens 1996.

21. Churchland and Sejnowski 1992, 36.

22. Sejnowski and Churchland 1988, Stufflebeam and Bechtel 1997.

23. McKeown 1997.

24. Quoted in Barinaga 1997.

25. A sampling of proponents of this view include Braitenberg 1984, Freeman 1991, Gallez and Babloyantz 1991, Glass and Mackey 1988, Henden, Horn, and Usher 1991, Kelso 1995, Mandel and Selz 1991, Mpitsos 1989, Skarda and Freeman 1987, Zak 1990; see also Van Gelder and Port 1995, Smith and Thelen 1993.

26. See discussion in Grush 1997, 234, Ashby 1952.

27. Katchalsky, Rowland, and Blumenthal 1974, 152, as quoted in Kelso 1995, 258.

28. Good introductions to dynamical systems theory and chaos (at varying degrees of difficulty) are Devaney 1987, Glass and Mackey 1988, Gleick 1987, Kellert 1993.

29. Agnati, Bjelke, and Fuxe 1992, Fuxe and Agnati 1991.

30. Cytowic 1996, 134–135.

31. Van Gelder and Port 1995, Van Gelder 1995.

32. As discussed in Bains 1997.

33. Hebb 1949.

34. Miller, Keller, and Stryker 1989, Obermayer, Ritter, and Schulten 1992.

35. Crair, Gillespie, and Stryker 1998.

36. For example, Britton and Skevington 1996, Lutzenberger, Flor, and Birbaumer 1997, Panescu, Webster, and Stratbucker 1994, Sviderskaya and Kovalev 1996.

37. The neurons in the dorsal horn keyed to a broad band of input are called "wide dynamic range" or "mulitreceptive" neurons. The experimental procedure and conditions are described in Sandkühler and Eblen-Zajjur 1994.

38. Debus and Sandkühler 1996; see also Sandkühler 1996.

39. The algorithm is found in Grassberger and Procaccia 1983.

40. Eckman and Ruelle 1985.

41. This too is the sort of perspective one might adopt using the imaging data. Here we find different areas of the brain responding to different sorts of pain, with the individual neuronal contributions washed out. Furthermore, this might be one way of cashing out what one means by "psychologically" caused pain. If the mental just is the higher or abstract or complex organization of some physical structure, then data such as EEG recordings and fMRI, PET, and SPECT scans might be indexing psychological variables.

42. I take this example from Garson 1996, 314–315.

43. Garson 1996, 314.

44. Eliasmith 1997, 450.

45. Robertson, Cohen, and Mayer-Kess 1993, 119.

Chapter 5   The Nature of Pain

1. Apkarian 1995.

2. This is known as the binding problem in psychology; see Hardcastle 1994 for discussion.

3. Dennett 1987.

4. Dretske 1981, 1988.

5. Lehky, and Sejnowski 1988.

6. Cytowic 1989, 1993, Hubbard 1996, Rizzo and Eslinger 1989, Victor 1989.

7. Kandel and Schwartz 1985.

8. P. S. Churchland 1986.

9. Wright 1973.

10. Emmers 1981 describes modality-specific firing patterns in thalamus.

11. Even the classic story is becoming more complicated; see Kandel, Schwartz, and Jessel et al. 1995, chap. 27.

12. I owe this vision of the classic view to Cross's 1994 excellent review article. See also Kandel and Schwartz 1985 and Roland 1992a, b.

13. Information traveling at the slower speeds would take about 8 seconds to reach the spinal column in a horse from its hoof.

14. Though see Schott 1994 for contrary evidence. Other neurons that show this sort of convergence are the "nociceptive-specific" neurons in lamina I and the "complex" neurons in laminae VII and VIII of the dorsal horn. The interaction of autonomic information with somatic appears to be quite common throughout our pain system.

15. A. D. Craig et al. 1994.

16. P. M. Churchland 1985a, b, Dennett 1978.

17. Armstrong 1981, Newton 1989, Pritcher 1970.

18. Gillett 1991, Grahek 1991, McGinn 1983.

19. Wittgenstein 1953.

20. Melzack and Wall 1965 and Hilgard and Hilgard 1994 both argue that there are three components to pain processing: the discriminative, the affective-emotional, and the evaluative. I find little physiological evidence to support these claims. Here I only discuss two components.

21. See Hilgard and Hilgard 1994 for discussion.

22. Gracely, Dubner, and McGrath 1982.

23. Davis et al. 1995, French, Chou, and Story 1966, Head and Holmes 1911, Roland 1992a, b.

24. Chudler and Dong 1995a, b.

25. Wall 1989a, b.

26. See discussion in Hilgard and Hilgard 1994, Jensen and Rasmussen 1989.

27. Davis et al. 1995, Keay et al. 1994.

28. As reported in Gamsa 1994a.

29. Melzack, Wall, and Ty 1982.

30. Beecher 1956.

31. Evoked potential recordings of painful stimuli under hypnosis indicate that at least activity in the frontal lobe is affected (Helen Crawford, personal conversation).

32. Evans 1974.

33. Exactly what processing algorithms are being executed is a more complicated story, and one heavily influenced by the pain inhibitory system. Accounting for the details of the computations is beyond the scope of this chapter.

34. Critchley 1956, Sternbach 1963, 1968.

35. See also Wall 1989a. This view too accounts for why our C-fiber systems might be so slow. General monitoring of bodily conditions should not often require a quick response.

36. Ingvar 1975, Ingvar et al. 1976, Apkarian et al. 1992, Casey et al. 1996, Coghill et al. 1994.

37. Cf. Apkarian 1995.

38. Casey et al. 1994a, Coghill et al. 1994, Davis et al. 1997, Derbyshire, Jones, Brown, et al. 1993, Jones et al. 1991, Talbot et al. 1991, Vogt, Derbyshire, and Jones 1996.

39. Casey et al. 1994b.

40. Apkarian et al. 1992, Backonja et al. 1991, Duncan et al. 1994, Hsieh et al. 1995.

41. Apkarian 1995, Apkarian et al. 1992.

42. Guyton 1991.

43. Davis et al. 1995, Evans, Meyer, and Marret 1992, Hsieh et al. 1995, Roland 1992a, b, Stea and Apkarian 1992.

44. Drevets et al. 1995.

45. LeDoux 1993, LeDoux et al. 1988, LeDoux, Farb, and Ruggiero 1990.

46. Chapman 1996.

47. All true things I know about Aristotle, I have learned from Mark Gifford.

48. Chapman 1996, 63; see also Merskey 1979, Scarry 1985.

49. Baron et al. 1986, Cesaro et al. 1991, Derbyshire et al. 1993, Di Piero et al. 1991, Hirato et al. 1991, Hosobuchi 1991, Iadarola et al. 1995, Katayama et al. 1986, LeTerre, De Volder, and Goffinet 1988, Rosen et al. 1994, Tran Dinh et al. 1991.

50. Hsieh et al. 1995.

51. Cf. discussion in Apkarian 1995; see also Mountz et al. 1995.

52. Apkarian 1995, 289.

53. Hsieh et al. 1995.

54. Pandya, Barnes, and Panksepp 1987.

55. Cf. Pribram 1980; Turner, Mishkin, and Knapp 1980.

56. Newman et al. 1994.

57. Bernard, Huang, and Besson 1992, Sikes and Vogt 1992, Snow, Lumb, and Cervero 1992.

58. Penfield and Boldrey 1937, White and Sweet 1969; see also Parrent et al. 1992.

59. Actually, the intralaminar and medial thalamic regions may be necessary for chronic pain processing, but the lateral thalamus is not. In addition, a cingulatomy does decrease chronic pain (Bouckoms 1994).

60. Coderre, Vaccarino, and Melzack et al. 1990, Cohen and Melzack 1993, McKenna and Melzack 1992, 1994, Vaccarino and Melzack 1992.

61. Fulton 1951.

62. Brand and Yancey 1993, 210.

63. Rainville et al. 1997.

64. Gray 1982, 1987, Isaacson 1982, Papez 1937. To simplify matters, I am setting to one side the influence that stress mechanisms have on pain. See Chapman 1986 for a useful discussion.

65. Korf, Bunney, and Aghajanian 1974, Stone 1975, Morilak, Fornal, and Jacobs 1987, Svensson 1987.

66. McNaughton and Mason 1980, Redmond and Huang 1979.

67. Amaral and Sinnamon 1977.

68. Butler et al. 1990, Elam, Svensson, and Thoren 1986a, Foote and Morrison 1987, Foote, Bloom, and Aston-Jones 1983, Gray 1987, Svensson 1987.

69. Cf. Chapman and Nakamura 1997.

70. Chapman and Nakamura 1998, Chapman (personal communication); see also Derbyshire et al. 1994.

71. Rumelhart et al. 1986.

72. Hill, Niven, and Knussen 1996; see also Katz and Melzack 1990.

73. See also Canavero 1994.

Chapter 6   When a Pain Isn't

1. Wall 1989b, Melzack and Wall 1986.

2. Kosambi 1967.

3. Melzack, Wall, and Ty 1982.

4. Anonymous personal reports by self-injurers in answer to the question of why they engage in self-injurious behavior posted to http://www.palace.net/~llama/psych/injury.html.

5. See discussion in Favazza 1987.

6. DeMoore and Robertson 1996, Favazza and Rosenthal 1993.

7. Favazza 1987, 1998, Miller 1994.

8. It is a live debate whether there is a good correspondence between the pattern of activity in the retina and a particular type of experience. How you answer that question depends upon how elastic you believe our visual "module" to be. Paul Churchland and Richard Gregory, for example, think that our visual system is cognitively penetrable from above; Jerry Fodor does not.

9. Cervero 1991, Jänig 1987.

10. Ruch 1965; see also Bonica 1990, Fields 1987.

11. Loeser 1990, Melzack 1989, 1992, Roth and Sugerbacker 1980.

12. Chapman and Stillman 1996.

13. Sherman, Sherman, and Parker 1984, Roth and Sugarbaker 1980.

14. Melzack 1992.

15. Fields 1987.

16. Wall 1964, Wall and Cronly-Dillon 1960, Wall and Sweet 1967; see also Willis and Coggeshall 1978, Yakshe 1986.

17. Willer, Boureau, and Albe-Fessard 1980.

18. Known as Thunberg's thermal grill illusion, this was first demonstrated in 1896.

19. Wall 1989a.

20. A. D. Craig and Bushnell 1994.

21. Apkarian, Stea, and Bolanowski 1994.

22. IASP 1986.

23. IASP 1986.

24. See also Apkarian 1995.

25. Wall 1964, 1989b, Melzack and Wall 1986, see also Britton and Skevington 1980. Several aspects of the original theory have been shown to be incorrect; see Nathan 1976 and Kandel and Schwartz 1985 for discussion. However, most accept the general outline of the view.

26. Canavero 1994, 203–207; see also Dray, Urban, and Dickenson 1994.

27. The influence of the psychological on the perception of pain has a long and venerable history; see Whytt 1786, Brodie 1837, and Carter 1853, as described in Merskey and Spear 1967.

28. Wall 1989a, 12.

29. Melzack 1990, 1991, 1992; see also discussion in Canavero 1994.

30. Apkarian 1995, 290.

31. Wang and Nakai 1994.

32. Fields 1981, Fields and Basbaum 1989; see also Sherman and Liebeskind 1980 for references and review.

33. Vaccarino and Chorney 1994.

34. Kandel and Schwartz 1985, Fields and Basbaum 1989.

35. Lopez, Young, and Cox 1991.

36. Cf. Fields and Basbaum 1989.

37. Pagni 1989.

38. Fields and Basbaum 1989, Mayer 1982.

39. Fields and Basbaum 1989, Maier, Drugan, and Grau 1982, Lewis, Cannon, and Leibeskind al. 1980, Lewis, Sherman, and Leibeskind 1981, Lewis et al. 1982.

40. Kandel and Schwartz 1985.

41. Bodnar 1990, Kandel and Schwartz 1985, Szekely 1990.

42. Dubo et al. 1987, Romans et al. 1995, Van der Kolk, Perry, and Herman 1991, Yeo and Yeo 1993.

43. Gilbody, House, and Owens 1997, Zlotnick et al. 1996.

44. Rusch, Guastello, and Mason 1992.

45. Favazza and Rosenthal 1993, Kahan and Pattison 1984.

46. Miller 1994.

47. Kemperman et al. 1997, Russ et al. 1996.

48. Glover, Lader, and Walker-O'Keefe 1995, Glover et al. 1997.

49. Kemperman, Russ, and Shearin 1997, Russ et al. 1992, Russ et al. 1993, Russ et al. 1994.

50. New et al. 1997, Sabo et al. 1995.

51. Roth, Ostroff, and Hoffman 1996, though see Russ et al. 1994 for contrary results.

52. Jacob, Tremblay, and Colombel 1974.

53. Levine, Gordon, and Fields 1979.

54. Dubo et al. 1997, Herpertz 1995, Pies and Popli 1995.

55. Shearer 1994.

56. Anonymous descriptions of self-injurious behavior.

57. Honigl et al. 1997.

58. Montaigne [1532–1592] 1930.

59. Livingstone 1860, as quoted in Nuland 1994, 134.

60. Thomas 1980, 102.

61. As quoted in Nuland 1994, 126–127.

62. Fields and Basbaum 1989.

63. Tantum and Whittaker 1992.

64. Orian 1989.

65. Haines et al. 1995.

66. Wickelgren 1997, 35.

67. Nestler and Agahajanian 1997, 58.

68. I owe much of this discussion to my student Rachel Hash.

69. Levine 1981, 116.

70. Rorabaugh 1979, 48, as discussed in Fingarette 1988.

71. Wadley, Smith, and Sheiff 1997.

Chapter 7   "But Is It Going to Hurt?"

1. Barber 1959.

2. Gracely, McGath, and Dubner 1978a, Merskey 1973.

3. Bruner and Goodman 1947.

4. Gracely, McGath, and Dubner 1978b, Gracely, Dubner, and McGath 1979, 1982.

5. Reading 1989.

6. Melzack 1975.

7. Fordyce 1978.

8. Cf. DeGood 1988.

9. One problem with the clinicians' approach, though, is that they use their detailed assessment techniques to focus almost exclusively on improving behavioral functioning in treatment. I discuss this aspect of clinical practice in the next chapter.

10. Tursky 1976.

11. T. Lewis 1942.

12. K. D. Craig 1989, 220.

13. Melzack and Dennis 1980.

14. P. M. Churchland 1981, 67.

15. Dennett 1987 makes this argument as well.

16. Cf. Stich 1992, 1996.

17. Jacoby 1985.

18. Haldane 1988.

19. Descartes [1641] 1970, 190.

20. Wittgenstein 1953, 178.

21. Wittgenstein 1967, § 225.

22. Horst 1995, O'Brien 1987; see also Double 1986, 1987.

23. G. Rey 1997, 86; see also Averill 1990.

24. P. M. Churchland 1985b.

25. Plantinga 1986 and G. Rey 1997 make a similar point as mine.

26. Double 1986, Greenwood 1991, 1992, Hannan 1990, Robinson 1985; see also Horgan 1993, Horgan and Graham 1993, Jackson and Pettit 1990.

27. K. D. Craig 1986, K. D. Craig and Prkachin 1982, Patrick, Craig, and Prkachin 1986.

28. Buss and Portnoy 1967, K. D. Craig 1986, K. D. Craig and Wyckoff 1987, Katon, Kleinman, and Rosen 1982, Sternbach and Tursky 1965, Zborowski 1952.

29. Bogdan 1993, Horgan and Woodward 1985, Kitcher 1984, Lahav 1992.

30. Hannan 1993, 171.

31. Davidson 1980, 253.

32. Baker 1987, 1988, Boghossian 1990, 1991, Cling 1989, Malcolm 1968, Reppert 1991, 1992, Trout 1991.

33. See also Clark 1993, Nelson 1991.

34. Bertolet 1994, Devitt 1990, Devitt and Rey 1991, Rosenberg 1991; though see Sterelny 1993, Taylor 1994.

35. Wittgenstein 1953, 294–307.

36. See also Ramsey 1990a, b.

37. Feyerabend 1963a, b, Rorty 1965, see also Melnyk 1991.

38. Feyerabend 1963a, 295.

39. Feyerabend 1963a, 295.

40. Gracely 1980, 111.

41. DeGood 1988, Lewis 1972, Mersky 1982.

42. DeGood 1988, 2.

43. Bickle 1993, Botterill 1994, Clapin 1991, Clark 1989, 1990, Egan 1995, Forster and Saidel 1994, Horgan and Tienson 1995, 1996, O'Brien 1991, O'Gorman 1989, 1990, O'Leary-Hawthorne 1994, Smolensky 1995.

44. Davies 1991, Fodor and Pylyshyn 1988, Ramsey 1990a, b, 1994, Ramsey, Stich, and Garon 1991, Stich 1991, Stich and Warfield 1995.

45. Marr 1982, 24.

46. Horgan and Tienson 1995, 1997.

47. Marr 1982, 24–25.

48. Horgan and Tienson 1996, 45.

49. Horgan and Tienson 1996, 46.

50. Horgan and Tienson 1997, 46.

51. Horgan and Tienson 1996, 46.

52. Freeman and Schneider 1982.

53. Patricia Kitcher pointed out to me a similar difficulty with Marr several years ago. See also Kitcher 1988.

54. Horgan and Tienson 1997, 47.

55. Snyder 1979.

56. Blitz and Dinnerstein 1971, Gelfand 1964, McKenna 1958, Neufield and Davidson 1971.

57. Anderson and Pennebaker 1980.

58. Silverman et al. 1997.

Chapter 8 What We Do Know about Treating Pain

1. Barkin et al. 1996b, Linton 1994.

2. Barkin et al. 1996a.

3. Cf. Loscalzo 1996, Rowbotham 1995.

4. Helme and Katz 1993.

5. Garcia and Altman 1997a, McFarlane et al. 1997.

6. E.g. Conner-Warren 1996.

7. Fedorczyk 1997.

8. Ahmedzai 1995.

9. Garcia and Altman 1997a.

10. Garcia and Altman 1997b.

11. Katz 1996.

12. Conigliaro 1996, Pappagallo and Heinberg 1997, though see Bedder 1996, Krames 1996.

13. Portenoy 1996, Sees and Clark 1993.

14. Cherny 1996, Lipman 1996, D. C. Turk 1996.

15. D. E. Turk and Meichenbaum 1989.

16. Holzman, Turk, and Kerns 1986, D. C. Turk and Rudy 1987, D. E. Turk, Meichenbaum, and Genest 1983, D. C. Turk, Holzman, and Kerns 1986.

17. Fordyce 1976, 1986, Fordyce et al. 1968, Fordyce et al. 1973.

18. D. C. Turk and Rudy 1987.

19. Ciccone and Grzesiak 1988, 134.

20. Sternbach 1989.

21. Roberts and Reinhardt 1980.

22. Turner and Chapman 1982.

23. Linton 1986.

24. Buchser et al. 1994, Dane 1996, Holroyd 1995, Houghton, Heymann, and Whorwell 1996, Lang et al. 1996, Mitchell 1995, Sutcher 1997.

25. Elton, Burrows, and Stanely 1980, Knox et al. 1981, Kuttner 1988, Malone and Strube 1988, Melzack and Perry 1975, Smith, Barabasz, and Barabasz 1994,

Spinhoven 1988, Stern et al. 1977, ter Kuile et al. 1994, Ulett et al. 1978, Zeltzer and LeBaron 1982, Zitman et al. 1992.

26. Jacobs, Kurtz, and Strube 1995.

27. Mairs 1995, Moore and Wisener 1996.

28. Baram 1995, Dillenburger and Keenan 1996.

29. Patterson and Ptacek 1997, Patterson, Goldberg, and Ehde 1996, Patterson, Adcock, and Bombardier 1997, though see Everett et al. 1993.

30. Burte, Burte, and Araoz 1994, Byrne 1996.

31. Genius 1995, Shum 1996.

32. Golan 1997.

33. Haanen et al. 1991.

34. Brown et al. 1996, Genuis 1995, Lambert 1996, Smith, Barabasz, and Barabasz 1996.

35. Dane 1996.

36. ter Kuile, Spinhoven, and Linssen 1995.

37. This section owes much to Braude 1995, Chaves and Dworkin 1997, Margolis 1997, R. Rey 1993.

38. Kroger 1977, 1.

39. Roux 1836, 346.

40. Smith 1847, 85.

41. Braid 1843, 32–33.

42. James [1890] 1981, 208.

43. Binet 1896, 302.

44. Binet 1896, 297.

45. Hilgard 1986, Hilgard and Hilgard 1994.

46. As quoted in Braude 1995, 18.

47. Cf., for example, Eastwood, Gaskovski, and Bowers 1998.

48. Morgan, Johnson, and Hilgard 1974.

49. Hilgard 1980.

50. Orne and Dinges 1989.

51. Bowers 1976.

52. West 1836, 351.

53. Barber and Mayer 1977, De Benedittis, Panerai, and Villamira 1989, Domangue et al. 1985, Goldstein and Hilgard 1975, Guerra, Guantieri, and Tagliaro 1985, Nasrallah, Holly, and Janowski 1979, Olness, Wain, and Lorenz 1980, Spiegel and Albert 1985.

54. Goldstein and Hilgard 1975, Moret et al. 1991, Spiegel and Albert 1985.

55. Cf. Spanos 1986, Spanos et al. 1990.

56. De Pascalis and Perrone 1996.

57. Crawford 1994a, b, De Pascalis et al. 1992, Galbraith, Cooper, and London 1972, Guerrero-Figueroa and Heath 1964; Hernandez-Peon and Donoso 1959, Holroyd 1992, Mészáros Bányai, and Greguss 1980, Sharev and Tal 1989, Speigel, Bierre, and Rootenberg 1989, Zachariae and Bjerring 1994, Zachariae et al. 1991.

58. Blum and Nash 1982, Speigel et al. 1985.

59. Arendt-Nielson, Zacharie, and Bjerring 1990, Saletu et al. 1975, Spiegel, Bierre, and Rootenberg 1989.

60. Zaslansky et al. 1996.

61. Barber 1963.

62. Chapman and Feather 1973, Greene and Reyher 1972, Knox, Morgan, and Hilgard 1974.

63. Orne and Dinges 1989.

64. Maurer, Santangelo, and Claiborn 1993.

65. Dahlgren et al. 1995.

66. Kiernan et al. 1995, Malone, Kurtz, and Strube 1989.

67. Zachariae and Bjerring 1994.

68. Meier et al. 1993.

69. Hilgard et al. 1978, McGlashan et al. 1969.

70. Zachariae and Bjerring 1994.

71. Kiernan et al. 1995; see also Hernandez-Peon et al. 1960, Sharev and Tal 1989.

72. Gracely 1995.

73. Crawford 1990, 1994a, b, Crawford et al. 1993, Gruzelier and Warren 1993; see also discussion in Holroyd 1995.

74. Crawford et al. 1998.

75. Cohen 1993, Duncan and Desimone 1995, Posner and Dehaene 1994, Posner and Petersen 1990.

76. Frith 1991, 186.

77. Christenfeld 1997, Farthing et al. 1997.

78. Graham 1975.

79. Klein and Speigel 1989, Whorwell, Prior, and Faragher 1984, Whorwell, Prior, and Colgan 1987.

80. Banks 1985.

81. Ewin 1986, Swirsky-Sacchetti and Margolis 1986.

82. Gonsalkorale 1996.

83. Crawford et al. 1993.

84. Crawford et al. 1993, 192.

85. Posner et al. 1988.

86. Kropotov, Crawford, and Polyakov 1997.

87. Lederhaas 1997.

88. Gaukroger, Tomkins, and van der Walt 1995.

89. Owens and Todt 1984, McGrath and Hillier 1989.

90. Barr 1989.

91. McGraw 1941.

92. Fisichelli et al. 1974, Kassowitz 1958, Levy 1960.

93. Craig et al. 1984, Izard et al. 1983, Izard, Hembree, and Huebner 1987.

94. Barr 1983, Haslam 1969, Heinild et al. 1959, Lollar et al. 1982.

95. Jay, Ozolins, and Elliot 1983, Katz, Kellerman, and Siegel 1980, Lavigne, Shulein, and Hahn 1986, LeBaron and Zeltzer 1984, Zachary et al. 1985.

96. Zeltzer et al. 1997.

97. McGrath and Hillier 1989.

98. Romsing et al. 1996.

99. Alshuler and Ruble 1989, Band and Weisz 1988, 1990, Brown et al. 1986, Reissland 1983.

100. Brown et al. 1986.

101. Berstein et al. 1991.

102. Eland and Anderson 1977; see also Beyer et al. 1983, Mather and Mackie 1983.

103. Gaukroger, Tomkins, and van der Walt 1989.

104. Perry and Heidrich 1982.

105. Lawson 1986a, 124–125; see also Lawson 1986b, 1987, 1988a, b, 1990.

106. Anders et al. 1972, Gunnar, Fisch, and Malone 1984, Harpin and Rutter 1982, Owens and Todt 1984, Rawlings, Miller, and Engel 1980, Talbert, Kraybill, and Potter 1976.

107. Anand, Sippell, and Aynsley-Green 1987; see also Anand and Hickey 1987, 1992, Anand et al. 1988, Williamson and Williamson 1983.

108. Guy and Abbott 1992, McLaughlin et al. 1990, Yi and Barr 1995.

109. Craig et al. 1993, Fitzgerald 1991, Giannakoulopoulos et al. 1994.

110. Zeltzer et al. 1997.

111. Anand and Craig 1996.

112. Hardcastle 1995.

113. Derbyshire 1998, Fitzgerald 1995, Lloyd-Thomas and Fitzgerald 1996.

114. Chugani and Phelps 1987.

115. Derbyshire 1996, 211 (italics his).

116. Fillion and Blass 1986.

117. Cf. Grunau, Whitfield, et al. 1994, Gunnar et al. 1995, Johnson and Stevens 1996.

118. Fitzgerald 1995.

119. Taddio et al. 1995.

120. Gazarian et al. 1995, Taddio et al. 1994, 1995, 1997.

121. Suzuki 1995.

122. Walco, Cassidy, and Schechter 1994; see also Anand and McGrath 1993. Regrettably, though, neglect of infants' and children's pain inexplicably continues; cf. Boey 1991, Fedorczuk 1997, Garcia and Altman 1997a, Godfrey 1996, Lipman 1996, McQuay et al. 1995, Walker, Garber, and Greene 1993.

Chapter 9   Epilogue: Pain as a Paradigm for Philosophical Psychopathology

1. Kanner 1943, 217–250.

2. Baron-Cohen and Bolton 1993.

3. Baron-Cohen 1995, 62–63.

4. Courchesne 1997, Courchesne et al. 1988, Haas et al. 1996.

5. Akshoomoff and Courchesne 1992, Akshoomoff, Courchesne, and Townsend 1997, Allen et al. 1997, Townsend, Harris, and Courchesne 1996.

6. Courchesne 1997.

7. Courchesne et al. 1994, Pierce, Glad, and Schreibman 1997, Wainwright-Sharp and Bryson 1993.

8. Yeung-Courchesne and Courchesne 1997, 389.

9. Nestler and Aghajanian 1997.

10. Koob and Moal 1997.

11. Leshner 1997, 45.

12. Leshner 1997, 45.

13. Merskey 1989b.

14. As quoted in Rapoport 1989, 27–29.

15. Rapoport 1989, 29.

References

Adelman, A., and Shank, J. 1988. The association of psychosocial factors with the resolution of abdominal pain. *Family Medicine* 20: 266–270.

Adler, R., Zlot, S., Hurny, C., and Minder, C. 1989. Engel's "Psychogenic Pain and the Pain-Prone Patient": A retrospective, controlled clinical study. *Psychosomatic Medicine* 51: 87–101.

Agnati, L. F., Bjelke, B., and Fuxe, K. 1992. Volume transmission in the brain. *American Scientist* 80: 362–373.

Ahles, T., Khan, S., Yunus, M., Spiegel, D., and Masi, A. 1991. Psychiatric status of patients with primary fibromyalgia, patients with rheumatoid arthritis, and subjects without pain: A blind comparison of DSM-III diagnoses. *American Journal of Psychiatry* 148: 1721–1726.

Ahmedzai, S. 1995. Recent clinical trials of pain control: Impact on quality of life. *European Journal of Cancer* 31A Suppl.: S2–S7.

Akshoomoff, N. A., and Courchesne, E. 1992. A new role for the cerebellum in cognitive operations. *Behavioral Neuroscience* 106: 731–738.

Akshoomoff, N. A., Courchesne, E., and Townsend, J. 1997. Attention coordination and anticipatory control. *International Review of Neurobiology* 41: 575–598.

Alfven, G. 1993. The pressure pain threshold (PPT) of certain muscles in children suffering from recurrent abdominal pain of non-organic origin. An algometric study. *Acta Paediatrica* 82: 481–483.

Allen, G., Buxton, R. B., Wong, E. C., and Courchesne, E. 1997. Attentional activation of the cerebellum independent of motor involvement. *Science* 28: 1940–1943.

Allodi, F., and Goldstein, R. 1995. Posttraumatic somatoform disorders among immigrant workers. *Journal of Nervous and Mental Disease* 183: 604–607.

Almay, B., Haggendal, J., von Knorring, L., and Orelan, L. 1987. 5-HIAA and HVA in CSF in patients with idiopathic pain disorders. *Biological Psychiatry* 22: 403–412.

Almay, B., von Knorring, L., and Wetterberg, L. 1987. Melatonin in serum and urine in patients with idiopathic pain syndromes. *Psychiatric Research* 22: 179–191.

Altshuler, J. L., and Ruble, D. N. 1989. Developmental changes in children's awareness of strategies for coping with uncontrollable stress. *Child Development* 60: 1337–1349.

Amaral, D. B., and Sinnamon, S. H. 1977. The locus coeruleus: Neurobiology of a central noradrenergic nucleus. *Progress in Neurobiology* 9: 147–196.

American Psychiatric Association. 1968. *Diagnostic and Statistical Manual of Mental Disorders, Second Edition.* Washington, DC: American Psychiatric Association.

American Psychiatric Association. 1980. *Diagnostic and Statistical Manual of Mental Disorders, Third Edition.* Washington, DC: American Psychiatric Association.

American Psychiatric Association. 1987. *Diagnostic and Statistical Manual of Mental Disorders, Third Edition-Revised.* Washington, DC: American Psychiatric Association.

American Psychiatric Association. 1994. *Diagnostic and Statistical Manual of Mental Disorders, Fourth Edition.* Washington, DC: American Psychiatric Association.

Anand, K. J. S., and Craig. K. D. 1996. New perspectives on the definition of pain. *Pain* 67: 3–6.

Anand, K. J. S., and Hickey, P. R. 1987. Pain and its effects in the human neonate and fetus. *New England Journal of Medicine* 317: 1321–1329.

Anand, K. J. S., and Hickey, P. R. 1992. Halothane-morphine compared with high-dose sufentanil for anesthesia and post-operative analgesia in neonatal cardiac surgery. *New England Journal of Medicine* 326: 1–9.

Anand. K. J. S., and McGrath, P. J. 1993. An overview of current issues and their historical background. In K. J. S., Anand and P. J. McGrath (eds.), *Pain in Neonates.* Amsterdam: Elsevier.

Anand, K. J. S., Sippell, W. G., and Aynsley-Green, A. 1987. Randomized trial of fentanyl anesthesia in preterm babies undergoing surgery: Effects on the stress response. *Lancet* i: 243–248.

Anand, K. J. S., Sippell, W. G., Schofield, N. M., et al. 1988. Does halothane anesthesia decrease the metabolic rate and endocrine stress responses of newborn infants undergoing operation? *British Medical Journal* 296: 668–672.

Anders, T. F., Sachar, E. J., Kream, J., Roffwarg, H., and Hellman, L. 1972. Behavioral state and plasma cortisol response in the human newborn. *Pediatrics* 49: 250–259.

Anderson, D., and Pennebaker, J. 1980. Pain and pleasure. Alternative interpretations of identical stimuliations. *European Journal of Social Psychology* 10: 207–210.

Anzai, A., and Merkin, T. 1996. Adolescent chest pain. *American Family Physician* 53: 1682–1690.

Apkarian, A. V. 1995. Functional imaging of pain: New insights regarding the role of the cerebral cortex in human pain perception. *Seminars in the Neurosciences* 7: 279–293.

Apkarian, A. V., Stea, R. A., and Bolanowski, S. J. 1994. Heat-induced pain diminishes vibrotactile perception: A touch gate. *Somatosensory Motor Research* 11: 259–267.

Apkarian, A. V., Stea, R. A., Mangos, S. H., Szeverenyi, N. M., King, R. B., and Thomas, F. D. 1992. Persistent pain inhibits contralateral somatosensory cortical activity in humans. *Neuroscience Letters* 140: 141–147.

Apley, J. 1975. *The Child with Abdominal Pains.* Oxford: Blackwell Scientific Publications.

Arendt-Neilsen, L., Zacharie, R., and Bjerring, P. 1990. Qualitative evaluation of hypnotically suggested hyperanesthesia and analgesia by painful laser stimulation. *Pain* 42: 243–251.

Armstrong, D. 1981. *The Nature of Mind and Other Essays.* Ithaca: Cornell University Press.

Arntz, A., and Peters, M. 1995. Chronic low back pain and inaccurate predictions of pain: Is being too tough a risk factor for the development and maintenance of chronic pain? *Behavioral Research Therapy* 33: 49–53.

Ashby, W. R. 1952. *Design for a Brain.* London: Chapman and Hall.

Asmundson, G. L. G., and Norton, G. R. 1995. Anxiety sensitivity in patients with physically unexplained chronic back pain: A preliminary report. *Behavior, Research, and Therapy* 33: 771–777.

Asnes, R., Santulli, R., and Bemporad, J. 1981. Psychogenic chest pain in children. *Clinical Pediatrics* 20: 788–791.

Averill, E. W. 1990. Functionalism, the absent qualia objection, and eliminativism. *Southern Journal of Philosophy* 63: 449–467.

Backonja, M., Howland, E. W., Wang, J., Smith, J., Salinsky, M., and Cleeland, C. S. 1991. Tonic changes in alpha power during immersion of the hand in cold water. *Electroencephalography and Clinical Neurophysiology* 79: 192–203.

Bains, S. 1997. A subtler silicon cell for neural networks. *Science* 277: 1935.

Baker, L. R. 1987. *Saving Belief.* Princeton, NJ: Princeton University Press.

Baker, L. R. 1988. Cognitive suicide. In R. Grimm and D. Merrill (eds.), *Contents of Thought.* Tucson: University of Arizona Press.

Band, E. B., and Weisz, J. R. 1988. How to feel better when it feels bad: Children's perspectives on coping with everyday stress. *Developmental Psychology* 24: 247–253.

Band, E. B., and Weisz, J. R. 1990. Developmental differences in primary and secondary control and adjustment of juvenile diabetes. *Journal of Clinical Child Psychology* 19: 150–158.

Banks, W. 1985. Hypnotic suggestion for the control of bleeding in the angiography suite. *Ericksonian Monographs* 1: 76–88.

Baram, D. A. 1995. Hypnosis in reproductive health care: A review and case reports. *Birth* 22: 37–42.

Barber, J., and Mayer, D. J. 1977. Evaluation of the efficacy and neural mechanism of a hypnotic analgesia procedure in experimental and clinical dental pain. *Pain* 4: 41–48.

Barber, T. X. 1959. Toward a theory of pain: Relief of chronic pain by prefrontal leuocotomy, optiate, placebos, and hypnosis. *Psychological Bulletin* 56: 430–460.

Barber, T. X. 1963. The effect of "hypnosis" on pain: A critical review of experimental and clinical findings. *Psychosomatic Medicine* 24: 303–333.

Barinaga, M. 1997. New imaging methods provide a better view into the brain. *Science* 276: 1974–1976.

Barker, A., and Mayou, R. 1992. Psychological factors in patients with non-specific abdominal pain acutely admitted to a general surgical ward. *Journal of Psychosomatic Research* 36: 715–722.

Barkin, R. L., Lubenow, T. R., Breuhl, S., Husfeldt, B., Ivankovich, O., and Barkin, S. J. 1996a. Management of chronic pain. Part I. *Disease Monthly* 42: 389–454.

Barkin, R. L., Lubenow, T. R., Breuhl, S., Husfeldt, B., Ivankovich, O., and Barkin, S. J. 1996b. Management of chronic pain. Part II. *Disease Monthly* 42: 457–507.

Baron, J. C., D'Antona, R., Pantono, P., Serudaru, M., Samson, Y., and Bousser, M. G. 1986. Effects of thalamic stroke on energy metabolism of the cerebral cortex—a positron tomography study in man. *Brain* 109: 1243–1259.

Baron-Cohen, S. 1995. *Mindblindness: An Essay on Autism and Theory of Mind.* Cambridge, MA: The MIT Press.

Baron-Cohen, S., and Bolton, P. 1993. *Autism: The Facts.* New York: Oxford University Press.

Barr, R. G. 1983. Recurrent abdominal pain syndrome. In M. D. Levine, W. B. Carey, A. C. Crocker, and R. T. Gross (eds.), *Challenges to Development Paradigms: Implications for Theory, Assessment, and Treatment.* New York: Erlbaum.

Barr, R. G. 1989. Pain in children. In P. D. Wall and R. Melzack (eds.), *Textbook of Pain, Second Edition.* New York: Churchill Livingstone.

Baum, N., and Defidio, L. 1995. Chronic testicular pain. A workup and treatment guide for the primary care physician. *Postgraduate Medicine* 98: 151–153, 156–158.

Bayer, T., Chiang, E., Coverdale, J., Bangs, M., et al. 1993. Anxiety in experimentally induced somatoform symptoms. *Psychosomatics* 34: 415–423.

Bechtel, W. 1982. Two common errors in explaining biological and psychological phenomena. *Philosophy of Science* 49: 549–574.

Bechtel, W. 1983. A bridge between cognitive science and neuroscience: The functional architecture of the mind. *Philosophical Studies* 44: 549–574.

Bechtel, W., and Richardson, R. C. 1993. *Discovering Complexity: Decomposition and Localization as Strategies in Scientific Research*. Princeton, NJ: Princeton University Press.

Bedder, M. D. 1996. Epidural opioid therapy for chronic nonmalignant pain: Critique of current experience. *Journal of Pain Symptom Management* 11: 353–356.

Beecher, H. K. 1956. Relationship of significance of wound to the pain experience. *Journal of the American Medical Association* 161: 1609–1613.

Behbehani, M. M. and Dollberg-Stolik, 1994. Partial sciatic nerve ligation results in an enlargement of the receptive field and enhancement of the response of dorsal horn neurons to noxious stimulation by an adenosine agonist. *Pain* 58: 421–428.

Benjamin, S., Barnes, D., Berger, S., Clarke, I., and Jeacock, J. 1988. The relationship of chronic pain, mental illness, and organic disorders. *Pain* 32: 185–195.

Benjamin, S., Mawer, J., and Lennon, S. 1992. The knowledge and beliefs of family care givers about chronic pain patients. *Journal of Psychosomatic Research* 36: 211–217.

Bernard, J. F., Huang, G. F., and Besson, J. M. 1992. Nucleaus centralis of the amygdala and the globus pallidus ventralis: Electrophysiological evidence for an involvement in pain processes. *Journal of Neurophysiology* 68: 551–569.

Bernstein, B., Schechter, N. L., Hickman, T., et al. 1991. Premedication for painful procedures in children: A national survey. *Journal of Pain Symptom Management* 6: 190.

Bertolet, R. 1994. Saving eliminativism. *Philosophical Psychology* 7: 87–100.

Beyer, J. E., DeGood, D. E., Ashley, L. C., et al. 1983. Patterns of post-operative analgesic use with adults and children following cardiac surgery. *Pain* 17: 71–81.

Bickle, J. 1993. Connectionism, eliminativism, and the semantic view of theories. *Erkenntnis* 39: 359–382.

Binet, A. 1896. *Alterations of Personality*. New York: D. Appleton and Company.

Blackwell, B., Mersky, H., and Kellner, R. 1989. Somatoform pain disorders. In *Treatments of Psychiatric Disorders: A Task Force Report of the American Psychiatric Association*. Washington, DC: American Psychiatric Association.

Blitz, B., and Dinnerstein, A. 1971. Role of attentional focus in pain perception: Manipulation of response to noxious stimulation by instruction. *Journal of Abnormal Psychology* 77: 42–45.

Block, N. 1986. Advertisement for a semantics in psychology. In P. A. French, T. E. Uehling, and H. K. Wettstein (eds.), *Midwest Studies in Philosophy, Volume IX: Studies in the Philosophy of Mind*. Minneapolis: University of Minnesota Press.

Blum, G. S., and Nash, J. K. 1982. Selective inattention to anxiety-linked stimuli. *Journal of Experimental Psychology: General* 108: 182–224.

Blumer, D., and Heilbronn, M. 1982. Chronic pain as a variant of depressive illness: The pain-prone disorder. *Journal of Nervous Mental Disorders* 170: 381–406.

Blumer, D., Zorick, F., Heilbronn, M., and Roth, T. 1982. Biological markers for depression in chronic pain. *Journal of Nervous Mental Disorders* 170: 425–428.

Bodnar, R. J. 1990. Effects of opioid peptides on peripheral stimulation and "stress"-induced analgesia in animals. *Critical Reviews in Neurobiology* 6: 39–49.

Boey, W. K. 1991. Pain control. *Annual Academy of Medicine, Singapore* 20: 118–126.

Bogdan, R. J. 1993. The architectural nonchalance of commonsense psychology. *Mind and Language* 8: 189–205.

Boghossian, P. 1990. The status of content. *Philosophical Review* 99: 157–184.

Boghossian, P. 1991. The status of content revisited. *Pacific Philosophical Quarterly* 71: 264–278.

Bonica, J. J. (ed.). 1990. *The Management of Pain, 2nd Edition*. Philadelphia: Lea and Febiger.

Botterill, G. 1994. Beliefs, functionally discrete states, and connectionist networks. *British Journal for the Philosophy of Science* 45: 899–906.

Bouckoms, J. A. 1994. Limbic surgery for pain. In P. D. Wall and R. Melzack (eds.), *Textbook of Pain*. New York: Churchill Livingstone.

Bowers, K. S. 1976. *Hypnosis for the Seriously Curious*. Monteray, CA: Brooks/Cole.

Braid, J. 1843. *Neurypnology or the Rationale of Nervous Sleep in Relation with Animal Magnetism*. London: Churchill.

Braitenberg, V. 1984. *Vehicles*. Cambridge, MA: The MIT Press.

Brand, P., and Yancey, P. 1993. *Pain: The Gift Nobody Wants*. New York: HarperCollins.

Braude, S. E. 1995. *First Person Plural: Multiple Personality and the Philosophy of Mind, Revised Edition*. Lanham, MD: Roman and Littlefield.

Bresler, D. E., and Trubo, R. 1979. *Free Yourself from Pain*. New York: Simon and Schuster.

Britton, N. F., and Skevington, S. M. 1980. A mathematical model of the gate control theory of pain. *Journal of Theoretical Biology* 137: 91–105.

Brodmann, K. 1909. *Vergleichende Lokalisationslehre der Grosshirnrinde in ihren Prinzipien Dargestellt auf Grund des Zellenbaues*. Leipzig: Barth.

Brown, C. 1992. What narrow content is not. Paper presented at the American Philosophical Association Pacific Division Sixty-Sixth Annual Meeting, 25–28 March, Portland, Oregon.

Brown, G. W., Summers, D., Coffman, B., Riddell, R., et al. 1996. The use of hypnotheraphy with school-age children: Five case studies. *Psychotherapy in Private Practice* 15: 53–65.

Brown, J., O'Keefe, J., Sanders, S. and Baker, B. 1986. Developmental changes in children's cognition to stressful and painful situations. *Journal of Pediatric Psychology* 11: 343–357.

Bruner, J. S., and Goodman, C. C. 1947. Value and needs as organizing factors in perception. *Journal of Abnormal Social Psychology* 42: 33–44.

Buchser, W., Burnand, B., Sprunger, A. L., Clemence, A., Lepage, C., Martin, Y., Chedel, D., Guex, P., Sloutskis, D., and Rumely, R. 1994. Hypnosis and self-hypnosis, administered and taught by nurses, for the reduction of chronic pain: A controlled clinical trial. *Schweiz Medicin Wochenschr Supplement* 62: 77–81.

Burge, T. 1979. Individualism and the mental. In P. French, T. E. Euhling, and H. Wettstein (eds.), *Midwest Studies in Philosophy, Volume X. Studies in the Philosophy of Mind*. Minneapolis: University of Minnesota Press.

Burge, T. 1986. Individualism and psychology. *Philosophical Review* 95: 3–45.

Burte, J. M., Burte, W. D., and Araoz, D. L. 1994. Hypnosis in the treatment of back pain. *Australian Journal of Clinical Hypnotherapy and Hypnosis* 15: 93–115.

Buss, A. H., and Portnoy, N. M. 1967. Pain tolerance and group identification. *Journal of Personality and Social Psychology* 6: 106–108.

Butler, P. D., Weiss, J. N., Stout, J. C., and Nemeroff, C. B. 1990. Corticotropin-releasing factor produces fear-enhancing and behavioral activating effects following infusion into the locus coeruleus. *Journal of Neuroscience* 10: 176–183.

Byrne, M. 1996. Hypnosis in the treatment of chronic back pain. *Australian Journal of Clnical and Experimental Hypnosis* 24: 46–52.

Canavero, S. 1994. Dynamic Reverberation. A unified mechanism for central and phantom pain. *Medical Hypotheses* 42: 203–207.

Carlsson, A. M. 1986. Personality characteristics of patients with chronic pain in comparison with normal controls and depressed patients. *Pain* 25: 373–382.

Carstens, E. 1996. Quantitive experimental assessment of pain and hyperalgesia in animals and underlying neural mechanisms. In G. Carli and M. Zimmerman (eds.), *Progress in Brain Research, Volume 10: Towards the Neurobiology of Chronic Pain*. New York: Elsevier Science B. V.

Carstens, E. 1997. Responses of rat spinal dorsal horn neurons to intracutaneous microinjection of histamine, capsaicin and other irritants. *Journal of Neurophysiology* 77: 2499–2514.

Carstens, E., and Campbell, I. G. 1992. Responses of motor units during hind limb flexion withdrawal reflex evoked by noxious skin heating: Phasic and prolonged suppression by midbrain stimulation and comparison with simultaneously recorded dorsal horn units. *Pain* 48: 215–226.

Carstens, E., and Douglass, D. K. 1995. Midbrain suppression of limb withdrawal and tail flick reflexes in the rat: Correlates with descending inhibition of sacral spinal neurons. *Journal of Neurophysiology* 73: 2179–2194.

Carstens, E., and Watkins, L. R. 1986. Inhibition of the responses of neurons in the rat spinal cord to noxious skin heating by stimulation in midbrain periaqueductal gray or lateral reticular formation. *Brain Research* 382: 266–277.

Casey, K. L., Minoshima, S., Berger, K. L., Koeppe, R. A., Morrow, T. J., and Frey, K. A. 1994. Positron emission tomographic analysis of cerebral structures activated specifically by repetitive noxious heat stimuli. *Journal of Neurophysiology* 71: 802–807.

Casey, K. L., Minoshima, S., Koeppe, R. A., Weeder, J., and Morrow, T. J. 1994. Temporal-spatial dynamics of human forebrain activity during noxious heat stimulation. *Society of Neuroscience Abstracts* 20: 1573.

Casey, K. L., Minoshima, S., Morrow, T. J., and Koeppe, R. A. 1996. Comparison of human cerebral activation pattern during cutaneous warmth, heat pain, and deep cold pain. *Journal of Neurophysiology* 76: 571–581.

Caton, D. 1985. The secularization of pain. *Anesthesiology* 62: 493–501.

Cervero, F. 1991. Mechanisms of acute visceral pain. *British Medical Bulletin* 47: 549–560.

Cervero, F., Handwerker, H. O., and Laird, J. M. A. 1988. Prolonged noxious stimulation of the rat's tail: Responses and encoding properties of dorsal horn neurons. *Journal of Physiology (London)* 404: 419–436.

Cesaro, P., Mann, M. W., Moretti, J. L., Defer, G., Roualdès, B., Nguyen, J. P., and Degos, J. D. 1991. Central pain and thalamic hyperactivity: A single photon emission computerized tomographic study. *Pain* 47: 329–336.

Chaney, H., Williams, S., Cohn, C., and Vincent, K. 1984. MMPI results: A comparison of trauma victims, psychogenic pain, and patients with organic disease. *Journal of Clinical Psychology* 40: 1450–1454.

Chapman, C. R. 1986. Pain, perception, and illusion. In R. A. Sternbach (ed.), *The Psychology of Pain*. New York: Raven Press.

Chapman, C. R. 1996. Limbic processes and the affective dimension of pain. In G. Carli and M. Zimmerman (eds.), *Progress in Brain Research, Volume 10*. New York: Elsevier.

Chapman, C. R., and Feather, B. W. 1973. Effects of diasepam on human pain tolerance and pain sensitivity. *Psychosomatic Medicine* 35: 330–340.

Chapman, C. R., and Nakamura, Y. 1998. Hypnotic analgesia: A constructivist framework. *International Journal of Clinical and Experimental Hypnosis* 46: 6–27.

Chapman, C. R., and Stillman, M. 1996. Pathological pain. In L. Kruger (ed.), *Pain and Touch*. New York: Academic Press.

Chaturvedi, S., and Michael, A. 1986. Chronic pain in a psychiatric clinic. *Journal of Psychosomatic Research* 30: 347–354.

Chaves, J. F., and Dworkin, S. F. 1997. Hypnotic control of pain: Historical perspectives and future prospects. *The International Journal of Clinical and Experimental Hypnosis* 45: 356–376.

Cherney, N. I. 1996. Opioid analgesics: Comparative features and prescribing guidelines. *Drugs* 51: 713–737.

Cherry, D. A., Gourlay, G. K., McLachlan, M., Cousins, M. J. 1985. Diagnostic epidural opioid blockade and chronic pain: Preliminary report. *Pain* 21: 143–152.

Chibnall, J., Duckro, P., and Richardson, W. 1995. Physician frustration with chronic pain patients can and should be avoided. *Headache Quarterly* 6: 123–125.

Christenfeld, N. 1997. Memory for pain and the delayed effects of distraction. *Health Psychology* 16: 327–330.

Chudler, E. H., and Dong, W. K. 1995. The role of the basal ganglia in nociception and pain. *Pain* 60: 3–85.

Chugani, H. T., and Phelps, M. E. 1987. Maturational changes in cerebral function in infants determined by 18FDG position emission tomography. *Science* 231: 840–843.

Chung, J. M., Denshalo, D. R., Gerhart, K. D. and Willis, W. D. 1979. Excitations of primate spinothalamic neurons by cutaneous C-fiber volleys. *Journal of Neurophysiology* 42: 1354–1369.

Churchland, P. M. 1981. Eliminative materialism and the propositional attitudes. *Journal of Philosophy* 78: 67–90.

Churchland, P. M. 1985a. On the speculative nature of our self-conception. *Canadian Journal of Philosophy Supplement* 11: 157–173.

Churchland, P. M. 1985b. Reduction, qualia, and the direct introspection of brain states. *Journal of Philosophy,* 82: 2–28.

Churchland, P. M. 1989. *A Neurocomputational Perspective.* Cambridge, MA.: The MIT Press.

Churchland, P. S. 1983. Consciousness: The transmutation of a concept. *Pacific Philosophical Quarterly* 64: 80–95.

Churchland, P. S. 1986. Epistemology in the age of neuroscience. *Journal of Philosophy* 83: 544–553.

Churchland, P. S., and Sejnowski, T. J. 1992. *The Computational Brain.* Cambridge, MA: The MIT Press.

Ciccone, D., Just, N., and Bandilla, E. 1996. Non-organic symptom reporting in patients with chronic non-malignant pain. *Pain* 68: 329–341.

Ciccone, D. S., and Grzesiak, R. C. 1988. Cognitive therapy: An overview of theory and practice. In N. T. Lynch and S. V. Vasudevan (eds.), *Persistent Pain: Psychosocial Assessment and Intervention.* Dordrecht: Kluwer.

Clapin, H. 1991. Connectionism isn't magic. *Minds and Machines* 1: 167–184.

Clark, A. 1989. Beyond eliminativism. *Mind and Language* 4: 251–279.

Clark, A. 1990. Connectionist minds. *Proceedings of the Aristotelian Society* 90: 83–102.

Clark, A. 1993. Varieties of eliminativism: Sentential, intentional, and cata-strophic. *Mind and Language* 8: 223–233.

Cling, A. D. 1989. Eliminative materialism and self-referential inconsistency. *Philosophical Studies* 56: 53–75.

Cobishley, M., Hendrickson, R., Beutler, L., and Engle, D. 1990. Behavior, affect, and cognition among psychogenic pain patients in group expressive psychother-apy. *Journal of Pain Symptom Management* 5: 241–248.

Coderre, T. J., and Katz, J. 1997. Peripheral and central hyperexcitibility: Differ-ential signs and symptoms in persistent pain. *Behavioral and Brain Sciences* 20: 404–419.

Coderre, T. J., Baccarino, A. L., and Melzack, R. 1990. Central nervous system plasticity in the tonic pain response to subcutaneous formalin injection. *Brain Research* 535: 155–158.

Coghill, R. C., Talbot, J. D., Evans, A. C., Meyer, E., Gjedde, A., Bushnell, M. C., and Duncan, G. H. 1994. Distributed processing of pain and vibration by the human brain. *Journal of Neuroscience* 14: 4095–4108.

Cohen, R. A. 1993. *The Neuropsychology of Attention.* New York: Plenum Press.

Cohen, S. R., and Melzack, R. 1993. The habenula and pain: Repeated electrical stimulation produces prolonged analgesia but lesions have no effect on formalin pain or morphine analgesia. *Behavior and Brain Research* 54: 171–178.

Collins, J. G., and Stone, L. A 1966. Family structure and pain reactivity. *Journal of Clinical Psychology* 33: 22.

Conigliaro, D. A. 1996. Opioids for chronic non-malignant pain. *Journal of Florida Medical Association* 83: 703–711.

Connee, E. 1984. A defense of pain. *Philosophical Studies* 46: 239–248.

Conner-Warren, R. L. 1996. Pain intensity and home pain management of chil-dren with sickle cell disease. *Issues in Comprehensive Pediatric Nursing* 19: 183–195.

Cook, A. J., Woolf, C. J., Wall, P. D., and McMahon, S. B. 1987. Dynamic receptive field plasticity in rat spinal dorsal horn following C-primary afferent input. *Nature* 325: 151–153.

Cooper, P. J., Hawden, H. N., Camfield, P. R., and Camfield, C. S. 1987. Anxiety and life events in childhood migraine. *Pediatrics* 79: 999–1004.

Courchesne, E. 1997. Brainstem, cerebellar and limbic neuroanatomical abnor-malities in autism. *Current Opinions in Neurobiology* 7: 269–278.

Courchesne, E., Yeung-Courchesne, R., Press, G. A., Hesselink, J. R., and Jerni-gan, T. L. 1988. Hypoplasia of cerebellar vermal lobules VI and VII in autism. *New England Journal of Medicine* 318: 1349–1354.

Cox, B., Kuch, K., Parker, J., Shulman, I., et al. 1994. Alexithymia in somatoform disorder patients with chronic pain. *Journal of Psychosomatic Research* 38: 523–527.

Cox, G., Chapman, C., and Black, R. 1978. The MMPI and chronic pain: The diagnosis of psychogenic pain. *Journal of Behavioral Medicine* 1: 437–443.

Craig, A. D., and Bushnell, M. C. 1994. The thermal grill illusion: Unmasking the burn of cold pain. *Science* 265: 252–255.

Craig, A. D., Bushnell, M. C., Zhang, E.-T., and Blomqvist, A. 1994. A thalamic nucleus specific for pain and temperature sensation. *Nature* 372: 770–773.

Craig, K. D. 1986. Modeling and social learning factors in chronic pain. In J. J. Bonica (ed.), *Advances in Pain Research and Therapy*. New York: Raven Press.

Craig, K. D. 1989. Emotional aspects of pain. In P. D. Wall and R. Melzack (eds.), *Textbook of Pain*. New York: Churchill Livingstone.

Craig, K. D., and Prkachin, K. M. 1982. Non-verbal measures of pain. In R. Melzack (ed.), *Pain Measurement and Assessment*. New York: Raven Press.

Craig, K. D., and Wyckoff, M. G. 1987. Cultural factors in chronic pain management. In G. D. Burrows, D. Elton, and G. Stanley (eds.), *Handbook of Chronic Pain Management*. Amsterdam: Elsevier.

Craig, K. D., McMahon, R. J., Morison, J. D., and Zaskow, C. 1984. Developmental changes in infant pain expression during immunization injections. *Social Science and Medicine* 19: 1331–1337.

Craig, K. D., Whitfield, M. F., Grunau, R. V. E., Linton, J., and Hadjistavropoulos, H. D. 1993. Pain in the preterm neonate: Behavioral and physiological indices. *Pain* 52: 287–299.

Craig, M. C., Gillespie, D. C., and Stryker, M. P. 1998. The role of visual experience in the development of columns in cat visual cortex. *Science* 279: 566–570.

Crane, T., and Mellor, D. H. 1990. There is no question of physicalism. *Mind* 90: 185–206.

Crawford, H. J. 1990. Cognitive and psychophysiological correlates of hypnotic responsiveness and hypnosis. In M. L. Fass and D. Brown (eds.), *Creative Mastery in Hypnosis and Hypnoanalysis: A Festschrift for Erika Fromm*. Hillsdale, NJ: Lawrence Erlbaum.

Crawford, H. J. 1994a. Brain dynamics and hypnosis: Attentional and disattentional processes. *International Journal for Clinical and Experimental Hypnosis* 42: 204–232.

Crawford, H. J. 1994b. Brain systems involved in attention and disattention (hypnotic analgesia) to pain. In K. H. Pribram (ed.), *Origins: Brain and Self Organization*. Hillsdale, NJ: Lawrence Erlbaum.

Crawford, H. J., Gur, R. C., Skolnick, B., Gur, R. E., and Benson, D. M. 1993. Effects of hypnosis on regional blood flow during ischemic pain with and without suggested hypnotic analgesia. *International Journal of Psychophysiology* 15: 181–195.

Crawford, H. J., Knebel, T., Kaplan, L., Vendemia, J. M. C., Xie, M., Jamison, S., and Pribram, K. H. 1998. Hypnotic analgesia: 1. Somatosensory event-related potential changes to noxious stimuli and 2. Transfer learning to reduce chronic low back pain. *International Journal of Clinical and Experimental Hypnosis* 46: 92–132.

Critchley, M. 1956. Congenital indifference to pain. *Annals of Internal Medicine* 45: 737–747.

Cross, S. A. 1994. Pathophysiology of pain. *Mayo Clinic Proceedings* 69: 375–383.

Cytowic, R. E. 1989. *Synesthesia: A Union of the Senses.* New York: Springer Verlag.

Cytowic, R. E. 1993. *The Man Who Tasted Shapes: A Bizarre Medical Mystery Offers Revolutionary Insights into Reasoning, Emotion, and Consciousness.* New York: Putnam.

Cytowic, R. E. 1996. *The Neurological Side of Neuropsychology.* Cambridge, MA: The MIT Press.

Dahlgren, L. A., Kurtz, R. M., Strube, M. J., and Malone, M. D. 1995. Differential effects of hypnotic suggestion on multiple dimensions of pain. *Journal of Pain and Symptom Management* 10: 464–470.

Dane, J. R. 1996. Hypnosis for pain and neuromuscular rehabilitation with multiple sclerosis: Case summary, literature review, and analysis of outcomes. *International Journal of Clinical and Experimental Hypnosis* 44: 208–231.

Davidson, D. 1980. *Essays on Actions and Events.* Oxford: Oxford University Press.

Davies, M. 1991. Concepts, connectionism, and the language of thought. In W. Ramsey, S. Stich, and D. Rumelhart (eds.), *Philosophy and Connectionist Theory.* Hillsdale, NJ: Lawrence Erlbaum.

Davis, K. D., Tasker, R. R., Kiss, Z. H. T., Hutchison, W. D., and Dostrovsky, J. O. 1995. Visceral pain evoked by thalamic microstimulation in humans. *Neuroreport* 6: 369–374.

Davis, K. D., Taylor, S. J., Crawley, A. P. Wood, M. L., and Mikulis, D. J. 1997. Functional MRI of pain- and attention-related activation in the human cingulate cortex. *Neuroreport* 77: 3370–3380.

Davis, K. D., Wood, M. L., Crawley, A. P. and Mikulis, D. J. 1995. fMRI of human somatosensory and cingulate cortex during painful electrical nerve stimulation. *Neuroreport* 7: 321–325.

Davis, L. 1982. Functionalism and absent qualia. *Philosophical Studies* 41: 231–249.

Debus, S., and Sandkühler, J. 1996. Low dimensional attractors in discharges of sensory neurons in the rat spinal dorsal horn neurons are maintained by supraspinal descending system. *Neuroscience* 70: 191–200.

DeGood, D. D. 1988. A rationale and format for psychosocial evaluation. In N. T. Lynch and S. V. Vasudevan (eds.), *Persistent Pain: Psychosocial Assessment and Intervention.* Dordrecht: Kluwer Academic Publishers.

De Moore, G. M., and Robertson, A. R. 1996. Suicide in the 18 years after deliberate self-harm: A prospective study. *British Journal of Psychiatry* 169: 489–494.

Dennett, D. C. 1971. Intentional systems. *The Journal of Philosophy* 68: 87–106.

Dennett, D. C. 1978. Why you can't make a computer that feels pain. *Synthese* 38: 449.

Dennett, D. C. 1987. *The Intentional Stance*. Cambridge, MA: The MIT Press.

De Pascalis, V., and Perrone, M. 1996. EEG asymmetry and heart rate during experience of hypnotic analgesia in high and low hypnotizables. *International Journal of Psychophysiology* 21: 163–175.

De Pascalis, V., Crawford, H. J., and Marucci, F. S. 1992. The modulation of pain by hypnotic analgesia: Effect on somatorsensory evoked potentials. *Communicazioni Scientifiche di Psicologie Generale*, 71–89.

Derbyshire, S. W. G. 1996. Comment on editorial by Anand and Craig. *Pain* 67: 210–211.

Derbyshire, S. W. G. 1998. Reply to N. Cunningham. *Pain* 74: 104–106.

Derbyshire, S. W. G., Jones, A. K. P., Brown, W. D., Devani, P., Friston, K. J., Qi, L. Y., Pearce, S., Frackowiak, R. S. J., and Jones, T. 1993. Cortical and subcortical responses to pain in male and female volunteers. *7th World Congress on Pain* 7: 500.

Derbyshire, S. W. G., Jones, A. K. P., Devani, P, Friston, K. J., Feinman, C., Harris, M., and Pearce, S. 1993. Cerebral responses to pain in patients with atypical facial pain. *7th World Congress on Pain* 7: 261–262.

Derbyshire, S. W. G., Jones, A. K. P., Devani, K. J., Friston, K. J., Feinmann, C., Harris, M., Pearce, S., Watson, J. D. G., and Frackowiak, R. S. J. 1994. Cerebral responses to pain with atypical facial pain measured by positron emission tomography. *Journal of Neurology, Neurosurgery, and Psychiatry* 57: 1166–1172.

Descartes, R. [1641] 1970. Meditations on first philosophy. In *The Philosophical Works of Descartes, Volume 1*. Trans. by E. S. Haldane and G. R. T. Ross. Cambridge: Cambridge University Press.

Desimone, R., and Duncan, J. 1995. Neural mechanisms of selective visual attention. *Annual Review of Neuroscience* 18: 193–222.

Devaney, R. L. 1987. *An Introduction to Chaotic Dynamical Systems*. New York: Addison-Wesley.

Devinsky, O. 1996. Psychogenic basilar migraine. *Neurology* 46: 1786–1787.

Devitt, M. 1990a. Transcendentalism about content. *Pacific Philosophical Quarterly* 71: 247–263.

Devitt, M. 1990b. A narrow representational theory of mind. In W. Lycan (ed.), *Mind and Cognition*, 371–398. Oxford: Basil Blackwell.

Devitt, M., and Rey, G. 1991. Transcending transcendentalism. *Pacific Philosophical Quarterly* 72: 87–100.

Deyo, R. A., and Tsui-Wu, Y-J. 1987. Descriptive epidemiology of low back pain and its related medical care in the United States. *Spine* 12: 264–268.

Dillenburger, K., and Keenan, M. 1996. Obstetric hypnosis: An experience. *Contemporary Hypnosis* 13: 202–204.

Di Piero, V., Jones, A. K. P., Iannotti, F., Powell, M., Perani, D., Lenzi, G. L., and Frackowiak, R. S. J. 1991. Chronic pain: A PET study of the central effects of percutaneous high cervical codotomy. *Pain* 46: 9–12.

Domangue, B. B., Margolis, C. G., Lieberman, D., and Kaji, H. 1985. Biochemical correlates of hypnoanalgesia in arthritic pain patients. *Journal of Clinical Psychiatry* 46: 235–238.

Double, R. 1986. On the very idea of eliminating the intentional. *Journal of the Theory of Social Behavior* 16: 209–216.

Double, R. 1987. More on the ineliminable intentional: A reply to Churchland's "Cognition and conceptual change: A reply to Double." *Journal of the Theory of Social Behavior* 17: 219–225.

Dougherty, P. M., and Willis, W. D. 1992. Enhanced responses of spinothalamic tract neurons to excitatory amino acids accompany capsaicin-induced sensitization in the monkey. *Journal of Neuroscience* 12: 883–894.

Dray, A., Urban, L., and Dickenson, A. 1994. Pharmacology of chronic pain. *Trends in Pharmacological Science* 15: 190–197.

Dretske, F. 1981. *Knowledge and the Flow of Information.* Cambridge, MA: The MIT Press.

Dretske, F. 1988. *Explaining Behavior: Reasons in a World of Causes.* Cambridge, MA: The MIT Press.

Drevets, W. C., Burton, H., Videen, T. O., Snyder, A. Z., Simpson, J. R., Jr., and Raichle, M. E. 1995. Blood flow changes in human somatosensory cortex during anticipated stimulation. *Nature* 373: 249–252.

Drossman, D. 1982. Patients with psychogenic abdominal pain: Six years' observation in the medical setting. *American Journal of Psychiatry* 139: 1549–1557.

Dubo, E. D., Zanarini, M. C., Lewis, R. E., and Williams, A. A. 1997. Childhood antecedents of self-destructiveness in borderline personality disorder. *Canadian Journal of Psychiatry* 42: 63–69.

Duncan, G. H., Morin, C., Coghill, R. C., Evans, A., Worsley, K. J., and Bushell, M. C. 1994. Using psychophysical ratings to map the human brain regression of regional blood flow (rCBF) to tonic pain perception. *Society of Neuroscience Abstracts* 20: 1572.

Dworkin, S. F. 1994. Somatization, distress and chronic pain. *Quality of Life Research* 3: S77–83.

Dworkin, S. F., and Burgess, J. A. 1987. Orofacial pain of psychogenic origin: Current concepts and classification. *Journal of American Dental Association* 115: 565–571.

Eckman, J. P., and Ruelle, D. 1985. Ergodic theory of chaos and strange attractors. *Review of Modern Physics* 57: 617–656.

Egan, F. 1995. Folk psychology and cognitive architecture. *Philosophy of Science* 62: 179–196.

Ekselius, L., Eriksson, M., von Knorring, L., and Linder, J. 1996. Personality disorders and major depression in patients with somatoform pain disorders and medical illnesses in relation to age at onset of work disability. *European Journal of Psychiatry* 10: 35–43.

Eland, J. M., and Anderson, J. E. 1977. The experience of pain in children. In A. Jacox (ed.), *Pain: A Sourcebook for Nurses and Other Health Professionals*. Boston: Little, Brown.

Eliasmith, C. 1996. The third contender: A critical examination of the dynamicist theory of cognition. *Philosophical Psychology* 9: 441–464.

Elton, D., Burrows, G. D., and Stanely, G. V. 1980. Chronic pain and hypnosis. In G. D. Burrows and L. Dennerstein (eds.), *Handbook of Hypnosis and Psychosomatic Medicine*. Amsterdam: Elsevier.

Emmers, R. 1981. *Pain: A Spike-Interval Coded Message in the Brain*. New York: Raven Press.

Engel, G. L. 1959. "Psychogenic" pain and the pain-prone patient. *American Journal of Medicine* 26: 899–918.

Etscheidt, M., Steger, H., and Braverman, B. 1995. Multidimensional pain inventory profile classifications and psychopathology. *Journal of Clinical Psychology* 51: 29–36.

Evans, A. C., Meyer, E., and Marret, S. 1992. Pain and activation in the thalamus. *Trends in Neuroscience* 15: 252.

Evans, F. J. 1974. The placebo response in pain reduction. In J. J. Bonica (ed.), *International Symposium on Pain, Advances in Neurology, Volume 4*. New York: Raven Press.

Everett, J. J., Patterson, D. R., Burns, G. L., Montgomery, B., and Heimbach, D. 1993. Adjunctive interventions for burn pain control: Comparison of hypnosis and ativan: The 1993 Clinical Research Award. *Journal of Burn Care and Rehabilitation* 14: 676–683.

Ewin, D. M. 1986. The effect of hypnosis and mental set on major surgery and burns. *Psychiatric Annals* 16: 115–118.

Faravelli, C., Salvatori, S., Galassi, F., Aiazzi, L., Drei, C., and Cabras, P. 1997. Epidemiology of somatoform disorders: A community survey in Florence. *Social Psychiatry and Psychiatric Epidemiology* 32: 24–29.

Farthing, G. W., Venturino, M., Brown, S. W., and Lazar, J. D. 1997. Internal and external distraction in the control of cold-pressor pain as a function of hypnotizability. *International Journal of Clinical and Experimental Hypnosis* 45: 433–446.

Favazza, A. R. 1987. *Bodies Under Siege: Self-Mutilation in Culture and Psychiatry.* Baltimore, MD: The Johns Hopkins University Press.

Favazza, A. R. 1998. The coming of age of self-mutilation. *Journal of Nervous and Mental Disease* 186: 259–268.

Favazza, A. R., DeRosear, L., and Conterio, K. 1989. Self-mutilation and eating disorders. *Suicide and Life-Threatening Behavior* 19: 352–361.

Favazza, A. R., and Rosenthal, R. J. 1993. Diagnostic issues in self-mutilation. *Hospital and Community Psychiatry* 44: 134–140.

Fedorczyk, J. 1997. The role of physical agents in modulating pain. *Journal of Hand Therapy* 10: 110–121.

Feyerabend, P. K. 1963a. Mental events and the brain. *The Journal of Philosophy* 60: 295–296.

Feyerabend, P. K. 1963b. Materialism and the mind-body problem. *Review of Metaphysics* 17: 49–67.

Field, J. 1978. Mental representation. *Erkenntnis* 13: 9–61.

Fields, H. L. 1981. An endorphin-mediated analgesia system: Experimental and clinical observations. In J. B. Martin, S. Reichlin, and K. L. Brick (eds.), *Neurosecretion and Brain Peptides: Implications for Brain Function and Neurological Disease.* New York: Raven Press.

Fields, H. L. (ed.). 1987. *Pain.* New York: McGraw-Hill.

Fields, H. L., and Basbaum, A. I. 1989. Endogenous pain control mechanisms. In P. H. Wall and R. Melzack (eds.), *Textbook of Pain, Second Edition.* New York: Churchill Livingstone.

Fillion, T. J., and Blass, E. M. 1986. Infantile experience with suckling odors determines adult sexual behavior in male rats. *Science* 231: 729–731.

Fingarette, H. 1988. *Heavy Drinking: The Myth of Alcoholism as a Disease.* Berkeley, CA: University of California Press.

Fishbain, D. A. 1996. Where have two DSM revisions taken us for the diagnosis of pain disorder in chronic pain patients? *American Journal of Psychiatry* 153: 137–138.

Fisichelli, V. R., Karelitz, R. M., Fisichelli, R. M., and Cooper, J. 1974. The course of induced crying activity in the first year of life. *Pediatric Research* 8: 921–928.

Fitzgerald, M. 1991. Development of pain mechanisms. *British Medical Bulletin* 47: 667–675.

Fitzgerald, M. 1995. Fetal pain: An update of current scientific knowledge. Paper for the Department of Health, London.

Fitzgerald, M. 1995. Pain in infancy: Some unanswered questions. *Pain Reviews* 2: 77–91.

Fodor, J. A. 1974. Special sciences. *Synthese* 28: 77–115.

Fodor, J. A. 1987. *Psychosemantics: The Problem of Meaning in the Philosophy of Mind.* Cambridge, MA: The MIT Press.

Fodor, J. A. 1990a. *A Theory of Content and Other Essays.* Cambridge, MA: The MIT Press.

Fodor, J. A. 1990b. Psychosemantics, or: Where do truth conditions come from? In W. Lycan (ed.), *Mind and Cognition.* Oxford: Basil Blackwell.

Fodor, J. A. 1990c. Roundtable discussion. In P. Hanson (ed.), *Information, Language, and Cognition.* Vancouver: University of British Columbia Press.

Fodor, J. A., and Pylyshyn, Z. 1988. Connectionism and cognitive architecture: A critical analysis. *Cognition* 28: 3–71.

Foote, S. L., and Morrison, J. H. 1987. Extrathalamaic modulation of cortico-function. *Annual Review of Neuroscience* 10: 67–95.

Foote, S. L., Bloom, F. E., and Aston-Jones, G. 1983. Nucleus locus coeruleus: New evidence of anatomical and physiological specificity. *Physiology Review* 63: 844–914.

Fordyce, W. E. 1976. *Behavioral Methods for Chronic Pain and Illness.* St. Louis, MO: C. V. Mosby.

Fordyce, W. E. 1978. Learning process in pain. In R. A. Sternbach (ed.), *The Psychology of Pain.* New York: Raven Press.

Fordyce, W. E. 1986. Learning processes in pain. In R. A. Sternbach (ed.), *The Psychology of Pain, Second Edition.* New York: Raven Press.

Fordyce, W. E., Fowler, S. R., Jr., Lehmann, J., and DeLateur, B. J. 1968. Some implications of learning in problems of chronic pain. *Journal of Chronic Diseases* 21: 179–190.

Fordyce, W. E., Fowler, R., Lehmann, J., DeLateur, B. J., Sand, P. L., and Treischmann, R. 1973. Operant conditioning in the treatment of chronic pain. *Archives of Physical Medicine and Rehabilitation* 54: 399–408.

Forster, M., and Saidel, E. 1994. Connectionism and the fate of folk psychology. *Philosophical Psychology* 7: 437–452.

Francis, A., First, M. D., and Pincus, H. A. 1995. *DSM-IV Guidebook.* Washington, DC: American Psychiatric Press.

Freeman, R. 1993. A psychotherapeutic case illustrating a psychogenic factor in burning mouth syndrome. *British Journal of Psychotherapy* 10: 220–225.

Freeman, W. 1991. The physiology of perception. *Scientific American* 264: 78–85.

Freeman, W. J., and Schneider, W. 1982. Changes in spatial patterns of rabbit olfactory EEG with conditioning to odors. *Psychophysiology* 19: 44–56.

French, L. A., Chou, S. N., and Story, J. L. 1966. *Clinical Orthopedics* 46: 83–86.

Fry, R., Crisp, A., and Beard, R. 1997. Sociopsychological factors in chronic pelvic pain: A review. *Journal of Psychosomatic Research* 42: 1–15.

Frymoyer, J. W., and Cats-Baril, W. L. 1991. An overview of the incidences and costs of low back pain. *Orthopedic Clinics of North America* 22: 263–271.

Fulton, J. E. 1951. *Frontal Lobotomy and Affective Behavior.* New York: W. W. Norton.

Fuxe, K., and Agnati, L. F. (eds.). 1991. *Volume Transmission in the Brain: Novel Mechanisms for Neural Transmission.* New York: Raven Press.

Galbraith, G. C., Cooper, L. M., and London, P. 1972. Hypnotic susceptibility and the sonsory evoked response. *Journal of Comparative and Physiological Psychology* 80: 509–514.

Galen. [1821] 1997. *Claudii Galeni opera omnia.* New York: Hildesheim.

Gallez, D., and Babloyantz, A. 1991. Predictability of human EEG: A dynamical approach. *Biological Cybernetics* 64: 381–391.

Gamsa, A. 1994a. The role of psychological factors in chronic pain. I. A half century of study. *Pain* 57: 5–15.

Gamsa, A. 1994b. The role of psychological factors in chronic pain. II. A critical reappraisal. *Pain* 57: 17–29.

Gamsa, A. 1990. Is emotional disturbance a precipitator or a consequence of chronic pain? *Pain* 42: 183–195.

Gamsa, A., and Vikis-Freibergs, V. 1991. Psychological events are both risk factors in, and consequences of, chronic pain. *Pain* 44: 271–277.

Garber, J., Zeman, J., and Walker, L. 1990. Recurrent abdominal pain in children: Psychiatric diagnoses and parental psychopathology. *Journal of American Academic Child Adolescent Psychiatry* 29: 648–656.

Garcia, J., and Altman, R. D. 1997a. Chronic pain states. *Seminars in Arthritis and Rheumatism* 27: 1–16.

Garcia, J., and Altman, R. D. 1997b. Chronic pain states: Invasive procedures. *Seminars in Arthritis and Rheumatism* 27: 156–160.

Garson, J. W. 1996. Cognition poised at the edge of chaos: A complex alternative to a symbolic mind. *Philosophical Psychology* 9: 301–322.

Gatchel, R., Polatin, P., and Kinney, R. 1995. Predicting outcome of chronic back pain using clinical predictors of psychopathology: A prospective analysis. *Health Psychology* 14: 415–420.

Gaukroger, P. B., Tomkins, D. P., and van der Walt, J. H. 1989. Patient-controlled analgesia in children. *Anaesthesia and Intensive Care* 17: 264–268.

Gazarian, M., Taddio, A., Klein, J., et al. 1995. Penile absorption of EMLA cream in piglets: Implications for use of EMLA in neonatal circumcision. *Biological Neonate* 68: 334–341.

Gelfand, S. 1964. The relationship of experimental pain tolerance to pain threshold. *Canadian Journal of Psychology* 18: 36–42.

Genuis, M. L. 1995. The use of hypnosis in helping cancer patients control anxiety, pain, and emesis: A review of recent empirical studies. *American Journal of Clinical Hypnosis* 37: 316–325.

Ghia, J., Duncan, G., Toomey, T., Mao, W., and Gregg, J. 1979. The pharmacologic approach in differential diagnosis of chronic pain. *Spine* 4: 447–451.

Ghia, J., Mueller, R., Duncan, G., Scott, D., and Mao, W. 1981. Serotonergic activity in man as a function of pain, pain mechanisms, and depression. *Anesthesiology and Analgesia* 60: 854–861.

Giannakoulopoulos, X., Sepulveda, W., Pourtis, P., Glover, V., and Fisk, N. M. 1994. Fetal plasma cortisol and β-endorphin response to intrauterine needling. *Lancet* 344: 77–80.

Gilbody, S., House, A., and Owens, D. 1997. The early repetition of deliberate self-harm. *Journal of the Royal College of Physicians London* 31: 171–172.

Giles, L. G. F., and Crawford, C. M. 1997. Shadows of the truth in patients with spinal pain: A review. *Canadian Journal of Psychiatry* 42: 44–48.

Giles, L. G. F., and Kaveri, M. J. P. 1990. Some osseous and soft tissue causes of human intervertebral canal (foramen) stenosis. *Journal of Rheumatology* 17: 1471–1481.

Gillett, G. R. 1991. The neurophilosophy of pain. *Philosophy* 66: 191–206.

Glass, L. and Mackey, M. C. 1988. *From Clocks to Chaos: The Rhythms of Life.* Princeton, NJ: Princeton University Press.

Gleick, J. 1987. *Chaos: Making a New Science.* New York: Viking.

Glover, H., Lader, W., and Walker-O'Keefe, J. 1995. Vulnerability scale scores in female inpatients diagnosed with self-injurious behavior, dissociative identity disorder, and major depression. *Psychology Reports* 77: 987–993.

Glover, H., Lader, W., Walker-O'Keefe, J., and Goodnick. 1997. Numbing scale scores in female psychiatric inpatients diagnosed with self-injurious behavior, dissociative identity disorder, and major depression. *Psychiatry Research* 70: 115–123.

Godfrey, R. G. 1996. A guide to the understanding and use of tricyclic antidepressants in the overall management of fibromyalgia and other chronic pain syndromes. *Archives of Internal Medicine* 156: 1047–1052.

Godfrey-Smith, P. 1989. Misinformation. *Canadian Journal of Philosophy* 19: 533–550.

Golan, H. P. 1997. The use of hypnosis in the treatment of psychogenic oral pain. *American Journal of Clinical Hypnosis* 40: 89–96.

Goldstein, A. and Hilgard, E. R. 1975. Failure of opiate antagonist naloxone to modify hypnotic analgesia. *Proceedings of the National Academy of Sciences* 72: 2041–2043.

Gomez, J., and Dally, P. 1977. Psychologically mediated abdominal pain in surgical and medical outpatients clinics. *British Medical Journal* 1: 1451–1453.

Gonsalkorale, W. M. 1996. The use of hypnosis in medicine: The possible pathways involved. *European Journal of Gastroenterology and Heptology* 8: 520–524.

Gracely, R. H. 1980. Pain measurement in man. In J. J. Bonica (ed.), *Pain, Discomfort, and Humanitarian Care.* Amsterdam: Elsevier.

Gracely, R. H. 1995. Hypnosis and hierarchical pain control systems. *Pain* 60: 1–2.

Gracely, R. H., Dubner, R., and McGath, P. A. 1979. Narcotic analgesia: Fentanyl reduces the intensity but not the unpleasantness of painful tooth pulp sensations. *Science* 203: 1261–1263.

Gracely, R. H., Dubner, R., and McGath, P. A. 1982. Fentanyl reduces the intensity of painful tooth pulp sensations: Controlling for detection of active drugs. *Anesthesia and Analgesia* 61: 751–755.

Gracely, R. H., McGath, P., and Dubner, R. 1978a. Ratio scales of sensory and affective verbal pain descriptors. *Pain* 5: 5–18.

Gracely, R. H., McGath, P., and Dubner, R. 1978b. Validity and sensitivity of ratio scales of sensory and affective verbal pain descriptiors. *Pain* 5: 19–29.

Graham, G., and Stephens, G. L. 1985. Are qualia a pain in the neck for functionalists? *American Philosophical Quarterly* 22: 73–80.

Graham, G. W. 1975. Hypnotic treatment for migraine headaches. *International Journal of Clinical and Experimental Hypnosis* 23: 165–171.

Grahek, N. 1991. Objective and subjective aspects of pain. *Philosophical Psychology* 4: 249–266

Grassberger, P., and Procaccia, I. 1983. Characterization of strange attractors. *American Physics Society* 50: 346–349.

Gray, J. A. 1982. *The Neuropsychology of Anxiety: An Enquiry into the Functions of the Septo-hippocampal System.* New York: Oxford University Press.

Gray, J. A. 1987. *The Psychology of Fear and Stress.* New York: Cambridge University Press.

Greene, R. J., and Reyher, J. 1972. Pain tolerance in hypnotic analgesic and imagination states. *Journal of Abnormal Psychology* 79: 29–38.

Greenwood, J. D. 1991. Reasons to believe. In J. D. Greenwood (ed.), *The Future of Folk Psychology.* Cambridge, MA: Cambridge University Press.

Greenwood, J. D. 1992. Against eliminative materialism: From folk psychology to Volkerpsychologie. *Philosophical Psychology* 5: 349–368.

Grunau, R. V. S., Whitfield, M. F., et al. 1994. Early pain experience, child temperament and family characteristics as precursors of somatization: A prospective study of preterm and fullterm children. *Pain* 56: 353–359.

Grush, R. 1997. Review of *Mind as Motion: Exploration in the Dynamics of Cognition. Philosophical Psychology* 10: 233–242.

Grushka, M., Sessle, B. J., and Miller, R. 1987. Pain and personality profiles in burning mouth syndrome. *Pain* 28: 155–167.

Gruzelier, J. H., and Warren, K. 1993. Neurophyschological evidence of reductions on left frontal tests with hypnosis. *Psychological Medicine* 23: 93–101.

Grzesiak, R. C., and Ciccone, D. S. (eds). 1994. *Psychological Vulnerability to Chronic Pain*. New York: Springer.

Guerrero-Figueroa, R., and Heath, R. G. 1964. Evoked responses and changes during attentive factors in man. *Archives of Neurology* 10: 74–84.

Gunnar, M. R., Fisch, R. O., and Malone, S. 1984. The effects of a pacifying stimulus on behavioral and adrenocortical responses to circumcision. *Journal of American Academy of Child Psychiatry* 23: 34–38.

Gunnar, M. R., Porter, F. L., Wolf, C. M., Rigatuso, J., and Larson, M. C. 1995. Neonatal stress reactivity: Predictions to later emotional temperament. *Child Development* 66: 1–13.

Gustafson, R., and Kallmen, H. 1990. Psychological defense mechanisms and manifest anxiety as indicators of secondary psychosomatic body pain. *Psychology Reports* 66: 1283–1292.

Guy, E. R., and Abbott, F. V. 1992. The behavioral response to formalin pain in preweanling rats. *Pain* 51: 81–90.

Guyton, A. C. 1991. *Basic Neuroscience: Anatomy and Physiology*. Philadelphia: W. B. Saunders.

Haanen, H. C. M., Hoenderdos, H. T. W., Van Romunde, L. K. J., Hop, W. C. J., Malle, C., Terweil, J. P., and Hekster, G. B. 1991. Controlled trial of hypnotherapy in the treatment of refractory fibromyalgia. *Journal of Rheumatology* 18: 72–75.

Haas, R. H., Townsend, J., Courchesne, E., Lincoln, A. J., Schreibman, L., and Yeung-Courchesne, R. 1996. Neurologic abnormalities in infantile autism. *Journal of Child Neurology* 11: 84–92.

Haegerstam, G., and Allerbring, M. 1995. Lack of disability in patients with chronic orofacial pain. A retrospective study. *Acta Odontolica Scandanavia* 53: 345–348.

Haines, J., Williams, C. L., Brain, K. L., and Wilson, G. V. 1995. The psychophysiology of self-mutilation. *Journal of Abnormal Psychology* 104: 471–489.

Haldane, J. 1988. Understanding folk. *Aristotelian Society Supplement* 62: 222–246.

Hall, R. J. 1989. Are pains necessarily unpleasant? *Philosophy and Phenomenological Research* 49: 643–659.

Hannan, B. 1990. "Non-scientific" realism about propositional attitudes as a response to eliminativist arguments. *Behavior and Philosophy* 18: 21–31.

Hannan, B. 1993. Don't stop believing: The case against eliminative materialism. *Mind and Language* 8: 165–179.

Hardcastle, V. G. 1992. Reduction, explanatory extension, and the mind/brain sciences. *Philosophy of Science* 59: 408–428.

Hardcastle, V. G. 1994. Psychology's binding problem and possible neurobiological solutions. *Journal of Consciousness Studies* 1: 66–90.

Hardcastle, V. G. 1995. *Locating Consciousness.* Amsterdam: John Benjamins Press.

Hardcastle, V. G. 1996. *How to Build a Theory in Cognitive Science.* Albany, NY: SUNY Press.

Hardcastle, V. G. 1997. When a pain is not. *The Journal of Philosophy* 94: 381–409.

Harpin, V. A., and Rutter, N. 1982. Making heel pricks less painful. *Archives of Diseases in Childhood* 71: 226–228.

Haslam, D. 1969. Age and the perception of pain. *Psychonomic Science* 15: 86–87.

Hausotter, W. 1996. Die Begatuchtung der Eisenbahnunfälle am Beginn des Industriezeitalters: Ein medizinhistorischer Exkurs mit Bezug zur Gegenwart. *Versicherungsmedizin* 48: 138–142.

Head, H., and Holmes, G. 1911. Sensory disturbances from cerebral lesions. *Brain* 34: 102–254.

Hebb, D. O. 1949. *The Organization of Behavior.* New York: Wiley.

Heinild, S. V., Malner, E., Roelfaard, G., and Worning, B. 1959. A psychosomatic approach to RAP in childhood with particular reference to the X-ray appearances of the stomach. *Acta Pediatrica Scandinavica* 48: 361–370.

Helme, R. D., and Katz, B. 1993. Management of chronic pain. *Medical Journal* 158: 478–481.

Henden, O., Horn, D., and Usher, M. 1991. Chaotic behavior of a neural network with dynamical thresholds. *International Journal of Neural Systems* 1: 327–335.

Hendler, N., and Kozikowski, J. 1993. Overlooked physical diagnoses in chronic pain patients involved in litigation. *Psychosomatics* 34: 494–501.

Hendler, N., Bergson, C., and Morrison, C. 1996. Overlooked physical diagnoses in chronic pain patients involved in litigation, Part 2. The addition of MRI, nerve blocks, 3-D CT, and qualitative flow meter. *Psychosomatics* 37: 509–517.

Hendler, N., Zinreich, J., and Kozikowski, J. G. 1993. Three-dimensional CT validation of physical complaints in "psychogenic pain" patients. *Psychosomatics* 34: 90–96.

Hernandez-Peon, R., and Donoso, M. 1959. Influence of attention and suggestion upon subcortical evoked electric activity in the human brain. In L. Van Bobaert and J. Radermecker (eds.), *First International Congress of Neurological Sciences, Volume 3.* Oxford: Pergamon.

Hernandez-Peon, R., Dittborn, J., Borlone, M., and Davidovich, A. 1960. Changes in spinal excitabilitiy during hypnotically induced anesthesia and hyperesthesia. *American Journal of Clinical Hypnosis* 3: 64.

Herpertz, S. 1995. Self-injurious behavior. Psychopathological and nosological characteristics in subtypes of self-injurers. *Acta Psychiatry Scandanavia* 91: 57–68.

Hilgard, E. R. 1980. Hypnosis in the treatment of pain. In G. D Burrows and L. Dennerstein (eds.), *Handbook of Hypnosis and Psychosomatic Medicine*. Amsterdam: Elsevier.

Hilgard, E. R. 1986. *Divided Consciousness: Multiple Controls in Human Thought and Action*. New York: Wiley.

Hilgard, E. R., and Hilgard, J. R. 1994. *Hypnosis in the Relief of Pain, Revised Edition*. New York: Brunner/Mazel Publishers.

Hill, A., Niven, C. A., and Knussen, C. 1996. Pain memories in phantom limbs: A case study. *Pain* 66: 381–384.

Hirato, M., Kawashima, Y., Shibazaki, T., Shibasaki, T., and Ohye, C. 1991. Patholophysiology of central (thalamic) pain: A possible role of the intralaminar nuclei in superficial pain. *Acta Neuroschirugica* (Suppl.) 52: 133–136.

Hoheisel, U., and Mense, S. 1989. Long-term changes in discharge behavior of cat dorsal horn neurones following noxious stimulation of deep tissues. *Pain* 36: 231–247.

Holroyd, J. 1992. Hypnosis as a methodology in psychological research. In E. Fromm and M. R. Nash (eds.), *Contemporary Hypnosis Research*. New York: Guildford.

Holroyd, J. 1995. Hypnosis treatment of clinical pain: Understanding why hypnosis is useful. *International Journal of Clinical and Experimental Hypnosis* 44: 33–51.

Holzman, A. D., Turk D. C., and Kerns, R. D. 1986. The cognitive-behavioral approach in treating chronic pain. In A. D. Holzman and D. C. Turk (eds.), *Pain Management: A Handbook of Psychological Treatment Approaches*. Elmsford, NY: Pergamon Press.

Honigl, D., Kriechbaum, N., Zidek, D., Hasiba, K., and Zapotoczky, H. G. 1997. Self-injury behavior. *Acta Medical Austriaca* 24: 19–22.

Horgan, T. 1993. The austere ideology of folk psychology. *Mind and Language* 8: 282–297.

Horgan, T., and Graham, G. 1990. In defense of southern fundamentalism. *Philosophical Studies* 62: 107–134.

Horgan, T., and Tienson, J. 1995. Connectionism and the commitments of folk psychology. *Philosophical Perspectives* 9: 127–152.

Horgan, T., and Tienson, J. 1996. *Connectionism and the Philosophy of Psychology*. Cambridge, MA: The MIT Press.

Horgan, T., and Woodward, J. 1985. Folk psychology is here to stay. *Philosophical Review* 94: 197–225.

Horst, S. 1995. Eliminativism and the ambiguity of "belief." *Synthese* 104: 123–145.

Hosobuchi, Y. 1991. Treatment of cerebral ischemia with electrical stimulation of the cervical spinal cord. *Pace* 14: 122–126.

Houghton, L. A., Heyman, D. J., and Whorwell, P. J. 1996. Symptomatology, quality of life and economic features of irritable bowel syndrome—the effect of hypnotherapy. *Alimentary Pharmacological Therapy* 10: 91–95.

Hsieh, J., Belfrage, M., Stone-Elander, S., Hansson, P., and Ingvar, M. 1995. Central representation of chronic ongoing neuropathic pain studied by positron emission tomography. *Pain* 63: 225–236.

Hubbard, T. L. 1996. Synesthesia-like mappings of lightness, pitch, and melodic interval. *American Journal of Psychology* 109: 219–238.

Hubel, D. H., and Wiesel, T. N. 1972. Laminar and columnar distribution of geniculo-cortical fibers in the Macaque monkey. *Journal of Comparative Neurology* 158: 267–294.

Hubel, D. H., and Wiesel, T. N. 1977. Functional architecture of macaque monkey visual cortex. *Proceedings of the Royal Society of London B* 198: 1–59.

Hylden, J. L. K., Nahin, R. L., Traub, R. J., and Dubner, R. 1989. Expansion of receptive fields of spinal lamina 1 projection neurones in rats with unilateral adjuvant-induced inflammation: The contribution of dorsal horn mechanisms. *Pain* 37: 229–243.

Iadarola, M. J., Max, M. B., Berman, K. F., Byas-Smith, M. G., Coghill, R. C., Gracely, R. H., and Bennett, G. J. 1995. Unilateral decrease in thalamic activity observed with positron emission tomography in patients with chronic neuropathic pain. *Pain* 63: 55–64.

Ingvar, D. H. 1975. Patterns of brain activity revealed by measurements of regional cerebral blood flow. In D. H. Ingvar and N. A. Lassen (eds.), *Brain Work: The Coupling of Function, Metabolism, and Blood Flow in the Brain.* Copenhagen: Munksgaard.

Ingvar, D. H., Rosén, I., Eriksson, M., and Elmqvist, D. 1976. Activation patterns induced in the dominant hemisphere by skin stimulation. In Y. Zotterman (ed.), *Sensory Functions of the Skin.* London: Pergamon Press.

International Association for the Study of Pain (IASP). Subcommittee on Classification. 1986. Pain terms: A current list with definitions and notes on usage. *Pain* Supplement 3: 217.

Isaacson, R. L. 1982. *The Limbic System.* New York: Plenum Press.

Izard, C. E., Hembree, E. A., and Huebner, R. R. 1987. Infants' emotion expression to acute pain: Developmental change and stability of individual differences. *Developmental Psychology* 23: 105–113.

Izard, C. E., Hembree, E. A., Dougherty, L. M., and Spizzirri, C. C. 1983. Changes in facial expressions of 2- to 19-month-old infants following acute pain. *Developmental Psychology* 19: 418–426.

Jackson, F., and Petit, P. 1990. In defense of folk psychology. *Philosophical Studies* 59: 31–54.

Jacob, J. J., Tremblay, E. C., and Colombel, M-C. 1974. Facilitation de réactions nociceptives par le naloxone chez la souris et chez le rat. *Psychopharmacologia* 37: 217–223.

Jacobs, A. L., Kurtz, R. M., and Strube, M. J. 1995. Hypnotic analgesia, expectancy effects, and choice of design: A reexamination. *International Journal of Clinical and Experimental Hypnosis* 43: 55–69.

Jacoby, H. 1985. Eliminativism, meaning, and qualitative states. *Philosophical Studies*

James, W. [1890] 1981. *The Principles of Psychology.* Cambridge, MA: Harvard University Press.

Jänig, W. 1987. Neuronal mechanisms of pain with special emphasis on visceral and deep somatic pain. *Acta Neuroschirugica* (Suppl.) 38: 16–32.

Jay, S. M., Ozolins, M., and Elliot, C. H. 1983. Assessment of children's distress during painful medical procedures. *Health Psychology* 2: 133–147.

Jensen, J. 1988. Pain in non-psychotic psychiatric patients: Life events, symptomatology and personality traits. *Acta Psychiatrica Scandanavia* 78: 201–207.

Jensen, T. S., and Rasmussen, P. 1989. Phantom pain and related phenomena after amputation. In P. D. Wall and R. Melzack (eds.), *Textbook of Pain, 2nd Edition.* New York: Churchill Livingstone.

Johansson, F., Almay, B., von Knorring, L., Terenius, L., and Astrom, M. 1979. Personality traits in chronic pain patients related to endorphin levels in cerebrospinal fluid. *Psychiatry Research* 1: 231–239.

Johnson, C. C., and Stevens, B. 1996. The effect of postnatal age, perinatal factors, and repeated painful events on the response to pain from routine heelstick in preterm infants of 32 weeks gestational age. *Pediatrics.*

Jones, A. K. P., Brown, W. D., Friston, K. J., Qi, L. Y., and Frackowiak, R. S. J. 1991. Cortical and subcortical localization of response to pain in man using positron emission tomography. *Proceedings of the Royal Society London* 244: 39–44.

Joukamaa, M. 1987. Psychological factors in low back pain. *Annual Clinic Research* 19: 129–134.

Joukamaa, M. 1991. Low back pain and psychological factors. *Psychotherapy and Psychosomatics* 55: 186–190.

Joyce, P. R., and Walshe, J. W. B. 1980. A family with abdominal pain. *New Zealand Medical Journal* 92: 278–279.

Kahan, J., and Pattison, E. M. 1984. Proposal for a distinctive diagnosis: The deliberate self-harm syndrome. *Suicide and Life Threatening Behavior* 14: 17–35.

Kandel, E. R., and Schwartz, J. H. 1985. *Principles of Neural Science, Second Edition.* New York: Elsevier.

Kandel, E. R., Schwartz, J. H., and Jessel, J. J. 1995. *Principles of Neural Science, Third Edition.* New York: Elsevier.

Kanner, L. 1943. Autistic disturbance of affective contact. *Nervous Child* 2: 217–250.

Kassowitz, K. E. 1958. Psychodynamic reactions of children to the use of hypodermic needles. *American Medical Association Journal of Diseases in Childhood* 95: 253–257.

Katayama, Y., Tsubokawa, T., Hirayama, T., Kido, G., Tsukiyama, T., and Io, I. 1986. Response of regional cerebral blood flow and oxygen metabolism to thalamic stimulation in humans as revealed by positron emission tomography. *Journal of Cerebral Blood Flow Metabolism* 6: 637–641.

Katchalsky, A. K., Rowland, V., and Blumenthal, R. 1974. Dynamic patterns of brain cell assemblies. *Neuroscience Research Program Bulletin* 12: 152.

Katon, W., Egan, K., and Miller, D. 1985. Chronic pain: Lifetime psychiatric diagnoses and family history. *American Journal of Psychiatry* 142: 1156–1160.

Katon, W., Kleinman, A., and Rosen, G. 1982. Depression and somatization: A review (parts 1 and 2). *American Journal of Medicine* 72: 127–247.

Katz, E. R., Kellerman, J., and Siegel, S. E. 1980. Behavioral distress in children with cancer undergoing medical procedures: Developmental considerations. *Journal of Consulting and Clinical Psychology* 48: 356–365.

Katz, J., and Melzack, R. 1990. Pain "memories" in phantom limbs: Review and clinical observations. *Pain* 43: 319–336.

Katz, W. A. 1996. Approach to the management of nonmalignant pain. *American Journal of Medicine* 101: 54S–63S.

Kaufman, R. 1985. Is the concept of pain incoherent? *The Southern Journal of Philosophy* 23: 279–283.

Keay, K. A., Clement, C. I., Owler, B., Depaulis, A., and Bandelr, R. 1994. Convergence of deep somatic and visceral nociceptive-information onto a discrete ventrolateral midbrain periqueductal gray region. *Neuroscience* 61: 727–732.

Keel, P. 1984. Psychosocial criteria for patient selection: Review of studies and concepts for understanding chronic back pain. *Neurosurgery* 15: 935–941.

Kellert, S. 1993. *In the Wake of Chaos*. Chicago: University of Chicago Press.

Kelso, J. A. S. 1995. *Dynamic Patterns*. Cambridge, MA: The MIT Press.

Kemperman, I., Russ, M. J., and Shearin, E. 1997. Self-injurious behavior and mood regulation in borderline patients. *Journal of Personal Disorders* 11: 146–157.

Kemperman, I., Russ, M. J., Clark, W. C., Kakuma, T., Zanine, E., and Harrison, K. 1997. Pain assessment in self-injurious patients with borderline personality disorder using signal detection theory. *Psychiatry Research* 70: 175–183.

Kenshalo, D. R., Leanard, R. B., Chung, J. M., and Willis, W. D. 1979. Responses of primate spinothalamic neruons to graded and to repeated noxious heat stimuli. *Journal of Neurophysiology* 42: 1370–1389.

Kiernan, B. D., Dane, J. R., Phillips, L. H., and Price, D. D. 1995. Hypnotic analgesia reduces R-III nociceptive reflex: Further evidence concerning the multifactorial nature of hypnotic analgesia. *Pain* 60: 39–47.

King, S. A. 1995. Review: DSM-IV and pain. *Clinical Journal of Pain* 11: 171–176.

King, S. A., and Strain, J. J. 1996. Somatoform pain disorder. In T. A. Widiger, A. J. Frances, J. A. Pincus, R. Ross, M. B. First, and W. W. Davis (eds.), *DSM-IV Sourcebook, Volume 2.* Washington, DC: American Psychiatric Association.

Kisely, S., Creed, F., and Cotter, L. 1992. The course of psychiatric disorder associated with non-specific chest pain. *Journal of Psychosomatic Research* 36: 329–335.

Kitcher, P. S. 1984. In defense of intentional psychology. *Journal of Philosophy* 81: 89–106.

Kitcher, P. S. 1988. Marr's computational theory of vision. *Philosophy of Science.*

Klein, K. B., and Speigel, D. 1989. Modulation of gastric acid secretion by hypnosis. *Gastroenterology* 96: 1383–1387.

Knox, V. J., Gekoski, W. L., Shum, K., and McLaughlin, D. M. 1981. Analgesia for experimentally induced pain: Multiple session of acupuncture compare to hypnosis in high- and low-susceptible subjects. *Journal of Abnormal Psychology* 90: 28–34.

Kohler, T., and Kosanic, S. 1992. Are persons with migraine characterized by a high degree of ambition, orderliness, and rigidity? *Pain* 48: 321–323.

Koob, G. F., and Moal, M. L. 1997. Drug abuse: Hedonic hemeostatic dysregulation. *Science* 278: 52–58.

Korf, J., Bunney, B. S., and Aghajanian, G. K. 1974. Noradrenergic neurons: Morphine inhibition of spontaneous activity. *European Journal of Pharmacology* 25: 165–169.

Kosambi, D. D. 1967. Living prehistory in India. *Scientific American* 216: 105–114.

Krames, E. S. 1996. Intraspinal opioid therapy for chronic nonmalignant pain: Current practice and clinical guidelines. *Journal of Pain Symptom Management* 11: 333–352.

Kripke, S. 1979. Identity and necessity. In T. Honderich and M. Burnyeat (eds.), *Philosophy as It Is.* New York: Penguin Press.

Kroger, W. 1977. History of hypnosis. In *Clinical and Experimental Hypnosis, Second Edition.* Philadelphia: J. B. Lippincott.

Kropotov, J. D., Crawford, H. J., and Polyakov, Y. I. 1997. Somatosensory event-related potential changes to painful stimuli during hypnotic analgesia: Anterior cingulate cortex and anterior temporal cortex intracranial recordings. *International Journal of Psychophysiology* 27: 1–8.

Kupers, R. C., Koning, H., Adriaensen, H., and Gybels, J. 1991. Morphine differentially affects the sensory and affective pain rating in neurogenic and idiopathic forms of pain. *Pain* 47: 5–12.

Kuttner, L. 1988. Favorite stories: A hypnotic pain reduction technique for children in acute pain. *American Journal of Clinical Hypnosis* 30: 289–295.

Lahav, R. 1992. The amazing predictive power of folk psychology. *Australasian Journal of Philosophy* 70: 99–105.

Lambert, S. A. 1996. The effects of hypnosis/guided imagery on the postoperative course of children. *Journal of Developmental and Behavioral Pediatrics* 17: 307–310.

Lang, E. V., Joyce, J. S., Speigel, D., Hamilton, D., and Lee, K. K. 1996. Self-hypnotic relaxation during interventional radiological procedures: Effects on pain perception and intravenous drug use. *International Journal of Clinical and Experimental Hypnosis* 44: 106–119.

Lavigne, J. V., Schulein, M. J., and Hahn, Y. S. 1986. Psychological aspects of painful medical conditions in children. I. Developmental aspects and assessment. *Pain* 27: 133–146.

Lawson, J. R. 1986a. Letter to the editor. *Birth* 13: 124–125.

Lawson, J. R. 1986b. Letter to the editor. *Perinatal Press* 9: 141–142.

Lawson, J. R. 1987. Letter to the editor. *Lancet* ii: 1033.

Lawson, J. R. 1988a. Pain in the neonate and fetus. *New England Journal of Medicine* 318: 1398.

Lawson, J. R. 1988b. Standards of practice and the pain of premature infants. *Zero to Three* 9: 1–5.

Leavitt, F. 1985. The value of the MMPI conversion 'V' in the assessment of psychogenic pain. *Journal of Psychosomatic Research* 29: 125–131.

Leavitt, F., and Katz, R. 1989. Is the MMPI invalid for assessing psychological disturbance in pain related organic conditions? *Journal of Rheumatology* 16: 521–526.

LeBaron, S., and Zeltzer, L. 1984. Assessment of acute pain and anxiety in children and adolescents by self-reports, observer reports, and a behavior checklist. *Journal of Consulting and Clnical Psychology* 52: 729–738.

Lederhaas, G. 1997. Pediatric pain management. *Journal of Florida Medical Association* 84: 37–40.

LeDoux, J. E. 1993. Emotional memory: In search of systems and synapses. In F. M. Crinella and J. Yu (eds.), *Brain Mechanisms*.

LeDoux, J. E., Farb, C., and Ruggiero, D. A. 1990. Topographic organization of neurons in the acoustic thalamus that project to the amygdala. *Journal of Neuroscience* 10: 1043–1054.

LeDoux, J. E., Iwata, J., Cicchetti, P., and Reis, D. J. 1988. Different projections of the central amygdaloid nucleus mediate autonomic and behavioral correlates of conditioned fear. *Journal of Neuroscience* 8: 2517–2529.

Lee, J., Giles, K., and Drummond, P. 1993. Psychological disturbances and an exaggerated response to pain in patients with whiplash injury. *Journal of Psychosomatic Research* 37: 105–110.

Lehky, S. R., and Sejnowski, T. R. 1988. Network model of shape-from-shading: Neuron function arises from both receptive and projective fields. *Nature* 333: 452–454.

Lempert T., Dieterich M., Huppert D., and Brandt, T. 1990. Psychogenic disorders in neurology: Frequency and clinical spectrum. *Acta Neurologica Scandinavica* 82: 335–340.

Leshner, A. I. 1997. Addiction is a brain disease, and it matters. *Science* 278: 45–48.

Lesse, S. 1974. Atypical facial pain of psychogenic origin: A masked depressive syndrome. In S. Lesse (ed.), *Masked Depression*. New York: Jason Aronson.

Lesser, L. M., and Lesser, B. Z. 1983. Alexithymia: Examining the development of a psychological concept. *American Journal of Psychiatry* 140: 1305–1308.

LeTerre, E. C., De Volder, A. G., and Goffinet, A. M. 1988. Brain glucose metabolism in thalamic syndrome. *Journal of Neurosurgery and Psychiatry* 51: 427–428.

Levine, H. A. 1981. The good creature of God and the demon rum: Colonial American and 19th-century ideas about alcohol, crime, and accidents. In R. Room and G. Collins (eds.), *Alcoholism and Disinhibition: Nature and Meaning of the Link*. Rockville, MD: Department of Health and Human Services, National Institute of Alcohol Abuse and Alcoholism.

Levine, J. D., Gordon, N. C., and Fields, H. L. 1979. Naloxone dose dependently produces analgesia and hyperanalgesia in postoperative pain. *Nature* 278: 740–741.

Levitan, Z., Eibschitz, I., de Vries, K., Hakim, M., and Sharf, M. 1985. The value of laparoscopy in women with chronic pelvic pain and a "normal pelvis." *International Journal of Gynacology and Obstetrics* 23: 71–74.

Levy, D. M. 1960. The infant's earliest memory of inoculation: A contribution of public health procedures. *Journal of Genetic Psychology* 96: 3–46.

Lewis, A. 1972. Psychogenic: A word and its mutations. *Psychological Medicine* 2: 209–215.

Lewis, J. W., Cannon, J. T., and Leibeskind, J. C. 1980. Opioid and non-opioid synapse mediates the interaction of spinal and brain stem sites in morphine analgesia. *Brain Research* 236: 85–91.

Lewis, J. W., Sherman, J. E., and Leibeskind, J. C. 1981. Opioid and non-opioid stress analgesia: Assessment of tolerance and cross tolerance with morphine. *Journal of Neuroscience* 1: 358–363.

Lewis, J. W., Tordoff, M. G., Sherman, J. E., and Liebeskind, J. C. 1982. Adrenal medullary enkephalin-like peptides may mediate opioid stress analgesia. *Science* 217: 557–559.

Lewis, T. 1942. *Pain*. London: Macmillan.

Lim, L. 1994. Psychogenic pain. *Singapore Medical Journal* 35: 519–522.

Lindal, E. 1990. Interaction between constant levels of low back pain and other psychological parameters. *Psychology Reports* 67: 1223–1234.

Liniger, H., and Molineus, G. 1930. Der Unfallmann. *2. Ausflage*. Leipzig: Johann Ambrosius Barth Verlag.

Linton, S., and Gotestam, K. 1985. Relations between pain, anxiety, mood and muscle tension in chronic pain patients. A correlation study. *Psychotherapy and Psychosomatics* 43: 90–95.

Linton, S. J. 1986. Behavioral remediation of chronic pain: A status report. *Pain* 24: 125–141.

Linton, S. J. 1994. The role of psychological factors in back pain and its remediation. *Pain Reviews* 1: 231–243.

Lipman, A. G. 1996. Analgesic drugs for neuropathic and sympathetically maintained pain. *Clinical Geriatric Medicine* 12: 501–515.

Lipowski, Z. 1990. Chronic idiopathic pain syndrome. *Annual Medicine* 22: 213–217.

Livingstone, D. 1860. *Missionary Travels and Researches in South Africa: Including a Sketch of Sixteen Years' Residence in the Interior of Africa, and a Journey from the Cape of Good Hope to Loanda on the West Coast; Thence across the Continent, down the River Zambesi, to the Eastern Ocean, 25th Edition*. New York: Harper and Brothers.

Lloyd-Thomas, A. R., and Fitzgerald, M. 1996. Reflex responses do not necessarily signify pain. *British Medical Journal* 313: 797–798.

Loar, B. 1981. *Mind and Meaning*. Cambridge: Cambridge University Press.

Loeser, J. D. 1990. Pain after amputation: Phantom limb and stump pain. In J. J. Bonica (ed.), *The Management of Pain, 2nd Edition*. Philadelphia: Lea and Febiger.

Lollar, D. J., Smits, S. J., and Patterson, D. L. 1982. Assessment of pediatric pain: An empirical perspective. *Journal of Pediatric Psychology* 7: 267–277.

Lorente de Nó, R. 1943. Cerebral cortex: Architecture, intracortical connections, motor projections. In J. F. Fulton (ed.), *Psychology of the Nervous System, Second Edition*. Oxford: Oxford University Press.

Loscalzo, M. 1996. Psychological approaches to the management of pain in patients with advanced cancer. *Hematology and Oncology Clnics in North America* 10: 139–155.

Love, A. W., and Peck, C. L. 1987. The MMPI and psychological factors in chronic low back pain: A review. *Pain* 49: 337–347.

Lucas, P., Leaker, B., Murphy, M., and Neild, G. 1995. Loin pain and haematuria syndrome: A somatoform disorder. *The Quarterly Journal of Medicine* 88: 703–709.

Lutzenberger, W., Flor, H., and Birbaumcr, M. 1997. Enhanced dimensional complexity of the EEG during memory for personal pain in chronic pain patients. *Neuroscience Letters* 226: 167–170.

Lycan, W. G. 1981. Form, function, and feel. *Journal of Philosophy* 77: 24–50.

Lycan, W. G. 1988. *Judgment and Justification*. Cambridge: Cambridge University Press.

Magni, G., Andreoli, C., de Leo, D., Martinotti, G., and Rossi, C. 1986. Psychological profile of women with chronic pelvic pain. *Archives Gynecology* 237: 165–168.

Magni, G., de Bertolini, C., Dodi, G., and Infantino, A. 1986. Psychological findings in chronic anal pain. *Psychopathology* 19: 170–174.

Magni, G., Schifano, F., and de Leo, D. 1985. Pain as a symptom in elderly depressed patients. Relationship to diagnostic subgroups. *European Archives of Psychiatric and Neurological Sciences* 235: 143–145.

Maier, S. F., Drugan, R. C., and Grau, J. W. 1982. Controllability, coping behavior, and stress-induced analgesia in the rat. *Pain* 12: 47–56.

Mairs, D. A. E. 1995. Hypnosis and pain in childbirth. *Contemporary Hypnosis* 12: 111–118.

Malcolm, N. 1968. The conceivability of mechanism. *Philosophical Review* 77: 45–72.

Malone, M. D., and Strube, M. J. 1988. Meta-analysis of non-medical treatment for chronic pain. *Pain* 34: 231–234.

Malone, M. D., Kurtz, and Strube, M. J. 1989. The effects of hypnotic suggestion on pain report. *American Journal of Clinical Hypnosis* 31: 221–229.

Mandel, A., and Selz, K. 1991. Is the EEG a strange attractor? In C. Grebogi and J. Yorke (eds.), *The Impact of Chaos on Science and Technology*. Tokyo: United Nations University Press.

Margolis, C. G. 1997. Hypnotic trance: Old and new. *Primary Care* 24: 809–823.

Marr, D. C. 1982. *Vision: A Computational Investigation into the Human Representation and Processing of Visual Information*. San Francisco: Freeman.

Mather, L. and Mackie, J. 1983. The incidence of postoperative pain in children. *Pain* 15: 271–282.

Mavromichalis, I., Zaramboukas, T., Richman, P. I., and Slavin, G. 1992. Recurrent abdominal pain of gastro-intestinal origin. *European Journal of Pediatrics* 151: 560–563.

Maurer, C., Santangelo, M., and Claiborn, C. D. 1993. The effects of direct versus indirect hypnotic suggestion on pain in a cold pressor task. *International Journal of Clinical and Experimental Hypnosis* 41: 305–316.

Mayer, M. L. 1982. Periaqueductal gray neuronal activity: Correlation with EEG arousal evoked by noxious stimuli in the rat. *Neuroscience Letters* 28: 297–301.

Mayr, E. 1982. *The Growth of Biological Thought: Evolution, Diversity, and Inheritance*. Cambridge, MA: Harvard University Press.

McCulloch, W. S., and Pitts, W. 1943. A logical calculus of the ideas immanent in nervous activity. *Bulletin of Mathematical Biophysics* 5: 115–133.

McFarlane, B. V., Wright, A., O'Callaghan, J., and Benson, H. A. 1997. Chronic neuropathic pain and its control. *Pharmocological Therapy* 75: 1–19.

McGinn, C. 1983. *The Subjective View*. Oxford: Oxford University Press.

McGrath, P., Goodman, J., Firestone, P., Shipman, R., and Peters, S. 1983. Recurrent abdominal pain: A psychogenic disorder? *Archives of Disorders in Children* 58: 888–890.

McGrath, P. A., and Hillier, L. M. 1989. The enigma of pain in children: An overview. *Pediatrician* 16: 6–15.

McGraw, M. B. 1941. Neural maturation as exemplified in the changing reactions of the infant to pin prick. *Child Development* 12: 31–42.

McKenna, A. 1958. The experimental approach to pain. *Journal of Applied Psychology* 13: 449–456.

McKenna, J. E., and Melzack, R. 1992. Analgesia produced by lidocaine microinjection into the dentate gyrus. *Pain* 49: 105–112.

McKenna, J. E., and Melzack, R. 1994. Bilateral VB thalamotomy does not reduce pain in the formalin test. *Society of Neuroscience Abstracts* 20: 1572.

McKeown, M. J. 1997. Methods and models in interpreting fMRI: The case of independent components of fMRI images. Paper presented at the 19th Annual Cognitive Science Meeting.

McLaughlin, C. R., Lichtman, A. H., Fanselow, M. S., and Cramer, C. P. 1990. Tonic nociception in neonatal rats. *Pharmacological Biochemical Behavior* 36: 859–862.

McMahan, S. B., and Wall, P. D 1984. Receptive fields of rat lamina 1 projection cells move to incorporate nearby region of injury. *Pain* 19: 235–247.

McNaughton, N., and Mason, S. T. 1980. The neuropsychology and neuropharmacology of the dorsal ascending noradrenergic bundle—a review. *Progress in Neurobiology* 14: 157–219.

McQuay, H., Carroll, D., Jadad, A. R., Wiffen, P., and Moore, A. 1995. Anticonvulsant drugs for management of pain: A systematic view. *British Medical Journal* 311: 1047–1052.

Meade, T. W., Dyer, S., Brown, W., and Frank, A. O. 1995. Randomised comparison of chiropractic and hospital outpatient management for low back pain: Results from extended follow up. *British Medical Journal* 311: 349–351.

Meade, T. W., Dyer, S., Brown, W., Townsend, T., and Frank A. O. 1990. Low back pain of mechanical origins: Randomised comparison of chiropractic and hospital outpatient treat. *British Medical Journal* 300: 1431–1437.

Melnyk, A. 1991. Physicalism: From supervenience to elimination. *Philosophy and Phenomenological Research* 573–587.

Melzack, R. 1975. The McGill pain questionnaire: Major properties and scoring methods. *Pain* 1: 275–299.

Melzack, R. 1989. Phantom limbs, the self, and the brain. The D. O. Hebb Memorial Lecture. *Canadian Psychology* 30: 1–16.

Melzack, R. 1990. Phantom limbs and the concept of a neuromatrix. *Trends in Neuroscience* 13: 88–92.

Melzack, R. 1991. Central pain syndromes and theories of pain. In Casey (ed.),

Melzack, R. 1992. Phantom limbs. *Scientific American* 266: 120–126.

Melzack, R., and Dennis, S. G. 1980. Phylogenetic evolution of pain expression in animals. In H. W. Kosterlitz, and T. Y. Terenius (eds.), *Pain and Society*. Weinheim: Verlag Chemie.

Melzack, R., and Perry, C. 1975. Self-regulation of pain: The use of alpha feedback and hypnotic training for the control of pain. *Experimental Neurology* 46: 452–469.

Melzack, R., and Wall, P. D. 1965. Pain mechanisms: A new theory. *Science* 150: 971–979.

Melzack, R., and Wall, P. D. 1986. *The Challenge of Pain*. New York: Penguin Books.

Melzack, R., Wall, P. D., and Ty, T. C. 1982. Acute pain in an emergency clinic: Latency of onset and descriptor patterns related to different injuries. *Pain* 14: 33–43.

Menges, L. 1983. Chronic low back pain: A medical-psychological report. *Social Science Medicine* 17: 747–753.

Merskey, H. 1965a. The characteristics of persistent pain in psychological illness. *Journal of Psychosomatic Research* 9: 291–298.

Merskey, H. 1965b. Psychiatric patients with persistent pain. *Journal of Psychosomatic Research* 9: 299–309.

Merskey, H. 1973. The perception and measurement of pain. *Journal of Psychosomatic Research* 17: 251–255.

Merskey, H. 1979. Pain terms: A list with definitions and a note on usage. Recommended by the International Association for the Study of Pain (IASP) Subcommittee on Taxonomy. *Pain* 6: 249–252.

Merskey, H. 1984. Symptoms that depress the doctor. Too much pain. *British Journal of Hospital Medicine* (Jan.): 63–66.

Merskey, H. 1989a. Pain and psychological medicine. In P. D. Wall and R. Melzack (eds.), *Textbook of Pain, Second Edition*. New York: Churchill Livingstone.

Merskey, H. 1989b. Psychiatry and chronic pain. *Canadian Journal of Psychiatry* 34: 329–335.

Merskey, H., and Spear, F. G. 1967. *Pain: Psychological and Psychiatric Aspects*. London: Baillière, Tindall, and Cassel.

Merskey, H., Brown, J., Brown, A., Malhotra, D., Morrison, D., and Ripley, C. 1985. Psychological normality and abnormality in persistent headache patients. *Pain* 23: 35–47.

Mersky, H. 1982. Body-mind dilemma in chronic pain. In R. Royand and E. Tunks (eds.), *Chronic Pain: Psychosocial Factors in Rehabilitation*. Baltimore, MD: Williams and Wilkins.

Mészáros, I., Bányai, É. I., and Greguss, A. C. 1980. Evoked potential, reflecting hypnotically altered state of consciousness. In G. Ádám, I. Mészáros, and É. I. Bányai (eds.), *Advances in Physiological Sciences, Volume 17: Brain and Behavior*. Oxford: Pergamon.

Miller, D. 1994. *Women Who Hurt Themselves: A Book of Hope and Understanding*. New York: Basic Books.

Miller, K. D., Keller, J. B., and Stryker, M. P. 1989. Ocular dominance column development: Analysis and simulation. *Science* 245: 605–615.

Millikan, R. G. 1984. *Language, Thought, and Other Biological Categories*. Cambridge, MA: The MIT Press.

Milov, D., and Kantor, R. 1990. Chest pain in teenagers. When is it significant? *Postgraduate Medicine* 88: 153–154.

Mitchell, M. 1995. The use of hypnosis in the treatment of chornic ostereoarthritic pain: A case study. *Australian Journal of Clinical and Experimental Hypnosis* 23: 41–50.

Montaigne, N. [1532–1592] 1930. *The Essays of Michel de Montaigne*. London: G. Bell.

Moore, L. W., and Wiesner, S. L. 1996. Hypnotically-induced vasodilation in the treatment of repetitive strain injuries. *American Jorunal of Clinical Hypnosis* 39: 97–104.

Moret, V., Forster, A., Laverriere, M. C., Lambert, J., Gaillard, R. C., Bourgeois, P., Haynal, A., Gemperle, M., and Buchser, E. 1991. Mechanism of analgesia induced by hypnosis and acupuncture: Is there a difference? *Pain* 45: 135–140.

Morgan, A. H., Johnson, D. L., and Hilgard, E. R. 1974. The stability of hypnotic susceptibility: A longitudinal study. *International Journal of Clinical and Experimental Hypnosis* 22: 249–257.

Morilak, D. A., Fornal, C. A., and Jacobs, B. L. 1987. Effects of physiological manipulations of locus coeruleus neuronal activity in freely moving cats. II. Cadiovascular challenge. *Brain Research* 422: 42–31.

Mountcastle, V. N. 1957. Modality and topographic properties of single neurones of cat's somatic sensory cortex. *Journal of Neurophysiology* 20: 408–434.

Mountz, J. M., Bradley, L. A., Modell, J. G., Alexander, R. W., Triana-Alexander, M., Aaron, L. A., Stewart, K. E., Alarcan, G. S., and Mountz, J. D. 1995. Fibromyalgia in women: Abnormalities of regional cerebral blood flow in the thalamus and the caudate nucleus are associated with low pain threshold levels. *Arthritis and Rheumatism* 38: 926–938.

Mpitsos, G. 1989. Chaos in brain function and the problem of nonstationarity: A commentary. In E. Basar and T. Bullock (eds.), *Brain Dynamics: Progress and Perspectives*. Berlin: Springer-Verlag.

Muhs, A., and Schepank, H. 1995. Influence of hereditary factors in psychogenic disorders. *Psychopathology* 28: 177–184.

Murtagh, J. E. 1994. The non-pharmacological treatment of back pain. *Australian Prescriber* 17: 9–12.

Naidoo, P., and Patel, C. 1993. Stress, depression and left-sided psychogenic chest pain. *Acta Psychiatrica Scandinavica* 88: 12–15.

Naliboff, B., Cohen, M., and Yellen A. 1982. Does the MMPI differentiate chronic illness from chronic pain? *Pain* 32: 207–213.

Nasrallah, H. A., Holley, T., and Janowsky, D. S. 1979. Opiate antagonism fails to reverse hypnotic-induced analgesia. *Lancet* i: 1355.

Nathan, P. W. 1976. The gate-control theory: A critical review. *Brain* 99: 123–158.

Nelkin, N. 1986. Pain and pain sensations. *Journal of Philosophy* 83: 129–148.

Nelkin, N. 1994. Reconsidering pain. *Philosophical Psychology* 7: 325–343.

Nelson, M. T. 1991. Eliminative materialism and substantive commitments. *International Philosophical Quarterly* 39–49.

Nestler, E. J., and Aghajanian, G. K. 1997. Molecular and cellular basis of addiction. *Science* 278: 58–63.

Neufield, R., and Davidson, P. 1971. The effect of vicarious and cognitive rehearsal on pain tolerance. *Journal of Psychosomatic Research* 15: 329–335.

New, A. S., Trestman, R. L., Mitropoulou, V., Benishay, D. S., Coccaro, E., Silverman, J., and Siever, L. J. 1997. Serotonergic function and self-injurious behavior in personality disorder patients. *Psychiatry Research* 69: 17–26.

Newman, H. M., Stevens, R. T., Pover, C. M., and Apkarian, A. V. 1994. Spinal-suprathalamic projections form the upper cervical and the cervical enlargement in rat and squirrel monkey. *Society of Neuroscience Abstracts* 20: 118.

Newton, N. 1989. On viewing pain as a secondary quality. *Nous* 23: 569–598.

Nuland, S. B. 1994. *On How We Die: Reflections on Life's Final Chapter*. New York: Alfred A. Knopf.

O'Brien, G. 1987. Eliminative materialism and our psychological self-knowledge. *Philosophial Studies* 52: 49–70.

O'Brien, G. 1991. Is connectionism commonsense? *Philosophical Psychology* 4: 165–178.

O'Gorman, P. F. 1989. Mentalism-cum-physicalism vs. elminative materialism. *Irish Philosophy Journal* 6: 133–147.

O'Gorman, P. F. 1990. The naturalization of epistemology and eliminative materialism. *Irish Philosophy Journal* 7: 79–103.

O'Leary-Hawthorne, J. 1994. On the threat of eliminativism. *Philosophical Studies* 74: 325–346.

Ochoa, J. L., and Verdugo, R. J. 1995. Reflex sympathetic dystrophy: A common clinical avenue for somatoform expression. *Neurologic Clinics* 13: 351–363.

Olness, K., Wain, H. J., and Lorenz, N. G. 1980. A pilot study of blood endorphin levels in children using self-hypnosis to control pain. *Journal of Developmental and Behavioral Pediatrics* 4: 187–188.

Orian, C. 1989. Self-injurious behavior as a habit and its treatment. *American Journal of Clinical Hypnosis* 32: 84–89.

Orne, M. T., and Dinges, D. F. 1989. Hypnosis. In P. D. Wall and R. Melzack (eds.), *Texbook of Pain, Second Edition*. New York: Churchill Livingstone.

Owens, M. E., and Todt, E. H. 1984. Pain in infancy: Neonatal reaction to a heel lance. *Pain* 20: 213–230.

Pagni, C. A. 1989. Central pain due to spinal cord and brain stem damage. In P. D. Wall and R. Melzack (eds.), *Textbook of Pain*. New York: Churchill Livingstone.

Pandya, D. N., Barnes, C. L., and Panksepp, J. 1987. Architecture and connections of the frontal lobe. In E. Perecman (ed.), *The Frontal Lobes Revisited*. Hillsdale, NJ: Lawrence Erlbaum.

Panescu, D., Webster, J. G., and Stratbucker, R. A. 1994. A nonlinear electrical-thermal model of the skin. *IEEE Trans Biomedical Engineering* 41: 672–680.

Papez, J. W. 1937. A proposed mechanisms of emotion. *Archives of Neurology and Psychology* 38: 725–743.

Papineau, D. 1987. *Reality and Representation*. Oxford: Basil Blackwell.

Pappagallo, M., and Heinberg, L. J. 1997. Ethical issues in the management of chronic nonmalignent pain. *Seminars in Neurology* 17: 203–211.

Parrent, A. G., Lozano, A. M., Dostrovsky, J. O., and Tasker, R. R. 1992. Central pain in the absence of functional sensory thalamus. *Sterotact Functional Neurosurgery* 59: 9–14.

Patrick, C. J., Craig, K. D., and Prkachin, K. M. 1986. Observer judgments of acute pain: Facial action determinants. *Journal of Personality and Social Psychology* 50: 1291–1298.

Patterson, D. R., Adcock, R. J., and Bombardier, C. H. 1997. Factors predicting hypnotic analgesia in clinical burn pain. *International Journal of Clinical and Experimental Hypnosis* 45: 377–395.

Patterson, D. R., and Ptacek, J. T. 1997. Baseline pain as a moderator of hypnotic analgesia for burn injury treatment. *Journal of Consulting and Clinical Psychology* 65: 60–67.

Patterson, D. R., Goldberg, M. L., and Ehde, D. M. 1996. Hypnosis in the treatment of patients with severe burns. *American Journal of Clinical Hypnosis* 38: 200–213.

Penfield, W., and Boldrey, W. 1937. Somatic motor and sensory representation in the cerebral cortex of man as studied by electrical stimulation. *Brain* 60: 389–443.

Perl, E. R. 1976. Sensitization of nociceptors and its relation to sensation. In J. J. Bonica, D. Albe-Fessard (eds.), *Advances in Pain Research and Therapy, Vol. 1.* New York: Raven Press.

Perry, S., and Heidrich, G. 1982. Management of pain during debridement: A survey of U.S. burn units. *Pain* 13: 267–280.

Petit, M-A. [1499] 1502. Discours sur la douleur. Paper given at the opening of the lectures on anatomy and surgery at the Hospice général des malades de Lyon, 28 brumaire, year VII. Reprinted in *Ortus Sanitatis: Translate de Latin en Francois.* Paris: Anthoine Verard.

Peveler, R., Edwards, J., Daddow, J., and Thomas, E. 1996. Psychosocial factors and chronic pelvic pain: A comparison of women with endometriosis and with unexplained pain. *Journal of Psychosomatic Research* 40: 305–315.

Peyrot, M., Moody, P., and Wiese, H. 1993. Biogenic, psychogenic, and sociogenic models of adjustment to chronic pain: An exploratory study. *International Journal of Psychiatry Medicine* 23: 63–80.

Phillips, H., and Grant, L. 1991. The evolution of chronic back pain problems: A longitudinal study. *Behavior, Research, and Therapy* 29: 435–441.

Pierce, K., Glad, K. S., and Schreibman, L. 1997. Social perception in children with autism: An attentional deficit? *Journal of Autism and Developmental Disorders* 27: 265–282.

Pies, R. W., and Popli, A. P. 1995. Self-injurious behavior: pathophysiology and implications for treatment. *Journal of Clnical Psychiatry* 56: 580–588.

Pillay, A., and Lalloo, M. 1989. Psychogenic pain disorder in children. *South African Medical Journal* 76: 195–196.

Plantinga, A. 1986. On taking the belief in God as basic. In J. Runzo and C. Ihara (eds.), *Religious Experience and Belief.* Pittsburgh: University Press of America.

Portenoy, R. K. 1996. Opioid therapy for chronic nonmalignant pain: A review of the critical issues. *Journal of Pain and Symptom Management* 11: 203–217.

Posner, M. I., and Dehaene, S. 1994. Attentional networks. *Trends in Neuroscience* 17: 75–79.

Posner, M. I., and Petersen, S. W. 1990. The attention system of the human brain. *Annual Review of Neuroscience* 13: 25–42.

Posner, M. I., Petersen, S. W., Fox, P. T., and Raichle, M. E. 1988. Localization of cognitive operations in the human brain. *Science* 240: 1627–1631.

Potts, S., and Bass, C. 1995. Psychological morbidity in patients with chest pain and normal or near-normal coronary arteries: A long-term follow-up study. *Psychological Medicine* 25: 339–347.

Pribram, K. 1980. The biology of emotions and other feelings. In R. Plutchik and H. Kellerman (eds.), *Emotion: Theory, Research, and Experience, Volume 1.* New York: Academic Press.

Price, D. D., Hayes, R. L., Ruda, M., and Dubner, R. 1978. Spatial and temporal transformations of input to spinothalamic tract neurons and their relation to somatic sensations. *Journal of Neurophysiology* 41: 933–946.

Pritcher, G. 1970. Pain perception. *The Philosophical Review* 79: 368–393.

Putnam, H. 1979. The meaning of "meaning." In K. Gunderson (ed.), *Language, Mind, and Knowledge, Volume VII. Minnesota Studies in the Philosophy of Science.* Minneapolis: University of Minnesota Press.

Putnam, H. 1992. *Renewing Philosophy.* Cambridge, MA: Harvard University Press.

Quine, W. V. 1960. *Word and Object.* Cambridge, MA: The MIT Press.

Quine, W. V. 1966. On mental entities. Reprinted in *Ways of Paradox and Other Essays.* New York: Random House.

Rainville, P., Duncan, G. H., Price, D. D., Carrier, and Bushnell, M. C. 1997. Pain affect encoded in human anterior cingulate but not somatosensory cortex. *Science* 277: 968–971.

Ramsey, W. 1990a. Connectionism, eliminativism and the future of folk psychology. *Philosophical Perspectives, 4: Action Theory and Philosophy of Mind.* Atascadero, CA: Ridgeview.

Ramsey, W. 1990b. Where does the self-refutation objection take us? *Inquiry* 33: 453–465.

Ramsey, W. 1994. Distributed representation and causal modularity: A rejoinder to Forster and Saidel. *Philosophical Psychology* 7: 453–461.

Ramsey, W., Stich, S. P., and Garon, J. 1991. Connectionism, eliminativism, and the future of folk psychology. In W. Ramsey, S. Stich, and D. Rumelhart (eds.), *Philosophy and Connectionist Theory.* Hillsdale, NJ: Lawrence Erlbaum.

Rapoport, J. L. 1989. *The Boy Who Couldn't Stop Washing: The Experience and Treatment of Obsessive-Compulsive Disorder.* New York: Signet.

Rawlings, D. J., Miller, P. S., and Engel, R. R. 1980. The effect of circumcision on transcutaneous PO_2 in term infants. *American Journal of Diseases in Childhood* 134: 676–678.

Reading, A. E. 1989. Testing pain mechanisms in persons in pain. In P. D. Wall and R. Melzack (eds.), *Textbook of Pain.* New York: Churchill Livingstone.

Redmond, D. E. J., and Huang, Y. G. 1979. Current concepts. II. New evidence for a locus coeruleus-norepinephrin connection with anxiety. *Life Sciences* 25: 2149–2162.

Reissland, N. 1983. Cognitive maturity and the experience of fear and pain in hospital. *The Social Science of Medicine* 17: 1389–1395.

Reiter, R., Shakerin, L., Gambone, J., and Milburn, A. 1991. Correlation between sexual abuse and somatization in women with somatic and nonsomatic chronic pelvic pain. *American Journal of Obstetrics and Gynecology* 165: 104–109.

Report of the Panel on Pain to the National Advisory Neurological and Communicative Disorder and Stroke Council. 1979. NIH Publication No. 81: 1812.

Reppert, V. 1991. Ramsey on eliminativism and self-refutation. *Inquiry* 34: 499–508.

Reppert, V. 1992. Eliminative materialism, cognitive suicide, and begging the question. *Metaphilosophy* 23: 378–392.

Rey, G. 1997. *Contemporary Philosophy of Mind.* Oxford: Blackwell.

Rey, R. 1993. *History of Pain.* Trans. by L. E. Wallace, J. A. Cadden, and S. W. Cadden. Paris: Éditions la Découverte.

Rizzo, M., and Eslinger, P. J. 1989. Colored hearing synthesthesia: An investigation of neural factors. *Neurology* 39: 1409–1410.

Roberts, A. H., and Reinhardt, L. 1980. The behavioral management of chronic pain: Long-term follow-up with comparison groups. *Pain* 8: 151–162.

Robertson, S. S., Cohen, A. H., and Mayer-Kess R. G. 1993. Behavioral chaos: Beyond the metaphor. In L. B. Smith, and E. Thelen (eds.), *A Dynamical Systems Approach to Development: Applications.* Cambridge, MA: The MIT Press.

Robinson, W. S. 1985. Toward eliminating Churchland's eliminativism. *Philosophical Topics* 13: 60–67.

Rogers, M., Weinshenker, N., Warshaw, M., Goisman, R., et al. 1996. Prevalence of somatoform disorders in a large sample of patients with anxiety disorders. *Psychosomatics* 37: 17–22.

Roland, P. E. 1992a. Cortical representations of pain. *Trends in Neuroscience* 15: 3–5.

Roland, P. E. 1992b. Reply. *Trends in Neuroscience* 15: 252–253.

Roll, M., and Theorell, T. 1987. Acute chest pain without obvious organic cause before age 40—Personality and recent life events. *Journal of Psychosomatic Research* 31: 215–221.

Romans, S. E., Martin, J. L., Anderson, J. C., Herbison, G. P., and Mullen, P. E. 1995. Sexual abuse in childhood and deliberate self-harm. *American Journal of Psychiatry* 152: 1336–1342.

Romsing, J., Moller-Sonnergaard, J., Hertel, S., and Rasmussen, M. 1996. Postoperative pain in children: Comparison between ratings of children and nurses. *Journal of Pain and Symptom Management* 11: 42–46.

Rook, J., Pesch, R., and Keeler, E. 1981. Chronic pain and the questionable use of the Minnesota Multiphasic Personality Inventory. *Archives of Physical Medicine Rehabilitation* 62: 373–376.

Rorabaugh, W. J. 1979. *The Alcoholic Republic.* Oxford: Oxford University Press.

Rorty, R. 1965. Mind-body identity, privacy, and categories. *Review of Metaphysics* 19: 24–54.

Rosch, E. 1973. On the internal structure of perceptual and semantic categories. In T. Moore (ed.), *Cognitive Development and the Acquisition of Language*. New York: Academic Press.

Rosch, E. 1978. Principles of categorization. In E. Rosch and B. B. Lloyd (eds.), *Cognition and Categorization*. Hillsdale, NJ: Lawrence Erlbaum.

Rosch, E. 1981. Prototype classification and logical classification: The two systems. In E. Scholnick (ed.), *New Trends in Cognitive Representation: Challenges to Piaget's Theory*. Hillsdale, NJ: Lawrence Erlbaum.

Rosch, E., and Mervis, C. 1975. Family resemblances: Studies in the internal structure of categories. *Cognitive Psychology* 7: 573–605.

Rosen, S. D., Paulesu, E., Frith, C. D., Frackowiak, R. S. J., Davis, G. J., and Jones, T. 1994. Central nervous pathways mediating angina pectoris. *Lancet* 344: 147–150.

Rosenberg, A. 1991. How is eliminative materialism possible? In R. Bogdan (ed.), *Mind and Common Sense*. Cambridge, MA: Cambridge University Press.

Rosenthal, R. 1993. Psychology of chronic pelvic pain. *Obstetrics and Gynecology Clinics in North America* 20: 627–642.

Rossi, L. N., Cortinovis, I., and Bellettini, G. 1992. Diagnostic criteria for migraine and psychogenic headache in children. *Developmental Medicine and Child Neurology* 34: 516–523.

Roth, A. S., Ostroff, R. B., and Hoffman, R. E. 1996. Naltrexone as a treatment for repetitive self-injurious behavior: An open-label trial. *Journal of Clinical Psychiatry* 57: 233–237.

Roth, Y. F., and Sugarbaker, P. H. 1980. Pains and sensations after amputation: Character and clinical significance. *Archives of Physical Medicine and Rehabilitation* 61: 490.

Roux, P. M. 1836. *Bulletin de l'Académie de Médicine*.

Rowbotham, M. C. 1995. Chronic pain: From theory to practical management. *Neurology* 45: S5–S10.

Rowe, M. L. 1969. Low back pain in industry: A position paper. *Journal of Occupational Medicine* 11: 161–169.

Roy, R. 1982. Pain-prone patient: A revisit. *Psychotherapy and Psychosomatics* 37: 202–213.

Roy, R. 1985. Engel's pain-prone disorder patient: 25 years after. *Psychotheraphy and Psychosomatics* 43: 126–135.

Rumelhart, D., and McClelland, J. L. 1986. *Parallel Distributed Processing, Volume 1: Foundations*. Cambridge, Massachusetts: The MIT Press.

Rumelhart, D. E., Smolensky, P., McClelland, J. L., and Hinton, G. E. 1986. Schemata and sequential thought processes in PDP models. In J. L. McClelland and D. E. Rumelhart (eds.), *Parallel Distributed Processing: Explorations in the*

Microstructure of Cognition, Volume 2: Psychological and Biological Models. Cambridge, MA: The MIT Press.

Rusch, K. M., Guastello, S. J., and Mason, P. T. 1992. Differentiating symptom clusters of borderline personality disorder. *Journal of Clinical Psychology* 48: 730–738.

Russ, M. J., Roth, S. D., Kakuma, T., Harrison, K., and Hull, J. W. 1994. Pain perception in self-injurious borderline patients: Naloxone effects. *Biological psychiatry* 35: 207–209.

Russ, M. J., Roth, S. D., Lerman, A., Kakuma, T., Harrison, K., Shindledecker, R. D., Hull, J., and Mattis, S. 1992. Pain perception in self-injurious patients with borderline personality disorder. *Biological Psychiatry* 32: 501–511.

Russ, M. J., Shearin, E. N., Clarkin, J. F., Harrison, K., and Hull, J. W. 1993. Subtypes of self-injurious patients with borderline personality disorders. *American Journal of Psychiatry* 150: 1869–1871.

Ryden, O., Lindal, E., Uden, A., and Hansson, S. 1985. Differentiation of back pain patients using a pain questionnaire. *Scandanavian Journal of Rehabilitation Medicine* 17: 155–161.

Sabo, A. N., Gunderson, J. G., Najavita, L. M., Chauncey, D., and Kisiel, C. 1995. Changes in self-destructiveness of borderline patients in psychotherapy. A prospective follow-up study. *Journal of Nervous Mental Disorders* 183: 370–376.

Saletu, B., Saletu, M., Brown, M., Stern, J., Sletten, I, and Ulett, G. 1975. Hypno-alagesia and acupuncture analgesia: A neurophysiological reality? *Neuropsychobiology* 1: 218–242.

Salter, M., Brooke, R. I., Merskey, H., Fichter, G. F., and Kapusianyk, D. H. 1983. Is the temporomandibular and dysfunction syndrome a disorder of mind? *Pain* 17: 151–166.

Sanchez-Villasenor, F., Devinsky, O., Hainline, B., Weinreb, H., et al. 1995. Psychogenic basilar migraine: Report of four cases. *Neurology* 45: 1291–1294.

Sandkühler, J. 1996. Neurobiology of spinal nociception: New concepts. In G. Carli and M. Zimmerman (eds.), *Progress in Brain Research, Volume 110: Towards the Neurobiology of Chronic Pain.* New York: Elsevier.

Sandkühler, J., and Eblen-Zajjur, A. 1994. Identification and characterization of rhythmic nociceptive and non-nociceptive spinal dorsal horn neurons in the rat. *Neuroscience* 61: 991–1006.

Scarry, E. 1985. *The Body in Pain: The Making and Unmaking of the World.* New York: Oxford University Press.

Schiffer, S. 1982. Intention based semantics. *Notre Dame Journal of Formal Logic* 23: 119–156.

Schmidt, J., and Wallace, R. 1982. Factorial analysis of the MMPI profiles of low back pain patients. *Journal of Personal Assessment* 46: 366–369.

Schott, G. D. 1994. Visceral afferents: Their contribution to 'sympathetic dependent' pain. *Brain* 117: 397–413.

Schouenbourg, J., and Dickenson, A. H. 1985. The effects of a distant noxious stimulation on A and C fibre evoked flexion reflexes and neuronal activity in the dorsal horn of the rat. *Brain Research* 328: 23–32.

Sees, K. L., and Clark, H. W. 1993. Opioid use in the treatment of chonic pain: Assessment of addiction. *Journal of Pain Symptom Management* 8: 257–264.

Sejnowski, T. J., and Churchland, P. S. 1988. Brain and cognition. In M. I. Posner (ed.), *Foundations of Cognitive Science*. Cambridge, MA: The MIT Press.

Seltzer, Z. Dubner, R., and Shir, Y. 1990. A novel behavioral model of neuropathic pain disorders produced in rats by patrial sciatic nerve injury. *Pain* 43: 205–218.

Sharev, U., and Tal, M. 1989. Masseter inhibitory periods and sensations evoked by electrical tooth-pulp stimulation in subjects under hypnotic anesthesia. *Brain Research* 479: 247–254.

Shearer, S. L. 1994. Phenomenology of self-injury among inpatient women with borderline personality disorder. *The Journal of Nervous and Mental Disease* 182: 524–526.

Sherman, J. E., and Liebeskind, J. C. 1980. An endorphinergic, centrifugal substrate of pain modulation: Recent findings, current concepts, and complexities. In J. J. Bonica (ed.), *Pain*. New York: Raven Press.

Sherman, R. A., Sherman, C. J., and Parker, L. 1984. Chronic phantom and stump pain among American veterans: Results of a survey. *Pain* 18: 83–95.

Shoemaker, S. 1975a. Functionalism and qualia. *Philosophical Studies* 27: 291–315.

Shoemaker, S. 1975b. Phenomenal similarity. *Critica* 7: 3–37.

Shoemaker, S. 1981. Absent qualia are impossible. *Philosophical Review* 90: 581–599.

Shorter, E. 1997. Somatization and chronic pain in historic perspective. *Clinical Orthopedics* (Mar.): 52–60.

Shum, N. 1996. Hypnosis in the management of pain of oral muscositis associated with high dose therapy for cancer. *Australian Journal of Clinical and Experimental Hypnosis* 24: 120–124.

Sikes, R. W., and Vogt, B. A. 1992. Nociceptive neurons in area 24 of rabbit cingulate cortex. *Journal of Neurophysiology* 68: 1720–1732.

Silverman, D. H. S., Munakata, J. A., Ennes, H., et al. 1997. Regional cerebral activity in normal and pathological perception of visceral pain. *Gastroenterology* 12: 64–72.

Simone, D. A., Sorkin, L. S., Oh, U., Chung, J. M., Owens, C., LaMotte, R. H., and Willis, W. D. 1991. Neurogenic hyperalgesia: Central neural correlates in responses of spinothalamic tract neurons. *Journal of Neurophysiology* 66: 228–246.

Simpson, D. E., and Gjerdingen, D. K. 1989. Family physicians' and internists' consideration of psychosocial hypotheses during the diagnostic process. *Family Practice Research Journal* 8: 55–56.

Singer, M. T. 1977. Psychological dimensions in psychosomatic patients. *Psychotheraphy and Psychosomatics* 28: 13–27.

Sivik, T. 1991. Personality traits in patients with acute low-back pain. A comparison with chronic low-back pain patients. *Psychotherapy and Psychosomatics* 56: 135–140.

Skarda, C., and Freeman, W. 1987. How brains make chaos in order to make sense of the world. *Behavioral and Brain Sciences* 10: 161–195.

Slocumb, J., Kellner, R., Rosenfeld, R., and Pathak, D. 1989. Anxiety and depression in patients with the abdominal pelvic pain syndrome. *General Hospital Psychiatry* 11: 48–53.

Smith, G. R. 1992. The epidemiology and treatment of depression when it coexists with somatoform disorders, somatization, or pain. *General Hospital Psychiatry* 14: 265–272.

Smith, J. T., Barabasz, A. F., and Barabasz, M. 1996. Comparison of hypnosis and distraction in severely ill children undergoing painful medical procedures. *Journal of Counseling Psychology* 43: 187–195.

Smith, J. V. C. 1847. Mesmeric examinations. *Boston Medical and Surgical Journal* 37: 85.

Smith, L. B., and Thelen, E. (eds.). 1993. *A Dynamic Systems Approach to Development: Applications.* Cambridge, MA: The MIT Press.

Smolensky, P. 1995. On the projectable predicates of connectionist psychology: A case for belief. In C. Macdonald (ed.), *Connectionism: Debates on Psychological Explanation.* New York: Blackwell.

Smyth, H. 1984. Problems with the MMPI. *Journal of Rheumatology* 11: 417–418.

Snow, P. J., Lumb, B. M., Cervero, F. 1992. The representation of prolonged and intense, noxious somatic and visceral stimuli in the ventrolateral orbital cortex of the cat. *Pain* 48: 89–99.

Snyder, M. 1979. Self-monitoring processes. In L. Berkowitz (ed.), *Advances in Social Psychology, Volume 2.* New York: Academic.

Spanos, N. 1986. Hypnotic behavior: A social-psychological interpretation of amnesia, analgesia, and "trance logic." *Behavioral and Brain Sciences* 9: 449–502.

Spanos, N. P., Perlini, A. H., Patrick, L., and Bell, S. 1990. Imaginal dispositions and situational-specific alterations in strategy-induced pain reductions. *Imagination, Cognition, and Personality* 9: 147–156.

Speigel, D., Cutcomb, S., Ren, C., and Pribram, K. 1985. Hypnotic hallucination alters evoked potentials. *Journal of Abnormal Psychology,* 94: 249–265.

Spiegel, D., and Albert, L. H. 1985. Naloxone fails to reverse hypnotic alleviation of chronic pain. *Psychopharmacology* 81: 140–143.

Spinhoven, P. 1988. Similarities and dissimilarities in hypnotic and nonhypnotic procedures for headache control: A review. *American Journal of Clinical Hypnosis* 30: 183–194.

Sriram, T., Chaturvedi, S., Gopinath, P., and Shanmugam, V. 1987. Controlled study of alexithymic characteristics in patients with psychogenic pain disorder. *Psychotherapy and Psychosomatics* 47: 11–17.

Stalnaker, R. 1984. *Inquiry.* Cambridge, MA: The MIT Press.

Stanley, D., Stockley, I., Davies, G., and Getty, C. 1993. A prospective study of diagnostic epidural blockade in the assessment of chronic back and leg pain. *Journal of Spinal Disorders* 6: 208–211.

Stea, R. A., and Apkarian, A. V. 1992. Pain and somatosensory activation. *Trends in Neuroscience* 15: 250–251.

Stephenson, D., and Leroux, J. A. 1994. Portrait of a creatively gifted child facing cancer. *Creativity Research Journal* 7: 71–77.

Sterelny, K. 1993. Refuting eliminative materialism on the cheap? *Mind and Language* 8: 306–315.

Stern, J. A., Brown, M., Ulett, G. A., and Sletten, I. 1977. A comparison of hypnosis, acupuncture, morphine, valium, aspirin, and placebo in the management of experimentally induced pain. *Annals of New York Academy of Sciences* 296: 175–193.

Sternbach, R. A. 1963. Congenital insensitivity to pain: A critique. *Psychological Bulletin* 60: 252–264.

Sternbach, R. A. 1968. *Pain: A Psychophysiological Analysis.* New York: Academic Press.

Sternbach, R. A. 1977. Psychological aspects of chronic pain. *Clinical Orthopedics* (Nov.–Dec.): 150–155.

Sternbach, R. A. 1989. Behavior therapy. In P. D. Wall and R. Melzack (eds.), *Textbook of Pain, Second Edition.* New York: Churchill Livingstone.

Sternbach, R. A., and Tursky, B. 1965. Ethnic differences among housewives in psychophysical and skin potential responses to electrical shock. *Psychophysiology* 1: 241–246.

Sthalekar, H. A. 1993. Hypnosis for relief of chronic phantom pain in a paralysed limb. A case study. *Australian Journal of Clinical Hypnotherapy and Hypnosis* 14: 75–80.

Stich, S. P. 1991. Causal holism and commonsense psychology: A reply to O'Brien. *Philosophical Psychology* 4: 179 181.

Stich, S. P. 1992. What is a theory of mental representation? *Mind* 101: 243–261.

Stich, S. P. 1993. Puritanical naturalism. In K. Neander and I. Ravenscroft (eds.), *Prospects for Intentionality, Working Papers in Philosophy, Volume 3,* Research School of Social Science, Australian National University.

Stich, S. P. 1996. *Deconstructing the Mind.* New York: Oxford University Press.

Stich, S. P., and Laurence, S. 1994. Intentionality and naturalism. In P. A. French, T. E. Uehling, and H. K. Wettstein (eds.), *Midwest Studies in Philosophy, Volume XIX, Philosophical Naturalism.* Notre Dame, IN: University of Notre Dame Press.

Stich, S. P., and Warfield, T. 1995. Reply to Clark and Smolensky: Do connectionist minds have beliefs? In C. Macdonald (ed.), *Connectionism: Debates on Psychological Explanation.* New York: Blackwell.

Stone, E. A. 1975. Stress and catecholamines. In A. J. Friedhoff (ed.), *Catecholamines and Behavior, Volume 2.* New York: Plenum Press.

Stufflebeam, R. S., and Bechtel, W. 1997. PET: Exploring the myth and the method. In L Darden (Ed.) *PSA96, Volume 2.* Philosophy of Science Association.

Sullivan, M. 1995. Key concepts: Pain. *Philosophy, Psychiatry, and Psychology* 2: 277–280.

Sullivan, M. I. L., Reesor, K., Mikail, S., and Fisher, R. 1992. The treatment of depression in chronic low back pain. *Psychosomatics* 14: 52–57.

Sutcher, J. 1997. Hypnosis as adjunctive therapy for multiple scloerosis: A progress report. *American Journal of Clinical Hypnosis* 39: 283–290.

Suzuki, H. 1995. Recent topics in the management of pain: Development of the concept of preemptive analgesia. *Cell Transplant* 4 Suppl. 1: S3–S6.

Svensson, T. H. 1987. Peripheral, autonomic regulation of locus coeruleus noradrenergic neurons in brain: Putative implications for psychiatry and psychopharmacology. *Psychopharmacology* 92: 1–7.

Sviderskaya, N. E., and Kovalev, A. A. 1996. Effect of unconscious interoceptive afferentation on the spatial organization of electrical activity in the human cerebral cortex. *Neuroscience Behavioral Psychiology* 26: 532–538.

Swirsky-Sacchetti, T., and Margolis, C. C. 1986. The effects of a comprehensive self hypnosis training program on the use of factor VIII in severe hemophilia. *International Journal of Clinical and Experimental Hypnosis* 34: 71–83.

Szekely, J. I. 1990. Opioid peptides and stress. *Critical Reviews in Neurobiology* 6: 1–12.

Taddio, A., Gazarian, M., Klein, J., et al. 1994. Systemic exposure to lidocaine and prilocain from EMLA application to the penile region in pigs: Implications for use in neonatal circumcision. *Clinical Investigations in Medicine* 17: B17.

Taddio, A., Goldbach, M. Ipp, M., Stevens, B., and Koren, G. 1995. Effect of neonatal circumcision on pain responses during vaccination in boys. *Lancet* 345: 291–299.

Taddio, A., Katz, J., Ilersich, A. L., et al. 1997. Effect of neonatal circumcision on pain response during subsequent routine vaccination. *Lancet* 349: 599–603.

Takaishi, D., Eisele, H., and Carstens, E. 1996. Behavioral and electrophysiological assessment of hyperalgesia and changes in dorsal horn responses following partial sciatic nerve ligation in rats. *Pain* 66: 297–306.

Talbert, L. M., Kraybill, E. N., and Potter, H. D. 1976. Adrenal cortical response to circumcision in the neonate. *Obstetrics and Gynecology* 48: 208–210.

Talbot, J. D., Marrett, S., Evans, A. C., Meyer, E., Bushnell, M. C., and Duncan, G. H. 1991. Multiple representations of pain in human cerebral cortex. *Science* 251: 1355–1358.

Taylor, A., Skelton, J., and Butcher, J. 1984. Duration of pain condition and physical pathology as determinants of nurses' assessments of patients in pain. *Nursing Research* 33: 4–8.

Taylor, K. A. 1994. How not to refute eliminative materialism. *Philosophical Psychology* 7: 101–125.

ter Kuile, M. M., Spinhoven, P., Linssen, A. C. G., Zitman, G. F., Van Dyck, R., and Rooijmans, H. G. M. 1994. Autogenic training and cognitive self-hypnosis for the treatment of recurrent headaches in three subject groups. *Pain* 58: 331–340.

Thomas, L. 1980. *The Medusa and the Snail—More Notes of a Biological Watcher.* London: Allen Lane.

Torebjörk, H. E., LaMotte, R. H., and Robinson, C. J. 1992. Central changes in processing of mechanoreceptive input in capsaicin-induced secondary hyperalgesia in humans. *Journal of Physiology* 448: 765–780.

Townsend, J., Harris, N. S., and Courchesne, E. 1996. Visual attention abnormalities in autism: Delayed orienting to location. *Journal of the International Neuropsychology Society* 2: 541–550.

Tran Dinh, Y. R., Thurel, C., Serrie, A., Cunin, G., and Seylaz, J. 1991. Glyceral injection into the trigeminal ganglion provokes a selective increase in human cerebral blood flow. *Pain* 46: 13–16.

Trief, P., Elliott, D., Stein, N., and Frederickson, B. 1987. Functional vs. organic pain: A meaningful distinction? *Journal of Clinical Psychology* 43: 219–226.

Trout, J. D. 1991. Belief attribution in science: Folk psychology under theoretical stress. *Synthese* 379–400.

Tuke, D. H. 1884. *Illustrations of the Influence of the Mind upon the Body in Health and Disease Designed to Elucidate the Imagination, Second Edition.* Philadelphia: Henry C. Lee's.

Turk, D. C. 1994. Perspectives on chronic pain: The role of psychological factors. *Current Directions in Psychological Science* 3: 45–48.

Turk, D. C. 1996. Clinicians' attitudes about prolonged use of opioids and the issue of patient heterogeneity. *Journal of Pain and Symptom Management* 11: 218–230.

Turk, D. C., and Rudy, T. E. 1987. An integrated approach to pain treatment: Beyond the scalpel and syringe. In C. D. Tollison (ed.), *Handbook of Chronic Pain Management.* Baltimore: Williams and Wilkins.

Turk, D. E., and Meichenbaum, D. H. 1989. A cognitive-behavioral approach to pain management. In P. D. Wall and R. Melzack (eds.), *Textbook of Pain, Second Edition.* New York: Churchill Livingstone.

Turk, D. E., Meichenbaum, D. H., and Genest, M. 1983. *Pain and Behavioral Medicine: A Cognitive-Behavioral Perspective.* New York: Guilford Press.

Turner, B. H., Mishkin, M., and Knapp, M. 1980. Organization of the amydalopedal projections from modality-specific cortical association areas in the monkey. *Journal of Comparative Neurology* 19: 515–543.

Turner, J. A., and Chapman, C. R. 1982. Psychological interventions for chronic pain: A critical review. I. Operant conditioning, hypnosis, and cognitive behavioral therapy. *Pain* 12: 23–46.

Tursky, B. 1976. The development of a pain perception profile: A psychophysical approach. In M. Weisenberg, and B. Tursky (eds.), *Pain, New Perspective in Therapy and Research.* New York: Plenum Press.

Tye, M. 1994a. A representational theory of pains and their phenomenal character? *Philosophical Perspectives, Volume 9.* Atascadero, CA: Ridgeview Publishing.

Tye, M. 1994b. Naturalism and the problem of intentionality. In P. A. French, T. E. Uehling, and H. K. Wettstein (eds.), *Midwest Studies in Philosophy, Volume XIX, Philosophical Naturalism.* Notre Dame, IN: University of Notre Dame Press.

Tye, M. 1995. *Ten Problems of Consciousness: A Representational Theory of the Phenomenal Mind.* Cambridge, MA: The MIT Press.

Ulett, G. A., Parwatiker, S. D., Stern, J. A., and Brown, M. 1978. Acupuncture, hypnosis, and experimental pain. II. Study with patients. *Acupuncture and Electro-Therapeutive Research International Journal* 3: 191–201.

Unruh, A. 1996. Gender variations in clinical pain experience. *Pain* 65: 123–167.

Vaccarino, A. L., and Chorney, D. A. 1994. Descending modulation of central neural plasticity in the formalin pain test. *Brain Research* 666: 104–108.

Vaccarino, A. L., and Melzack, R. 1992. Temporal processes of formalin pain: Differential role of the cingulum bundle, fornix pathway and medial bulboreticular formation. *Pain* 49: 257–271.

Valdes, M., Garcia, L., Treserra, J., de Pablo, J., and de Flores, T. 1989. Psychogenic pain and depressive disorders: An empirical study. *Journal of Affective Disorders* 16: 21–25.

Valdes, M., Treserra, J., Garcia, L., de Pablo, J., and de Flores, T. 1988. Psychogenic pain and psychological variables: A psychometric study. *Psychotherapy and Psychosomatics* 50: 15–21.

Van Gelder, T. 1995. What is cognition, if not computation? *Journal of Philosophy* 91: 345–381.

Van Gelder, T., and Port, R. 1995. It's about time: An overview of the dynamaical approach to cognition. In R. Port and T. Van Gelder (eds.), *Mind as Motion.* Cambridge, MA: The MIT Press.

Van Houdenhove, B., and Joostens, P. 1995. Burning mouth syndrome: Successful treatment with combined psychotherapy and psychopharmacotherapy. *General Hospital Psychiatry* 17: 385–388.

Victor, J. D. 1989. Colored hearing synesthesia. *Neurology* 39: 1409–1410.

Vogt, B. A., Derbyshire, S., and Jones, A. K. 1996. Pain processing in four regions of human cingulate cortex localized with co-registered PET and MR imaging. *European Journal of Neuroscience* 8: 1461–1473.

von Knorring, L., and Ekselius, L. 1994. Idiopathic pain and depression. *Quality of Life Research* 3: S57–68.

Wade, J. B., Dougherty, L. M., Hart, R. P., and Cook, D. B. 1992. Patterns of normal personality structure among chronic pain patients. *Pain* 48: 37–43.

Wadley, J. P., Smith, G. T., and Sheiff, C. 1997. Self-trephination of the skull with an electric power drill. *British Journal of Neurosurgery* 11: 156–158.

Wainwright-Sharp, J. A., and Bryson, S. E. 1993. Visual orienting deficits in high-functioning people with autism. *Journal of Autism and Developmental Disorders* 23: 1–13.

Walco, G. A., Cassidy, R. C., and Schechter, N. L. 1994. Pain, hurt, and harm: The ethics of pain control in infants and children. *New England Journal of Medicine* 331: 541–544.

Walker, E., Katon, W., Hansom, J., Harrop-Griffiths, J., Holm, L., Jones, M., Hickok, L., and Russo, J. 1995. Psychiatric diagnoses and sexual victimization in women with chronic pelvic pain. *Psychosomatics* 36: 531–540.

Walker, E., Katon, W., Harrop-Griffiths, J., Holm, L., Russo, J., and Hickok, L. 1988. Relationship of chronic pelvic pain to psychiatric diagnoses and childhood sexual abuse. *American Journal of Psychiatry* 145: 75–80.

Walker, E., Katon, W., Neraas, K., Jemelka, R., and Massoth, D. 1992. Dissociation in women with chronic pelvic pain. *American Journal of Psychiatry* 149–534–537.

Walker, L., and Greene, J. 1989. Children with recurrent abdominal pain and their parents: More somatic complaints, anxiety, and depression than other patient families? *Journal of Pediatric Psychology* 14: 231–243.

Walker, L., Garber, J., and Greene, J. 1991. Somatization symptoms in pediatric abdominal pain patients: Relation to chronicity of abdominal pain and parent somatization. *Journal of Abnormal Child Psychology* 91: 379–394.

Walker, L., Garber, J., and Greene, J. 1993. Psychosocial correlates of recurrent childhood pain: A comparison of pediatric patients with recurrent abdominal pain, organic illness, and psychiatric disorders. *Journal of Abnormal Psychology* 102: 248–258.

Walker, W. A., Sullican, M. D., and Stenchever, M. A 1993. Use of antidepressants in the management of women with chronic pelvic pain. *Obstetrics and Gynecology Clinics of North America* 20: 743–751.

Wall, P. D. 1964. Presynaptic control of impulses at the first central synapse in the cutaneous pathway. *Physiology of Spinal Neurons. Progress in Brain Research 12.* New York: Elsevier.

Wall, P. D. 1989a. Introduction. In P. D. Wall and R. Melzack (eds.), *Textbook of Pain, Second Edition.* New York: Churchill Livingstone.

Wall, P. D. 1989b. The dorsal horn. In P. D. Wall and R. Melzack (eds.), *Textbook of Pain, Second Edition*. New York: Churchill Livingstone.

Wall, P. D., and Cronly-Dillon. 1960. Pain, itch, and vibration. *Archives of Neurology* 2: 365–375.

Wall, P. D., and Sweet, W. H. 1967. Temporary abolition of pain in man. *Science*, 155: 108–109.

Walling, M., O'Hara, M., Reiter, R., Milburn, A., Lilly, G., and Vincent, S. 1994. Abuse history and chronic pain in women: II. A multivariate analysis of abuse and psychological morbidity. *Obstetrics and Gynecology* 84: 200–206.

Wang, Q-P., and Nakai, Y. 1994. The dorsal raphe: An important nucleus in pain modulation. *Brain Research Bulletin* 6: 575.

Watson, D. 1982. Neurotic tendencies among chronic pain patients: An MMPI item analysis. *Pain* 14: 365–385.

West, B. H. 1836. Experiments in animal magnetism. *Boston Medical and Surgical Journal* 14: 349–351.

White, J. C., and Sweet, W. H. 1969. *Pain and the Neurosurgeon*. Springfield, IL: C. Thomas.

Whorwell, P. J., Prior, A., and Faragher, E. B. 1984. Controlled trial of hypnotherapy in the treatment of severe refractory irratable bowel syndrome. *Lancet* ii: 1232–1233.

Whorwell, P. J., Prior, A., Colgan, A. M. 1987. Hypnotherapy in severe irritable bowel syndrome: Further experience. *Gut* 28: 423–425.

Wickelgren, I. 1997. Getting the brain's attention. *Science* 278: 35–37.

Wigley, R. 1994. Occupation neuroses and the psychogenic connotation of "repetition strain injury": The misconstruction of neurosis. *Integrative Psychiatry* 10: 179–180.

Wilkes, K. 1977. *Physicalism*. London: Routledge and Kegan Paul.

Willer, J. C., Boureau, F. and Albe-Fessard, D. 1980. Human nociceptive reactions: Effects of spatial summation of afferent input from relatively large diameter fibers. *Brain Research* 201: 465–470.

Williamson, P. S., and Williamson, M. L. 1983. Physiologic stress reduction by a local anesthetic during circumcision. *Pediatrics* 71: 36–40.

Willis, W. D., and Coggeshall, R. E. 1978. *Sensory Mechanisms in the Spinal Cord*. New York: Plenum Press.

Wimsatt, W. C. 1976. Reductionism, levels of organization, and the mind-body problem. In G. Globus, G. Maxwell, and I. Savodnik (eds.), *Consciousness and the Brain*. New York: Plenum Press.

Winchel, R. M., and Stanley, M. 1991. Self-injurious behavior: A review of the behavior and biology of self-mutilation. *American Journal of Psychiatry* 148: 306–17.

Wittchen, H., Essau, C., Rief, W., and Fichter, M. 1993. Assessment of somatoform disorders and comorbidity patterns with the CIDI: Findings in psychosomatic inpatients. *International Journal of Methods in Psychiatric Research* 3: 87–99.

Wittgenstein, L. 1967. *Zettel.* Ed. by G. E. M. Anscombe and G. H. von Wright. Oxford: Blackwell.

Wittgenstein, L. 1953. *Philosophical Investigations.* Trans. by G. E. M. Anscombe. New York: Macmillan.

Wood, D., Wiesner, M., and Reiter, R. 1990. Psychogenic chronic pelvic pain: Diagnosis and management. *Clinical Obstetrics and Gynecology* 33: 179–195.

Woolf, C. J., and King, A. E. 1990. Dynamic alterations in the cutaneous mechanoreceptive fields of dorsal horn neurons in the rat spinal cord. *Journal of Neuroscience* 10: 2717–2726.

Wright, L. 1973. Functions. *The Philosophical Review* 82: 139–182.

Yakshe, T. L. 1986. *Spinal Afferent Processing.* New York: Plenum Press.

Yeo, H. M., and Yeo, W. W. 1993. Repeat deliberate self-harm: A link with childhood sexual abuse? *Archives of Emergency Medicine* 10: 161–166.

Yeung-Courchesne, R., and Courchesne, E. 1997. From impasse to insight in autism research: From behavioral symptoms to biological explanations. *Developmental Psychopathology* 9: 389–419.

Yi, D. K., and Barr, G. A. 1995. The induction of fos-like immunoreactivity by noxious thermal, mechanical, and chemical stimuli in the lumbar spinal cord of infant rats. *Pain* 27: 257–265.

Zachariae, R., and Bjerring, P. 1994. Laser-induced pain-related brain potentials and sensory pain ratings in high and low hypnotizable subjects during hypnotic suggestions of relaxation, dissociated imagery, focused analgesia, and placebo. *International Journal of Clinical and Experimental Hypnosis* 42: 56–80.

Zachary, R. A., Friedlander, S. Huang, L. N., Silverstein, S. and Leggot, P. 1985. Effects of stress-relevant and -irrelevant filmed modeling on children's responses to dental treatment. *Journal of Pediatrics and Psychology* 10: 383–401.

Zak, M. 1990. Creative dynamics approach to neural intelligence. *Biological Cybernetics* 64: 15–23.

Zaslansky, R., Sprecher, E., Katz, Y., Rozenberg, B., et al. 1996. Pain-evoked potentials: What do they really measure? *Electroencephalography and Clinical Neurophysiology: Evoked Potentials* 100: 384–392.

Zborowski, M. 1952. Cultural components in responses to pain. *Journal of Social Issues* 4: 16–30.

Zeisat, H. A. 1978. Are family patterns related to the development of chronic low back pain? *Perception and Motor Skills* 46: 1062.

Zeltzer, L. K., and LeBaron, S. 1982. Hypnosis and nonhypnotic techniques for reduction of pain and anxiety during painful procedures in children and adolescents with cancer. *Journal of Pediatrics* 101: 1032–1035.

Zeltzer, L. K., Bush, J. P., Chen, E., and Riveral, A. 1997. A psychobiologic approach to pediatric pain: Part I. History, physiology, and assessment strategies. *Current Problems in Pediatrics* 27:225–253.

Ziegler, D. K., and Schlemmer, R. B. 1994. Familial psychogenic blindness and headache: A case study. *Journal of Clinical Psychiatry* 55: 114–117.

Zitman, F. G., van Dyck, R., Spinhoven, P., Linssen, A. C. G., and Corrie, G. 1992. Hypnosis and autogenic training in the treatment of tension headaches: A two-phase constructive design study with follow-up. *Journal of Psychosomatic Research* 36: 219–228.

Index